Advances in Mental Health and Addiction

Series Editor
Masood Zangeneh, Richmond Hill, ON, Canada

Over the past several decades we have witnessed dramatic shifts in prevailing approaches to mental health and addiction. Significant scientific achievements have led to novel treatment options that impacted the experiences of individuals with mental disorders. In recent years, new perspectives have begun to influence the way we address mental health and substance dependencies, resulting in a greater emphasis on mental health promotion and prevention strategies. Despite these progressions, mental health care systems too often remain stagnant, fragmented, and peripheral.

More information about this series at https://link.springer.com/bookseries/13393

Ahmed Sayed Aboraya

Manual for the Standard for Clinicians' Interview in Psychiatry (SCIP)

A New Assessment Tool for Measurement-Based Care (MBC) and Personalized Medicine in Psychiatry (PMP)

Springer

Ahmed Sayed Aboraya
Morgantown, WV, USA

This work contains media enhancements, which are displayed with a "play" icon. Material in the print book can be viewed on a mobile device by downloading the Springer Nature "More Media" app available in the major app stores. The media enhancements in the online version of the work can be accessed directly by authorized users.

ISSN 2570-3390 ISSN 2570-3404 (electronic)
Advances in Mental Health and Addiction
ISBN 978-3-030-94929-7 ISBN 978-3-030-94930-3 (eBook)
https://doi.org/10.1007/978-3-030-94930-3

This Springer imprint is published by the registered company Springer Nature Switzerland AG
The registered company address is: Gewerbestrasse 11, 6330 Cham, Switzerland

Dedicated to my wife Salwa, my family and my patients.

SCIP Manual Preface

My personal experience with using measures in clinical practice inspired me to write this manual. After I finished a Master of Public Health (MPH) and a Doctor of Public Health (Dr.PH) from Johns Hopkins University in 1991, I started my psychiatry residency training with the aim of using psychiatric measures in clinical settings. After 10 years of trying to use almost all the relevant existing scales and standardized diagnostic interviews for adult psychiatric disorders, I concluded that existing measures were not practical for use in real-world of psychiatric practice. Consequently, I embarked on developing the Standard for Clinicians' Interview in Psychiatry (SCIP) as a tool to be used by clinicians in real clinical settings for assessment and clinical decision making.

My aim in writing this manual is to provide psychiatrists, mental health professionals, and researchers with a reference tool to facilitate understanding of how to use the measures and scales in clinical practice and research. Readers of the manual can learn the principles of psychopathology assessment and practice how to use the scales by watching 15 videotaped interviews. In doing so, readers can become qualified measurement-based care (MBC) trainers who can then teach modern psychopathology to future generations of mental health professionals and researchers.

Chapter 1 of the SCIP manual reviews the history of the development of rating scales, from review of Father Thomas V. Moore's first modern rating scales to discussion of the current status of measures in psychiatry, including advances and shortcomings. Chapters 2, 3, 4, and 5 describe the principles of psychopathology assessment and the development of the SCIP scales and the SCIP glossary. Chapter 6 describes the development of measurement-based care (MBC) as one of the advances in the twenty-first century. Chapter 7 explains the psychiatric interview component of MBC. Chapter 8 reviews basic epidemiological concepts including reliability, validity, and types of measures commonly used in psychiatry. Chapter 9 describes the first comprehensive training curriculum designed to teach clinicians and psychiatry residents to use scales in clinical settings. Chapter 10 includes the transcripts for 15 videotaped interviews, conducted with real patients by the author and colleagues at West Virginia University (WVU), and shows how to transform qualitative information from psychiatric interviews into quantitative data. Chapter

11 describes how the SCIP is a new assessment tool for personalized medicine in psychiatry (PMP).

I thank my colleagues at West Virginia University (WVU) and other institutions, my mentors all over the globe, and our patients for their contributions to this manual.

Morgantown, WV, USA Ahmed Sayed Aboraya

Manual Contributors

1. **Ahmed Sayed Aboraya, MD, DrPH**
   Chief of Psychiatry, William R. Sharpe, Jr. Hospital.
   Clinical Professor of Psychiatry,
   West Virginia School of Osteopathic Medicine.
   Adjunct Faculty, School of Public Health
   West Virginia University (WVU).
   936 Sharpe Hospital Road,
   Weston, WV 26452, USA
   W (304) 269-1210
   E-mail Ahmed.S.Aboraya@wv.gov
2. **Henry A. Nasrallah, MD**
   Vice Chair for Faculty Development and Mentorship
   Professor of Psychiatry, Neurology, & Neuroscience Director, Neuropsychiatry and Schizophrenia Programs
   Director, Psychiatry CME Programs University of Cincinnati College of Medicine
   Office: 513-558-5953
   Mobile: 513-407-0833
   Email: henry.nasrallah@uc.edu
   Editor, INSIGHT MATTERS, The Ohio Psychiatric Physicians Association (OPPA) Newsletter
   Founding Editor of the International Journal: Schizophrenia Research
   Editor-In-Chief: Biomarkers in Neuropsychiatry
   Editor-In-Chief of the U.S. Journal: Current Psychiatry
   President: American Academy of Clinical psychiatrists
   Founder: SIRS (Schizophrenia International Research Society) Co-Founder, Executive Vice-President & Scientific Director, CURESZ Foundation
3. **Daniel Elswick, MD, FACLP**
   Vice Chair for Education & Residency Director,
   Professor, Department of Behavioral Medicine & Psychiatry,
   West Virginia University School of Medicine

4. **James H. Berry, DO**
Professor and Chair,
Department of Behavioral Medicine and Psychiatry,
Rockefeller Neuroscience Institute,
West Virginia University School of Medicine
5. **Cheryl A. Hill, MD PhD**
Associate Professor, WVU Medicine, Department of Behavioral Medicine and Psychiatry
6. **Yasha Rastgar, MD**
Staff Psychiatrist in Redondo Beach, CA
7. **Jeremy D. Hustead, MD**
Assistant Professor, WVU Medicine, Department of Behavioral Medicine and Psychiatry
8. **Dilip Chandran, MD**
Associate Professor, WVU Medicine, Department of Behavioral Medicine and Psychiatry
9. **Joy Parks, MD**
Psychiatry Resident (PGY4), WVU Medicine, Department of Behavioral Medicine and Psychiatry
10. **Jawad Zafar, DO**
Staff Psychiatrist at Farhat Medical Clinic in Beckley WV
11. **Sheena Dohar, MD**
Attending Psychiatrist in Community Mental Health, Pittsburgh, PA
12. **John D. Justice, MD**
Chief Medical Officer, William R. Sharpe Jr. Hospital, Mildred Mitchell Bateman Hospital. State Forensic Medical Director, WV Department of Health and Human Resources
13. **Wanhong Zheng, MD, MS**
Associate Professor, WVU Medicine, Department of Behavioral Medicine and Psychiatry
14. **Sara Berzingi, BA**
Researcher and WVU School of Medicine MD Candidate 2022, West Virginia University
15. **Rachael Spalding, MS**
Doctoral Candidate in Clinical Psychology, West Virginia University

Contents

Chapter 1
Historical Perspectives on the History of Measurement in Psychiatry

Measurement was best defined by Nunnally as "rules for assigning numbers to objects in such a way as to represent quantities of attributes" [1]. Scientific measurements need to meet the standards of reliability and validity to be used in scientific research. Once scientifically reliable and valid measurements are created, testing hypotheses and research projects become feasible, leading to advances in science and medicine. Major advances in science are often preceded by breakthroughs in measurement methods. For example, in 1903, Alfred Binet (1857–1911) invented a measure for intelligence (intelligence quotient or "IQ") as the ratio between demonstrated performance (mental age) and chronological age [2]. Since the introduction of IQ and intelligence tests like the Binet-Simon scale, an enormous and important body of literature has been generated on the topic [1, 3–5].

Measurement-based care in psychiatry is the use of reliable and validated clinical measurement instruments to objectify assessment, treatment, and clinical outcomes, including diagnosis, efficacy, safety, tolerability, functioning, and quality of life in patients with psychiatric disorders [6]. A measurement-based care tool, whether a psychopathology measure (commonly known as a rating scale), an efficacy measure, a functioning measure, a quality of life measure, a prognosis measure, or any other clinical measure, must have two components: a number (whether a fraction measure, a binary measure, or a score) and a useful way to interpret that number (e.g., a severity of a symptom, a sign, or a disorder) so that the clinician can use the tool in decision-making regarding the care of patients.

The history of mental illness and description of mental symptoms are closely intertwined with the social history of humankind. Descriptions of individuals with "strange," "maladaptive," or "dangerous" behaviors have been documented in some of the first known written records [7]. The descriptions of King Saul's homicidal and suicidal thoughts in the Old Testament (in about 1000 B.C.) suggest the extremes of a mood disorder. Greek philosophers Plato, Aristotle, Hippocrates, and Medieval physicians described various forms of madness: mania, hysteria, paranoia,

A. S. Aboraya, *Manual for the Standard for Clinicians' Interview in Psychiatry (SCIP)*, Advances in Mental Health and Addiction,
https://doi.org/10.1007/978-3-030-94930-3_1

melancholia, and dementia. At the turn of the nineteenth century, the main diagnostic categories of mental disorders such as melancholia, mania, delirium, dementia, and paranoia relied on the observation of what the individual did, looked like, and said, rather than on how the individual felt [8]. In other words, scientific measurement as defined today did not really exist or have any important role in the care of patients with mental illness prior to the nineteenth century.

Compared to the history of mental illness, the science of measurement in psychiatry is relatively recent and can be traced back to the beginning of the nineteenth century. Measurement in psychiatry has been used for two important tasks: the first is the identification and enumeration of who is and who is not "a person with mental illness" and the second is how to measure the nature and severity of psychopathology of the individual, otherwise known as the science of descriptive psychopathology (DP). This chapter describes the history of measurement in psychiatry from the nineteenth century and afterwards. Revolutionary advances in information technology that characterized the twenty-first century, such as the use of electronic health records (EHR), software programs, handheld devices, web-based training, and videos, have had an important impact on the development of measured-based care (MBC). Along with the development of MBC, new imaging techniques, experimental psychopathology research, and new innovative measures led to the birth of personalized medicine in psychiatry (PMP) in the twenty-first century.

Identification and Enumeration of Patients with Mental Illness

The Retreat, commonly known as the York Retreat, was established by the Society of Friends (Quakers), for the use and treatment of the insane members of their own community near York, England. The Retreat opened in 1796 with 30 patients and gradually expanded to accommodate 100 patients. Originally, the Retreat served only the Quakers but gradually became open to the public. The Retreat is famous for the "moral treatment" of patients with mental illness and became a model for asylums around the world. John Thurnam, the resident surgeon of the Retreat, wrote a detailed account, "The Statistics of the Retreat," in 1841 which describes the activities and patients residing there from 1796 to 1840 [9]. The classifications of mental disorders inherited by the nineteenth century alienists as depicted in the book were the following: mania, hysterical mania, mania alternating with melancholy (mania predominating), melancholy, hypochondriacal melancholy, melancholy alternating with mania (melancholy predominating), suicidal melancholy, monomania (partial insanity), monomania of suspicion and fear, moral insanity, dementia, congenital idiotcy, congenital imbecility, delirium tremens, and delirium of fever. Table 1.1 shows the outcome of the treatment for all patients: whether they recovered, improved, unimproved, or died.

Epidemiological methods at the same time continued to advance, and researchers were aware of the confounding factors such as age and gender. In 1844, the opinion among professionals was that insanity was more prevalent among women than men.

Table 1.1 Shewing the admissions, discharges, and deaths, for the 44 years, 1796–1840

		Males	Females	Total
Admitted		**282**	**333**	**615**
Discharged				
	Recovered	121	170	291
	Improved	41	24	65
	Unimproved	11	18	29
	Died	70	69	139
Total discharged during the 44 years		**243**	**281**	**524**
Remaining mid-summer, 1840		**39**	**52**	**91**
Average numbers resident during the 44 years		**28.30**	**38.65**	**67.15**

Source: Thurnam [9]

John Thurnam refuted this opinion and provided evidence to the contrary. He cited the need to consider the proportion of females in the general population (census data), incident versus prevalent cases, the mortality rates for males and females, the different communities, different social classes, and other important epidemiological factors. John Thurnam pointed out that the mortality of insane men exceeded that of insane women by 50%. That explained why the existing number of female patients in asylums was greater than that of the male patient. Taking all factors together, he concluded that women are actually less likely to suffer from "mental derangement" and are more likely to recover and less likely to die than men. However, the probability of relapse or recurrence of the disorder, after recovery from a first episode, is somewhat greater in women than in men [10, 11]. In addition to advances in epidemiological concepts, the causes of mental illness were discussed and debated. In a book titled "A manual of Psychological Medicine" published 1858 by J.C. Bucknill and D.H. Tuke, the causes of insanity were classified into predisposing causes (hereditary, seasons, marriage, age, sex) and exciting reasons (physical and moral) [12]. The exciting physical factors include, among others, epilepsy, head injuries, inflammation of brain, childbearing, old age, and mercury. The exciting moral factors include disappointed affections, domestic troubles, grief, wounded feelings, religious anxiety, and excitement.

A discussion on the epidemiological advances in the nineteenth century would not be complete without William Far, a founder, or perhaps *the* founder of modern epidemiology [13]. William Farr (1807–1883) was born at Kenley, a small village of Shropshire, England. He was a statistician for 40 years at the General Registrar Office, beginning in 1839. Farr studied the distributions and determinants of health disorders in populations, including the prevention and control of diseases. He provided tabulations of cholera mortality by source of water supply in his 1848 cholera report. On the basis of these data, John Snow precisely formulated his hypothesis that the cause of cholera was a self-reproducing organism excreted by victims of the disease and spread by fouled water supplies. John Snow anticipated the germ theory of cholera by 20 years. The selections from the reports and writings of William Farr published in 1885 represent the foundations of modern epidemiology and had significant public health impact [13].

In 1825, in the kingdom of Norway, a royal commission was issued to enumerate and measure the condition of the insane in the kingdom of Norway. Professor Holst published the results of the survey which was repeated in 1835 and 1845. The survey results described patients with "mania, melancholia, dementia, idiotia, blind in one eye or two eyes, deaf, dumb and lepers," classified by gender and by rural and urban districts [14].

In the United States and around the same time, efforts to identify and enumerate patients with mental disorders were underway. The National Reporting Program for Mental Health Statistics had its origins in the decennial US census, with enumeration of the "insane and idiotic" in 1840. Frederick Howard Wines, with the help from psychiatrists and psychologists, classified mental illness in the 1880 census into seven distinct forms of insanity: "mania, melancholia, monomania, paresis, dementia, dipsomania, and epilepsia" [15]. It was noted that between 1850 and 1880, the population of the United States had a little more than doubled; but the number of "insane, idiots, blind, and deaf-mutes" appears to be nearly five times as great as it was 30 years ago [16]. Table 1.2 shows the number of "insane, idiots, blind, and deaf-mute" in the United States in the years named, respectively, according to the census.

At the turn of the twentieth century, Kraepelin conceptualized his famous "dichotomy theory" that divided the "insanities" broadly into two diseases: dementia praecox (later renamed schizophrenia by Eugen Bleuler) and manic-depressive illness (later renamed bipolar disorder by Karl Kleist). His classification model was enshrined in Western psychiatry for more than a century, even though Kraepelin himself revised his theory in 1920 [17]. In 1933, Jacob Kasanin coined the term "schizoaffective" to describe patients with equal measure of coexisting psychotic and manic and/or depressive symptoms [18]. As an example of the beginning of advancement in psychiatric nosology, a survey conducted in 1936 in the Eastern Health District of Baltimore by Paul Lemkau described the following types of psychosis: schizophrenia, manic-depressive, involutional, senile and arteriosclerotic, alcoholic, syphilitic, with epilepsy, with mental deficiency, and others. The same survey described the following types of psychoneurosis: hysteria, psychasthenia, neurasthenia, hypochondriasis, reactive depression, anxiety attacks, and mixed psychoneurosis [19]. The Eastern Health District Survey showed that there were 3337

Table 1.2 The number of insane, idiots, blind, and deaf-mute in the United States

Class	1880	1870	1860	1850
Insane	91,997	37,432	24,042	15,610
Idiots	76,895	24,527	18,930	15,787
Blind	48,928	20,320	12,658	9794
Deaf-mute	33,878	16,205	12,821	9803
Total	251,698	98,484	68,451	50,994

Source: Wines [16]

Table 1.3 The number of cases and rate per 1000 population of mental disorders in Eastern Health District Survey, Baltimore, Md., 1936 (Population: 55,129)

Leading classification	Number of cases	Rate per 1000
Psychosis:	367	6.7
Schizophrenia	158	2.9
Manic-depressive	41	0.7
Senile and arteriosclerotic	38	0.7
Alcoholic	15	0.3
Syphilitic	29	0.5
With mental deficiency	28	0.5
Other	27	0.5
Undiagnosed	31	0.6
Psychoneurosis	171	3.1
Psychopathic personality	30	0.5
Personality disorder in adults	218	4.0
Behavior disorder in children	449	8.1
Minor and possible disorder in adults and children	651	11.8
Epilepsy	75	1.4
Mental deficiency	375	6.8
School progress problems without mental deficiency	434	7.9
Adult delinquency without other information	567	10.3
Total active cases	3337	60.5

Source: Lemkau et al. [21]

active cases of mental disorder during the survey year in a population of 55,129, or 60.5 active cases per 1000 population. So, at any one time, at least 6% of the population was suffering from some type of serious mental disorder. Table 1.3 shows the rate per 1000 population of mental disorders in the Eastern Health District of Baltimore in 1936 survey (population of 55,129) [20, 21].

The second half of the twentieth century has witnessed advances in psychiatric nosology due to the efforts of the World Health Organization (WHO) and the American Psychiatric Association (APA). The World Health Organization (WHO) published the sixth revision of the International Classification of Diseases (ICD-6) in 1948, which included a mental disorders section [22]. Several editions of the International Classification of Diseases (ICD) followed, including the tenth (and latest), published in 1993 [23]. In the United States, the American Psychiatric Association Committee on Nomenclature and Statistics developed and published the first edition of the Diagnostic and Statistical Manual of Mental Disorders (DSM-I) in 1952 [24], followed by the DSM-II in 1968 [25], DSM-III in 1980 [26], DSM-III-R in 1987 [27], DSM-IV in 1994 [28], DSM-IV-TR in 2000 [29], and the DSM-5 in 2013 [30]. The number of psychiatric diagnoses has exploded from 106 in DSM-I to 265 in DSM-5. Between 1980 and 1984, the National Institute of Mental Health (NIMH) launched the Epidemiological Catchment Area (ECA)

Table 1.4 Lifetime prevalence rates of DIS/DSM-III disorders per 100 persons 18 years and older in the United States

Disorders	Rate, % (SE)
Any DIS disorder	32.2 (0.5)
Alcohol abuse/dependence	13.3 (0.4)
Drug abuse/dependence	5.9 (0.2)
Schizophrenia	1.3 (0.1)
Manic episode	0.8 (0.1)
Major depressive episode	5.8 (0.3)
Dysthymia	3.3 (0.2)
Anxiety disorders	14.6 (0.4)
Somatization disorder	0.1 (0.0)
Personality disorder, antisocial personality	2.5 (0.2)
Cognitive impairment (severe)	1.3 (0.1)

Source: Regier et al. [32]

Table 1.5 Annual incidence of DIS/DSM-III disorders per 100 person-years of risk (18 years and older) in the United States

Disorders	Per 100 person-years of risk, (SE)
Alcohol abuse/dependence	1.79 (0.22)
Drug abuse/dependence	1.09 (0.17)
Major depressive disorder	1.59 (0.17)
Panic disorder	0.56 (0.09)
Phobic disorder	3.98 (0.30)
Obsessive-compulsive disorder	0.69 (0.08)
Cognitive impairment (all ages)	1.18 (0.13)
Cognitive impairment (age 18–29)	0.4 (0.14)
Cognitive impairment (age 30–44)	0.81 (0.20)
Cognitive impairment (age 45–64)	0.94 (0.22)
Cognitive impairment (age ≥ 65)	4.64 (0.59)

Source: Eaton et al. [33]

survey with the goals of estimating the prevalence and incidence of mental disorders in five locations in the United States. The ECA survey was carried out by five university-based research teams in different locations: Baltimore, MD (Johns Hopkins University), St. Louis, MO (Washington University), Durham, NC (Duke University), Los Angeles, CA (University of California), and New Haven, CT (Yale University). The NIMH Diagnostic Interview Schedule (DIS), based on the DSM-III, was used as the case-identification instrument in the ECA survey [31]. Table 1.4 shows the prevalence mental disorders [32], and Table 1.5 shows the incidence of mental disorders in the United States based upon the DIS/DSM-III diagnoses [33]. Eaton and his colleagues at Johns Hopkins University continued to follow up with the Baltimore ECA cohort through the twenty-first century and described the trends in prevalence and incidence of mental disorders as well as the risk of death associated with mental disorders [34, 35].

Measurement of Psychopathology

The Nineteenth Century: The Birth of the Science of Descriptive Psychopathology

During the early nineteenth century, many asylums were built for the insane in various countries; the most famous is the York Retreat, established by the Society of Friends (Quakers) near York, England. Patients were confined in a physical space for years. That allowed the nineteenth century alienists to be in direct contact with patients of mental illness; examine and describe their behaviors, symptoms, and signs; and observe the changes of behaviors and actions over time. The asylum practice was an important factor in the development of the science of descriptive psychopathology. Mental phenomena such as hallucinations, pseudohallucinations, illusions, delusions, thought disorders, obsessions, compulsions, mental retardation, cognitive impairment, memory disorders, disorders of consciousness, disorientation, delirium, mood disorders, anxiety disorders, anhedonia, depression, mania, catalepsy, catatonia, stupor, and others were described and debated. The development of the science of mental symptoms and signs (descriptive psychopathology) in Europe in the nineteenth century paved the way for advances in the classification of mental disorders (psychiatric nosology) in the twentieth century.

Incorporating the subjective experiences of patients into the symptom-repertoire of psychopathology was a significant achievement of the science of descriptive psychopathology in the nineteenth century [8]. Patients' subjective feelings of anxiety, mood, melancholia, mania, paranoia, hallucinations, and other mental symptoms were described, analyzed, and classified. Alienists studied symptoms and signs as either present or absent and did not allow for graded presentations during the nineteenth century [8]. In other words, elaborate and detailed measurements of symptoms and signs did not find its way in descriptive psychopathology until the twentieth century.

The First Half of the Twentieth Century: The Birth of Reliable and Validated Rating Scales

The introduction of the intelligence quotient (IQ) measure and intelligence tests like the Binet-Simon scale at the dawn of the twentieth century highlighted the important impact of measures in psychiatric research. As indicated earlier, a rating scale must have a measure scientifically assessed for reliability and/or validity and a meaning of the measure so that clinicians can use the measure in decision-making. That is not to be confused with hospital charts which are designed to measure the progress of the patient. In 1895, the Kankakee State Hospital in Illinois devised chart with the purpose of recording the patient's behavior. In 1901, the State Hospital at Worcester, Massachusetts, devised hospital chart to record the behaviors of the patient. With the encouragement of Adolf Meyer, Edward Kempf (a resident physician at the Phipps Clinic at Johns Hopkins Hospital) developed the Behavior Chart in mental diseases in 1915 with the goals of observing and recording accurately the activities and ideas of the patient in the chart and extend its use in research [36]. The Kempf Behavior Chart is completed by nurses and gives a graphic picture of the progress of the patient. Words used in the chart were simple and self-explanatory, such as irritable, impulsive, angry, combative, suicidal, delusions, and hallucinations, without specific definitions of the terms. In 1922, with the main goal of improving the nurses' notes in psychiatric hospitals, James Plant (a physician at Harvard Medical School) devised the rating scheme for conduct which included 19 categories: 3 physical (weight, sleep and physical exercise) and 16 mental ("attitude towards taking food, room and attire, reaction toward the nurses, care of self, general knowledge, emotional reaction, ingenuity, rapidity of habit formation, span of attention, hallucinations, delusions, orientation, insight, recent memory, reactions to visitors and judgment") [37]. Each category was subdivided into several subcategories. For example, attention ranged from 1 (stuporous) to 10 ("patient can plan and carry a piece of work requiring a long period of time, such as weaving a rug or making a piece of pottery"). Simply, the nurse entered 19 numbers in the chart for each patient evaluated at one point in time. The frequency of evaluation of the patient depended upon the recency of admission and the severity of illness. Plant Rating Scheme was developed at McLean hospital; however, it was never demonstrated to be reliable and was never published in full. Nurses constructed graphs in the chart that showed the progress of the patient. The Plant Rating Scheme was also designed to save time for the nurses, increase the nurse's interest in work, and improve the cooperation between the medical staff and nurses. Interestingly, Plant referred to the Kempf Behavior Chart used at Henry Phipps Psychiatric Clinic at Johns Hopkins Hospital and emphasized the difference between his rating scheme for conduct and the Kempf Behavior Chart. Our opinion is that neither the Kempf Behavior Chart nor Plant Rating Scheme met the standard of reliability and validity for rating scales, although were important precursors to their development.

In 1926, Emerson challenged the generous successes of family case work (social work) due to the lack of objective measures [38]. In a response to Emerson's critique, Wilcox and other researchers all agreed upon the need for developing standard "measuring sticks" and the ability to repeat the measures year by year or decade by decade in order to assess progress or lack thereof toward goals [39, 40]. Researchers acknowledged the difficulties of measuring intangible attributes, but the success of measuring intelligence with IQ was an important motivating factor because intelligence was considered immeasurable before the invention of IQ. A few years later, significant advances in measuring symptoms and signs were achieved by Father Thomas Verner Moore (TV Moore).

Father Thomas Verner Moore (TV Moore) was born in Louisville, Kentucky, on October 22, 1877, and died at the age of 92 in Cartuja de Miraflores, Burgos, Spain. He was ordained as a Roman Catholic priest in 1901. Father Moore was a dedicated man of God, and his extraordinary spiritual life is the subject of other books. TV Moore had extraordinary achievements in psychology and psychiatry and was ahead of his time in psychiatric research. He received the first doctorate in psychology granted in the District of Columbia from the Catholic University of America in 1903. He also received his medical degree from Johns Hopkins in 1915. TV Moore retired in 1947 as the head of the department of psychology and psychiatry at the Catholic University [41, 42]. TV Moore worked in the laboratory of Wilhelm Wundt, the founder of psychometrics, in Leipzig, Germany, where he met Charles Spearman, the founder of Spearman factor analysis. He also worked under Emil Kraepelin in Munich in 1914 and Adolf Meyer in Baltimore in 1915.

TV Moore can lay claim to three major achievements in psychiatry. First is the creation of the first rating scales in psychiatry, second is the use of factor analysis to decompose psychosis, and third is providing specific definitions of symptoms and signs. TV Moore quantitatively measured 48 symptoms and recorded the presence, absence, or a rating or test measure for each symptom. TV Moore used factor analysis to identify eight syndromes and their relationship to dementia praecox group and manic-depressive insanity:

1. The syndrome of cognitive defect
2. The catatonic syndrome
3. The uninhibited syndrome
4. The non-euphoric manic syndrome
5. The euphoric manic syndrome
6. The delusional hallucinatory syndrome
7. The syndrome of constitutional hereditary depression
8. The syndrome of retarded depression

TV Moore book "The Essential Psychoses and Their Fundamental Syndromes: Studies in Psychology and Psychiatry from the Catholic University of America" outlined the details of the rating scales used in his research [43].

Examples of Symptom Definitions

Hypochondriacal Delusions "This symptom was termed positive if the patient's delusions had to do with ideas about impossible pathological conditions, e.g., that his heart was gone, that his brain had wasted away to nothing, etc."

Bizarre Delusions "This symptom was termed positive if the patient's delusions referred to things clearly and palpably impossible, e.g., 'the man upstairs is using my brain so much that I have no chance to use it myself.' If the hypochondriacal delusions were peculiarly absurd and impossible they were also rated as bizarre."

Emotional symptoms were rated on a numerical scale. A schema for the quantitative measurement of each symptom was determined and recorded during the live interview or observed on the word. Symptoms were measured quantitatively, then transformed to present, or absent to allow the adoption of tetrachoric method of correlation.

Examples of Items

Auditory Hallucinations

Talking to voices: does the patient mutter and mumble to himself?	Never	A few times in the examination	Every few minutes	Almost without interruption	Continuously
In interview	0	2	4	8	16
On ward	0	2	4	8	16

	Occasionally	Often
Does the patient talk to himself?	5	10
Does the patient carry on conversations aloud with invisible voices?	5	10
Does the patient gesticulate at invisible persons?	5	10

Anxiety

Facial expression	Not anxious	Distinctly worried	Very definite anxiety	Extremely anxious	Extremely frightened
In interview	0	2	4	8	16
On ward	0	2	4	8	16

Does the patient wring hands?	Zero	Once or twice	Every 10 minutes	Every few minutes	Continually
In interview	0	2	4	8	16
On ward	0	2	4	8	16

TV Moore measured the reliability of the schema by having two individuals rate the schema of a number of cases and were found to have very close agreement, i.e., reliable. The sophistication of the reliability and factor analyses of TV Moore's scales and the specificity of symptom definitions gives TV Moore the honor of being the first psychiatric researcher to create symptom rating scales in psychiatry.

Given TV Moore's significant achievements in psychiatry and psychology as outlined above, he is considered one of the most underrecognized legends in the history of modern psychiatry.

"Rating scales, diagnostic instruments, and psychometric tools are not created in a vacuum; rather, they are the products of their time, with input from culture, biases, and what is considered to be the state of the art in psychopathology and psychopharmacology at the time of their development [44]." Just as TV Moore's psychosis scales and dimensions reflected the era of Kraepelin dementia praecox and manic-depressive doctrine, *history has shown that scale development reflects the important clinical needs of the day: the need for patient care, the need to test the new innovations of the field, and the need to evaluate (validate or refute) current predominating ideas.* Prefrontal lobotomy was a new and important treatment for patients with severe mental illness during the first half of the twentieth century. By September 1950, there had been nearly 1500 prefrontal lobotomy operations performed within the Veterans Administration Hospitals alone [45]. Clinicians badly needed a prognostic scale to help in selecting patients for a treatment procedure such as lobotomy or insulin shock [46]. Between 1941 and 1944, Phyllis Wittman developed and tested a rating scale of prognosis with 343 subjects at Elgin State Hospital [47, 48]. The new scale, Elgin Prognosis Scale (EPS), was composed of 30 prognostic factors; each prognostic factor had a range with the negative sign indicating good prognosis and a positive sign indicating poor prognosis. For example: "defects of interest" versus "definite display of interests" was an item rated from +3 to −3. The prognostic score is the algebraic sum of the weighted measures. A reliability correlation coefficient was calculated for 61 patients that were rated by two different members of the staff and was +0.87. The validity of the prognosis scale was measured and compared with the subjective judgments of prognosis made by Elgin staff. For all the levels of improvement following therapy, the scale averages appear to give a definitely more accurate prediction as to prognosis than average medical staff member's judgment. *To our knowledge and with consultation with experts in the field, the Elgin Prognosis Scale is the first published reliable and validated scale that was developed and used in psychiatry.* After the publication of Elgin Prognosis Scale (EPS) and to the end of the 1940s, several additional scales were published along with data suggesting their reliabilities [49–56].

The Second Half of the Twentieth Century: A Plethora of Reliable and Validated Rating Scales

Researchers in psychiatry and psychology entered the second half of the twentieth century with advances in psychometrics and experience in developing reliable and validated rating scales. The motives to create and test new scales continued and reflected the needs of patient care. Just as there was an important need for a prognosis scale to decide which patients were appropriate for lobotomy, there was another important need to assess and measure the changes in patients who were lobotomized. Maurice Lorr developed the Multidimensional Scale for Rating Psychiatric Patients (MSRPP) to measure symptom severity and changes in patients with psychosis who had been lobotomized [57]. The scale describes 12 areas of psychopathology: depression, mania, compliance, agitation, paranoid projection, activity level, motor disturbance, perceptual disturbances, withdrawal, grandiosity, disorganization, and hysterical conversion. The MSRPP was modified to the Inpatient Multidimensional Psychiatric Scale (IMPS) which measures ten psychotic syndromes based on observations of the patient behavior and interviewing the patient [58]. The IMPS consists of 75 items and was designed to be administered by trained clinical interviewers. The ten syndromes of the IMPS are excitement, hostility, paranoid projection, grandiosity, perceptual disturbances, anxiety, apathy, disorientation, motor disturbance, and conceptual disorganization. The IMPS demonstrated good internal consistency and interrater reliability and was used in early studies of antipsychotic medications.

In December 1951, chlorpromazine was synthesized in the laboratories of Rhone-Poiulenc and became available on prescription in France in November 1952 [59]. The discovery and success of chlorpromazine was instrumental in the development of the psychopharmacology era. Thus, a new need emerged: the need to test the efficacy of the newly discovered psychotropic medications. Researchers found that the IMPS was not sensitive to changes induced by psychotropic medications. In the late 1950s, John Overall collaborated with clinical psychologist John Gorham to develop a rapid assessment technique suited to the evaluation of patient change due to psychotropic medications. Overall and Gorham used Lorr's MSRPP and IMPS as a starting point, and eventually they developed, tested, and modified the Brief Psychiatric Rating Scale (BPRS) [60–62].

Researchers continued to develop scales for different purposes, different populations, and different areas of psychopathology. In 1951, Saslow developed a brief self-administered screening test that correctly identified over 85% of studied subjects as having or not having a behavioral disorder [63]. Lucero and Meyer developed the Fergus Falls Behavior Rating Sheet to record the behaviors of patients who were mute, unintelligible, hyperactive, or seclusive. Eleven aspects of behaviors were rated from 1 (deviant) to 5 (normal), and the scale was shown to be reliable [64]. The Hamilton scales for anxiety and depression, still widely used today, were also developed in the 1950s and 1960s [65–67].

The 1970s was an era that gave great importance to the development of standardized and structural approaches to assessment and diagnosis [68]. In Europe, the Present State Examination (PSE), which uses a computer program to make diagnoses, was developed by Wing and his colleagues [69–73]. In the United States, the Schedule for Affective Disorders and Schizophrenia (SADS) was developed by Endicott and Spitzer and allowed a clinician to make diagnoses using the Research Diagnostic Criteria [74, 75]. The publication of the DSM-III in 1980s and its widespread acceptance and use all over the world led to another need: the need for diagnostic interviews to diagnose mental disorders according to DSM diagnoses [26]. Standardized Diagnostic Interviews (SDIs) were developed with the main goal of arriving at a diagnosis based on the existing classification systems. Some SDIs, such as the World Health Organization Composite International Diagnostic Interview (CIDI) and the Mini-International Neuropsychiatric Interview (M.I.N.I.), are fully structured [76, 77]. For clinicians, semi-structured interviews were designed to allow for considerable variation in the interviewing style, depth of probing, and clinical judgment as to whether a patient's description of a particular behavior meets the relevant diagnostic criterion [78]. Two widely used semi-structured interviews in the assessment literature are the Structured Clinical Interview for DSM-IV Axis I Disorders (SCID-I) and the Schedules for Clinical Assessment in Neuropsychiatry (SCAN) [78–80].

In the early 1980s, Timothy Crow, a British psychiatrist, proposed a new concept of schizophrenia based upon two distinct clusters of symptoms—the positive and negative symptoms—that reflect separate pathologic symptom domains [81, 82]. The concept of a two-disease syndrome or disease process of schizophrenia was widely accepted in the United States and all over the world. At that time, the Brief Psychiatric Rating Scale (BPRS), the "gold standard" of schizophrenia assessment, was not adequate to assess the negative symptoms of the schizophrenia disease. Again, there appeared a new need to assess the negative symptoms of schizophrenia, which led to the development of new scales to measure negative symptoms such as Nancy Andreasen's Scale for Assessing Negative Symptoms (SANS) [83]. Lewis Opler and Stanley Kay were active researchers in the 1980s, and they decided to add 12 items derived from Psychopathology Rating Schedule (PRS) developed by Kay to the 18 BPRS items and create a single measure named the Positive and Negative Symptom Scale (PANSS) [44]. The new scale addressed the limitations of existing instruments, such as the need to measure the negative symptoms. The PANSS is a 30-item rating scale that is comprised of 7 items for positive symptoms, 7 items for negative symptoms, and 16 items for general psychopathology. Kay's research group demonstrated the PANSS to be a reliable and valid instrument, and it has been one of the most widely used instruments in schizophrenia research and the most frequently used scale in FDA clinical trials [84–86]. Sadly, in the 1990s, Dr. Stanley R. Kay died at age 44 from a heart attack while attending a conference in Japan, and the PANSS remained unchanged since then. Limitations of the PANSS have been described elsewhere [87–90].

The development of new rating scales, modification of existing scales, and evaluation of those scales in both adult and child psychiatry continued in the 1990s [91–98]. By the end of the second half of the twentieth century, scales and diagnostic interviews with good psychometric properties, covering all aspects of human behaviors including child psychiatry, were published and readily available. The Handbook of Psychiatric Measures published in 2000 by the American Psychiatric Association Task Force chaired by A.J. Rush Jr. includes more than 240 measures covering diagnostic interviews for adults and children, general psychiatric symptoms measures, general health status and mental health status measures, functioning and disabilities measures, quality of life measures, adverse effects and patient perceptions of care measures, stress and life events measures, suicide and aggression measures, personality disorders, and personality traits measures, in addition to measures specific to diagnostic categories [99].

The Twenty-First Century Advances in Neurosciences, Technology, and Measurement

Along with the successes and plethora of psychiatric measures developed and published in the twentieth century, there have been shortcomings. One shortcoming is the failure to use psychiatric measures in clinical settings. Most clinicians do not use rating scales or diagnostic interviews in clinical settings [100–107] due to perceived time and training constraints and other reasons [100, 108]. Another shortcoming is the limited focus on the reliability of individual psychopathology items. In any science, the isolation of basic variables is essential to its advancement [109] and that applies to psychiatry in particular due to the subjective nature of mental health data. Since TV Moore's use of factor analysis to decompose dementia praecox and manic depressive into eight syndromes, much research has focused on psychiatric syndromes and dimensions with little attention given to the individual psychopathology items. The most comprehensive research on individual psychopathology items was done by Rodgers and Mann who studied the largest number of psychiatric symptoms for reliability in 1986. The index of association for its presence, *IA(p)*, was calculated for 48 anxiety and depressive questions derived from the Present State Examination [110].

Three important technological achievements accompanied the twenty-first century. First is the advances in neurosciences such as structural and functional neuroimaging, neurobiology, neurophysiology, molecular genetics, psychoneuroendocrinology, pharmacogenomics, and other branches of the neurosciences which highlight the importance of reliably measuring the individual psychopathology items. Second is the use of electronic health records (EHR) across clinical settings from big university institutions to solo practices. Third is the advances in health information technology such as software programs, handheld devices, web-based training, and videos, apps, and other technological innovations.

The shortcomings of the twentieth century measures and the new technological advances in the twenty-first century led to the development of new measures such as the Standard for Clinicians' Interview in Psychiatry (SCIP), which was designed to meet these new challenges and complement the evolution of experimental psychopathology (EP) and personalized medicine in psychiatry (PMP) as new concepts of the twenty-first century modern psychiatry. Experimental psychopathology (EP), the study of the relationship between the psychopathology of an individual and objective measures, such as magnetic resonance imaging, functional imaging, positron emission tomography, single photon emission computed tomography, or magnetic resonance spectroscopy, has become an important research area in modern psychiatry [111–115]. Measuring psychopathology reliably at the level of individual symptoms and signs, and correlating them with brain changes in vivo, is one of the best approaches to unraveling the causes of mental disorders [108, 116]. Finally, personalized medicine in psychiatry (PMP) is the latest new concept in modern psychiatry. Personalized medicine in psychiatry (PMP) is the science of systematic use of individual unique characteristics across four domains (life story, environmental factors, psychopathology assessment and translational neuroscience findings [e.g., brain imaging, genomics, pharmacogenomics, biomarkers, endophenotypes, or any newly developed technique or blood test]) to guide the clinician toward a person-centered diagnosis, person-centered prognosis, and person-centered therapeutics (e.g., personalized selection and personalized dosing of medications), with the ultimate goal of improving the outcome of the disease and eventually the prevention of the disease [108].

In conclusion, measurement in psychiatry is a dynamic and changing science that may have a beginning in the nineteenth century, but will never have an ending. As the science of medicine and psychiatry advances, the science of measurement will continue to evolve, change, and advance.

References

1. Nunnally, J. C. (1978). *Psychometric theory*. McGraw-Hill.
2. Binet A: Experimental studies of intelligence. 1903, Paris: Schleicher.
3. Wolf, T. H. (1969). The emergence of Binet's conceptions and measurement of intelligence: A case history of the creative process. Part II. *Journal of the History of the Behavioral Sciences, 5*, 207–237.
4. Wolf, T. H. (1969). The emergence of Binet's conception and measurement of intelligence: A case history of the creative process. *Journal of the History of the Behavioral Sciences, 5*, 113–134.
5. Silverman, H. L., & Krenzel, K. (1964). Alfred Binet: Prolific pioneer in psychology. *The Psychiatric Quarterly Supplement, 38*, 323–335.
6. Aboraya, A., Nasrallah, H. A., Elswick, D. E., Ahmed, E., Estephan, N., Aboraya, D., Berzingi, S., Chumbers, J., Berzingi, S., Justice, J., Zafar, J., & Dohar, S. (2018). Measurement-based care in psychiatry-past, present, and future. *Innovations of Clinical Neuroscience, 15*, 13–26.
7. Stone, M. (1977). *Healing the mind: A history of psychiatry from antiquity to the present*. Edited by Stone M.
8. Berrios, G. (1998). *The history of mental symptoms: Descriptive psychopathology since the nineteenth century*. Cambridge University Press.
9. Thurnam, J. (1841). *The statistics of the retreat*. York.
10. Thurnam, J. (1844). Essay I: On the relative liability of the two sexes to insanity. Quarterly Journal of the Statistical Society of London. Read before the Statistical Section of the British Association at York, September 28th, 1844 (pp. 145–155).
11. Thurnam, J. (1844). Essay II: On the relative liability to insanity, at different ages. Quarterly Journal of the Statistical Society of London. Read before the Statistical Section of the British Association at York, September 28th, 1844 (pp. 156–168).
12. Bucknill, J. C., & Tuke, D. H. (1858). *A manual of psychological medicine*. Blanchard and Lea.
13. Farr, W. (1885). *Vital statistics: A memorial volume of selections from the reports and writings of William Farr*. The Sanitary Institute of Great Britain.
14. Holst. (1852). On the statistics of the insane, blind, deaf and dumb, and lepers, of Norway. *Journal of the Statistical Society of London, 15*, 250–256.
15. Manderscheid, R. W., Witkin, M. J., Rosenstein, M. J., & Bass, R. D. (1986). The national reporting program for mental health statistics: History and findings. *Public Health Reports, 101*, 532–539.

16. Wines, F. (1888). *Report on the defective, dependent, and delinquent classes of the population of the United States, as returned at the Tenth Census (June 1, 1880)*. Government Printing Office.
17. Kraepelin, E. (1920). Die Erscheinungsformen des Irreseins. *Zeitschrift fur die gesamte Neurologie und Psichiatrie, 62*, 1.
18. Kasanin, J. (1994). The acute schizoaffective psychoses. 1933. *The American Journal of Psychiatry, 151*, 144–154.
19. Lemkau, P., Tietze, C., & Cooper, M. (1942). Mental hygiene problems in an urban sistrict, second paper. *Mental Hygiene, 26*, 100–119.
20. Felix, R. H., & Kramer, M. (1953). Extent of the problem of mental disorders. *The Annals of the American Academy, 286*, 5–14.
21. Lemkau, P., Tietze, C., & Cooper, M. (1943). A survey of statistical studies on the prevalence and incidence of mental disorder in sample populations. *Public Health Reports, 58*, 1909–1927.
22. WHO. (1948). Manual of the international classification of diseases, injuries and causes of death. Geneva, World Health Organization.
23. WHO. (1993). *The ICD-10 classification of mental and behaviorhal disorders: Diagnostic criteria for research* (10th ed.). World Health Organization.
24. American Psychiatric Association. (1952). *Diagnostic and statistical manual of mental disorders* (1st ed.), Washington, DC, American Psychiatric Association.
25. American Psychiatric Association. (1968). *Diagnostic and statistical manual of mental disorders* (2nd ed.), Washington, DC, American Psychiatric Association.
26. American Psychiatric Association. (1980). *Diagnostic and statistical manual of mental disorders* (3rd ed.). American Psychiatric Press, Inc.
27. American Psychiatric Association. (1987). *Diagnostic and statistical manual of mental disorders* (3rd, Revised ed.). American Psychiatric Association.
28. American Psychiatric Association (Ed.). (1994). *Diagnostic and statistical manual of mental disorders* (4th ed.). American Psychiatric Association.
29. American Psychiatric Association. (2000). *Diagnostic and statistical manual of mental disorders* (4th, Text Revised ed.). American Psychiatric Association.
30. American Psychiatric Association (Ed.). (2013). *Diagnostic and statistical manual of mental disorders* (5th ed.). American Psychiatric Association.
31. Robins, L. N., Helzer, J. E., Croughan, J., & Ratcliff, K. S. (1981). National Institute of Mental Health Diagnostic Interview Schedule. Its history, characteristics, and validity. *Archives of General Psychiatry, 38*, 381–389.
32. Regier, D. A., Boyd, J. H., Burke, J. D., Jr., Rae, D. S., Myers, J. K., Kramer, M., Robins, L. N., George, L. K., Karno, M., & Locke, B. Z. (1988). One-month prevalence of mental disorders in the United States. Based on five epidemiologic catchment area sites 3. *Archives of General Psychiatry, 45*, 977–986.
33. Eaton, W. W., Anthony, J. C., Dryman, A., Shapiro, S., & Locke, B. Z. (1989). The incidence of specific DIS/DSM-III mental disorders: Data from the NIMH epidemiologic catchment area program. *Acta Psychiatrica Scandinavica, 79*, 163–178.
34. Eaton, W. W., Kalaydjian, A., Scharfstein, D. O., Mezuk, B., & Ding, Y. (2007). Prevalence and incidence of depressive disorder: The Baltimore ECA follow-up, 1981-2004. *Acta Psychiatrica Scandinavica, 116*, 182–188.
35. Eaton, W. W., Roth, K. B., Bruce, M., Cottler, L., Wu, L., Nestadt, G., Ford, D., Bienvenu, O. J., Crum, R. M., Rebok, G., Anthony, J. C., & Munoz, A. (2013). The relationship of mental and behavioral disorders to all-cause mortality in a 27-year follow-up of 4 epidemiologic catchment area samples. *American Journal of Epidemiology, 178*, 1366–1377.
36. Kempf, E. J. (1915). The behavior chart in mental diseases. *American Journal of Insanity, 71*, 761–772.
37. Plant, J. S. (1922). Rating scheme for conduct. *American Journal of Psychiatry, 1*, 547–572.

38. Emerson, H. (1926). Cards on the table: I. A plea for the measurement of social reconstruction. *Theatre Survey, 55*, 465–466.
39. Ihlder, J. (1926). Cards on the table. II. Measuring sticks wanted. *The Survey, 55*, 466–467.
40. Wilcox, E. (1927). The measurement of achievement in family case work. *The Family, 8*, 46–49.
41. Stafford, J. W. (1970). Thomas Verner Moore: 1877-1969. *The American Journal of Psychology, 83*, 286–288.
42. Noll, R., DeYoung, C. G., & Kendler, K. S. (2017). Thomas Verner Moore. *The American Journal of Psychiatry, 174*, 729–730.
43. Moore, T. (1933). In E. A. Pace (Ed.), *The essential psychoses and their fundamental syndromes: studies in psychology and psychiatry from the Catholic University of America*. Williams and Wilkins.
44. Liechti, S., Capodilupo, G., Opler, D. J., Opler, M., & Yang, L. H. (2017). A developmental history of the positive and negative syndrome scale (PANSS). *Innovations of Clinical Neuroscience, 14*, 12–17.
45. Jenkins, R. L., & Holsopple, J. Q. (1951). Criteria and experimental design for evaluating results of lobotomy. *Psychiatric Treatment Proceedings of the Association, 31*, 319–327.
46. Lorr, M., Wittman, P., & Schanberger, W. (1951). An analysis of the Elgin prognostic scale. *Journal of Child Psychology, 7*, 260–263.
47. Wittman, P., & Steinberg, L. (1944). Follow-up of an objective evaluation of prognosis in dementia praecox and manic-depressive psychosis. *Elgin Papers, Collected and Contributed, 5*, 216–227.
48. Wittman, P. (1941). A scale for measuring prognosis in schizophrenic patients. *Elgin Papers, 4*, 20–33.
49. Wilcox, P. H. (1942). The Gradner behavior chart. *Am J of Psychiatry, 98*, 874–880.
50. Cohen, L. H., Malmo, R. B., & Thale, T. (1944). Measurement of chronic psychotic overactivity by Norwich rating scale. *Journal of General Psychology, 30*, 65–74.
51. Malamud, W., Hoagland, H., & Kaufman, C. (1946). A new psychiatric rating scale. *Psychosomatic Medicine, 8*, 243–245.
52. Malamud, W., & Sands, S. (1947). A revision of the psychiatric rating scale. *American Journal of Psychiatry, 104*, 231–237.
53. Dollard, J., & Mowrer, O. H. (1947). A method of measuring tension in written documents. *Journal of Abnormal Psychology, 42*, 3–32.
54. Hunt, J. (1949). The problem of measuring the results of psychotherapy. *The Psychological Service Center Journal, 1*, 122–135.
55. Elizur, A. (1949). Content analysis of the Rorschach with regard to anxiety and hostility. *Rorschach Research Exchange and Journal of Projective Techniques, 13*, 247–284.
56. Abt, L. E. (1949). The analysis of structured clinical interviews. *Journal of Clinical Psychology, 5*, 364.
57. Lorr, M., Jenkins, R., & Holsopple, J. (1953). *Multidimensional scale for rating psychiatric patients, hospital form* (pp. 1–44). Veterans Administration Technical Bulletin.
58. Lorr, M., Klett, J., McNair, D., & Lasky, J. (1962). *Inpatient multidimensional psychiatric scale manual*. Consulting Psychologists Press.
59. Ban, T. A. (2007). Fifty years chlorpromazine: A historical perspective. *Neuropsychiatric Disease and Treatment, 3*, 495–500.
60. Overall, J. E., & Gorham, D. R. (1988). The brief psychiatric rating scale (BPRS): Recent developments in ascertainment and scaling. *Psychopharmacology Bulletin, 24*, 97–99.
61. Overall, J., & Gorham, D. (1962). The brief psychiatric rating scale. *Psychological Reports, 10*, 799–812.
62. Gorham, D. R., & Overall, J. E. (1960). Drug-action profiles based on an abbreviated psychiatric rating scale. *The Journal of Nervous and Mental Disease, 131*, 528–535.
63. Saslow, G., Counts, R. M., & DuBois, P. H. (1951). Evaluation of a new psychiatric screening test. *Psychosomatic Medicine, 13*, 242–253.

64. Lucero, R. J., & Meyer, B. T. (1951). A behavior rating scale suitable for use in mental hospitals. *Journal of Clinical Psychology, 7*, 250–254.
65. Hamilton, M. (1960). A rating scale for depression. *Journal of Neurology, Neurosurgery, and Psychiatry, 23*, 56–62.
66. Hamilton, M. (1959). The assessment of anxiety states by rating. *The British Journal of Medical Psychology, 32*, 50–55.
67. Hamilton, M. (1967). Development of a rating scale for primary depressive illness. *The British Journal of Social and Clinical Psychology, 6*, 278–296.
68. Hirsch, S. R., & Weinberger, D. R. (1996). *Schizophrenia*. Blackwell Science Ltd.
69. Wing, J., Nixon, J., von Cranach, M., & Strauss, A. (1977). Further developments of the 'present state examination' and CATEGO system. *Archiv für Psychiatrie und Nervenkrankheiten, 224*, 151–160.
70. Wing, J. K., Nixon, J. M., Mann, S. A., & Leff, J. P. (1977). Reliability of the PSE (ninth edition) used in a population study. *Psychological Medicine, 7*, 505–516.
71. Wing, J. K., Cooper, J. E., & Sartorius, N. (1974). *The measurement and classification of psychiatric symptoms: An instruction manual for the PSE and Catego program*. Cambridge University Press.
72. Wing, J. K., Birley, J. L., Cooper, J. E., Graham, P., & Isaacs, A. D. (1967). Reliability of a procedure for measuring and classifying "present psychiatric state". *The British Journal of Psychiatry: the Journal of Mental Science, 113*, 499–515.
73. Kendell, R. E., Everett, B., Cooper, J. E., Sartorius, N., & David, M. E. (1968). The reliability of the "present state examination". *Social Psychiatry, 3*, 123–129.
74. Endicott, J., & Spitzer, R. L. (1978). A diagnostic interview: The schedule for affective disorders and schizophrenia. *Archives General Psychiatry, 35*, 837–844.
75. Spitzer, R. L., Endicott, J., & Robins, E. (1978). Research diagnostic criteria: Rationale and reliability. *Archives General Psychiatry, 35*, 773–782.
76. WHO. (1990). *Compsite International Diagnostic Interview (CIDI)*. World Health Organization.
77. Sheehan, D. V., Lecrubier, Y., Sheehan, K. H., Amorim, P., Janavs, J., Weiller, E., Hergueta, T., Baker, R., & Dunbar, G. C. (1998). The Mini-International Neuropsychiatric Interview (M.I.N.I.): the development and validation of a structured diagnostic psychiatric interview for DSM-IV and ICD-10. *Journal of Clinical Psychiatry, 59*(Suppl 20), 22–33; quiz 34–57.
78. Williams, J. B., Gibbon, M., First, M. B., Spitzer, R. L., Davies, M., Borus, J., Howes, M. J., Kane, J., Pope, H. G., Jr., Rounsaville, B., et al. (1992). The structured clinical interview for DSM-III-R (SCID). II. Multisite test-retest reliability. *Archives of General Psychiatry, 49*, 630–636.
79. Spitzer, R. L., Williams, J. B., Gibbon, M., & First, M. B. (1992). The structured clinical interview for DSM-III-R (SCID). I: History, rationale, and description. *Archives of General Psychiatry, 49*, 624–629.
80. Wing, J., Babor, T., Brugha, T., Burke, J., Cooper, J. E., Giel, R., Jablenski, A., Regier, D., & Sartorius, N. (1990). SCAN. Schedules for clinical assessment in neuropsychiatry. *Archives of General Psychiatry, 47*, 589–593.
81. Crow, T. (1980). Positive and negative schizophrenic symptoms and the role of dopamine. *British Journal of Psychiatry, 137*, 383–386.
82. Crow, T. (1980). Regular review: Molecular pathology of schizophrenia: More than one disease process? *BMJ, 280*, 66–68.
83. Andreasen, N. (1989). The scale for the assessment of negative symptoms (SANS): Conceptual and theoretical foundations. *British Journal of Psychiatry, 155*, 49–52.
84. Kay, S. R., Fiszbein, A., & Opler, L. A. (1987). The positive and negative syndrome scale (PANSS) for schizophrenia. *Schizophrenia Bulletin, 13*, 261–276.
85. Kay, S. R., Opler, L. A., & Fiszbein, A. (1987). San Rafael. In *The positive and negative syndrome scale (PANSS) rating manual*. Social and Behavioral Sciences Documents.

86. Kay, S. R., Opler, L. A., & Lindenmayer, J. P. (1989). The positive and negative syndrome scale (PANSS): Rationale and standardisation. *The British Journal of Psychiatry. Supplement, 155*, 59–67.
87. Aboraya, A., & Nasrallah, H. A. (2016). Perspectives on the Positive and Negative Syndrome Scale (PANSS): Use, misuse, drawbacks, and a new alternative for schizophrenia research. *Annals of Clinical Psychiatry, 28*, 125–131.
88. Levine, S. Z., Rabinowitz, J., & Rizopoulos, D. (2011). Recommendations to improve the positive and negative syndrome scale (PANSS) based on item response theory. *Psychiatry Research, 188*, 446–452.
89. Leucht, S., Kissling, W., & Davis, J. M. (2010). The PANSS should be rescaled. *Schizophrenia Bulletin, 36*, 461–462.
90. Obermeier, M., Mayr, A., Schennach-Wolff, R., Seemuller, F., Moller, H. J., & Riedel, M. (2010). Should the PANSS be rescaled? *Schizophrenia Bulletin, 36*, 455–460.
91. Spitzer, R. L., Williams, J. B., Kroenke, K., Linzer, M., deGruy, F. V., 3rd, Hahn, S. R., Brody, D., & Johnson, J. G. (1994). Utility of a new procedure for diagnosing mental disorders in primary care. The PRIME-MD 1000 study. *Journal of the American Medical Association, 272*, 1749–1756.
92. Becker, M., Diamond, R., & Sainfort, F. (1993). A new patient focused index for measuring quality of life in persons with severe and persistent mental illness. *Quality of Life Research: An International Journal of Quality of Life Aspects of Treatment, Care and Rehabilitation, 2*, 239–251.
93. Endicott, J., Nee, J., Harrison, W., & Blumenthal, R. (1993). Quality of life enjoyment and satisfaction questionnaire: A new measure. *Psychopharmacology Bulletin, 29*, 321–326.
94. Frisch, M. B., Cornell, J., & Villaneuva, M. (1992). Clinical validation of the quality of life inventory: A measure of life satisfaction for use in treatment planning and outcome assessment. *Psychological Assessment, 4*, 92–101.
95. Ascher, B. H., Farmer, E. M. Z., Burns, B. J., et al. (1996). The child and adolescent services assessment (CASA): Description and psychometrics. *Journal of Emotional and Behavioral Disorders, 4*, 12–20.
96. Ambrosini, P., & Dixon, M. (1996). *The schedule for affective disorders and schizophrenia, childhood version* (4th ed.).
97. Jensen, P., Roper, M., Fisher, P., Piacentini, J., Canino, G., Richters, J., Rubio-Stipec, M., Dulcan, M., Goodman, S., Davies, M., et al. (1995). Test-retest reliability of the diagnostic interview schedule for children (DISC 2.1). Parent, child, and combined algorithms. *Archives of General Psychiatry, 52*, 61–71.
98. Conners, C. K. (1997). *Conners' rating scales-revised: Technical manual*. Multi-Health Systems.
99. John Rush Jr., A. (2000). *Handbook of psychiatric measures*. American Psychiatric Association.
100. Aboraya, A. (2009). Use of structured interviews by psychiatrists in real clinical settings: Results of an open-question survey. *Psychiatry (Edgmont), 6*, 24–28.
101. Duffy, F. F., Chung, H., Trivedi, M., Rae, D. S., Regier, D. A., & Katzelnick, D. J. (2008). Systematic use of patient-rated depression severity monitoring: Is it helpful and feasible in clinical psychiatry? *Psychiatric Services, 59*, 1148–1154.
102. Gilbody, S. M., House, A. O., & Sheldon, T. A. (2002). Psychiatrists in the UK do not use outcomes measures. National survey. *The British Journal of Psychiatry: The Journal of Mental Science, 180*, 101–103.
103. Bastiaens, L. (2011). Poor practice, managed care, and magic pills: Have we created a mental health monster? *Psychiatric Times, 28*, 1–4.
104. Morrison, J. (2008). *The first interview* (3rd ed.). The Guilford Press.
105. Rettew, D. C., Lynch, A. D., Achenbach, T. M., Dumenci, L., & Ivanova, M. Y. (2009). Meta-analyses of agreement between diagnoses made from clinical evaluations and standard-

ized diagnostic interviews. *International Journal of Methods in Psychiatric Research, 18*, 169–184.
106. Busner, J., Kaplan, S. L., Greco, N., & Sheehan, D. V. (2011). The use of research measures in adult clinical practice. *Innovations in Clinical Neuroscience, 8*, 19–23.
107. Nasrallah, H. A. (2009). Long overdue: Measurement-based psychiatric practice. *Current Psychiatry, 8*, 14–16.
108. Aboraya, A., Nasrallah, H., Muvvala, S., El-Missiry, A., Mansour, H., Hill, C., Elswick, D., & Price, E. C. (2016). The standard for clinicians' interview in psychiatry (SCIP): A clinician-administered tool with categorical, dimensional, and numeric output-conceptual development, design, and description of the SCIP. *Innovations in Clinical Neuroscience, 13*, 31–77.
109. Lorr, M., Rubinstein, E., & Jenkins, R. L. (1953). A factor analysis of personality ratings of outpatients in psychotherapy. *Journal of Abnormal Psychology, 48*, 511–514.
110. Rodgers, B., & Mann, S. A. (1986). The reliability and validity of PSE assessments by lay interviewers: A national population survey. *Psychological Medicine, 16*, 689–700.
111. Oertel-Knochel, V., Knochel, C., Rotarska-Jagiela, A., Reinke, B., Prvulovic, D., Haenschel, C., Hampel, H., & Linden, D. E. (2013). Association between psychotic symptoms and cortical thickness reduction across the schizophrenia spectrum. *Cerebral Cortex, 23*, 61–70.
112. Barta, P. E., Pearlson, G. D., Powers, R. E., Richards, S. S., & Tune, L. E. (1990). Auditory hallucinations and smaller superior temporal gyral volume in schizophrenia. *The American Journal of Psychiatry, 147*, 1457–1462.
113. Palaniyappan, L., Balain, V., Radua, J., & Liddle, P. F. (2012). Structural correlates of auditory hallucinations in schizophrenia: A meta-analysis. *Schizophrenia Research, 137*, 169–173.
114. Jardri, R., Pouchet, A., Pins, D., & Thomas, P. (2011). Cortical activations during auditory verbal hallucinations in schizophrenia: A coordinate-based meta-analysis. *The American Journal of Psychiatry, 168*, 73–81.
115. Shenton, M. E., Kikinis, R., Jolesz, F. A., Pollak, S. D., LeMay, M., Wible, C. G., Hokama, H., Martin, J., Metcalf, D., Coleman, M., et al. (1992). Abnormalities of the left temporal lobe and thought disorder in schizophrenia. A quantitative magnetic resonance imaging study. *The New England Journal of Medicine, 327*, 604–612.
116. Ozomaro, U., Wahlestedt, C., & Nemeroff, C. B. (2013). Personalized medicine in psychiatry: Problems and promises. *BMC Medicine, 11*, 132.

Chapter 2
Rationale for the Development of the Standard for Clinicians' Interview in Psychiatry (SCIP)

Background

As described in Chap. 1, Father Thomas Verner Moore made extraordinary contributions to psychology and psychiatry. One of his achievements was creating modern rating scales in 1933 [1]. Since then, hundreds of rating scales with good psychometric properties have been created and published, such as the Positive and Negative Syndrome Scale (PANSS), Brief Psychiatric Rating Scale (BPRS), Hamilton Rating Scale for Depression (Ham-D), Yale-Brown Obsessive Compulsive Scale (Y-BOCS), and others [2–7]. Rating scales focus on narrow clusters of symptoms, which do not necessarily incorporate details of the entire clinical picture and have not been shown to have the same predictive utility as diagnoses [8]. Existing rating scales are mostly used by research psychiatrists and psychologists, while the vast majority of psychiatric practitioners rarely use them in clinical practice [9]. Chapter 6 further explains why existing scales are not used in clinical practice.

The science of the classification of mental disorders has expanded over the course of the second half of the twentieth century due to efforts by the World Health Organization (WHO) and the American Psychiatric Association (APA). The World Health Organization (WHO) published the International Classification of Diseases (ICD), with the latest version (ICD-10) in 1993 [10]. In the United States, the American Psychiatric Association published the Diagnostic and Statistical Manual of Mental Disorders (DSM), with the latest version (DSM-5) in 2013 [11]. Consequently, Standardized Diagnostic Interviews (SDIs) were developed with the main goal of diagnosing mental disorders based upon the existing classification systems. For clinicians, semi-structured interviews were designed to allow for variations in the interviewing style, depth of probing, and clinical judgment regarding whether a patient's behavior meets the relevant diagnostic criterion [12]. The two most widely used semi-structured interviews in the assessment literature are the Structured Clinical Interview for DSM-IV Axis I Disorders (SCID-I) and the

A. S. Aboraya, *Manual for the Standard for Clinicians' Interview in Psychiatry (SCIP)*, Advances in Mental Health and Addiction,
https://doi.org/10.1007/978-3-030-94930-3_2

Schedules for Clinical Assessment in Neuropsychiatry (SCAN) [12–14]. The Structured Clinical Interview for DSM-IV Axis I Disorders (SCID-I) was designed with a top-down approach. In this approach, questions are grouped by diagnosis and criteria. Within each diagnostic category, if a required criterion is not met, the interviewer skips the remaining questions that assess other criteria for that diagnosis [13]. The SCID-I has been used by researchers all over the world [15, 16]. However, the SCID-I is not practical for use in clinical settings because it is lengthy and cumbersome and can interfere with establishing rapport with patients. The Schedules for Clinical Assessment in Neuropsychiatry (SCAN) is another semi-structured interview developed by the World Health Organization (WHO). It utilizes a bottom-up approach. In this approach, after a comprehensive baseline symptom assessment, algorithms are used to make psychiatric diagnoses [14]. Similarly, the SCAN is not practical to use in clinical settings because it is lengthy and requires extensive training. The Mini-International Neuropsychiatric Interview (M.I.N.I.) was developed by Sheehan (1998) as a short structured diagnostic interview [17]. Overall, the M.I.N.I. is simpler and shorter than the SCID-I and the SCAN and is more widely accepted for use in clinical settings [18]. A drawback of the M.I.N.I. is that it is simply a checklist of symptoms, and the clinical approach of probing and exploring the symptoms is largely lost [19].

Despite efforts to modify popular existing rating scales and standardized diagnostic interviews (SDIs) for clinical use, the literature indicates that most psychiatrists do not use the existing structured interviews or rating scales in real clinical settings [9, 20–25]. The personal experience of the author of the manual found this to be true as well. After I finished my master and doctoral degrees at Johns Hopkins University in 1991, I started my psychiatry residency training with a determination to use psychiatric measures in clinical settings. After 10 years of trying to use almost all the relevant existing scales and standardized diagnostic interviews for adult psychiatric disorders, I concluded that existing measures were not practical for use in the real world of psychiatric practice. Consequently, I embarked on developing the Standard for Clinicians' Interview in Psychiatry (SCIP) as a tool to be used by clinicians in real clinical settings for assessment and decision-making. In other words, the SCIP was designed from the outset as a measurement-based care tool.

Design of the Standard for Clinicians' Interview in Psychiatry (SCIP) Project

The SCIP was developed and tested in an international multisite study in three countries (USA, Canada, and Egypt) between 2000 and 2016. The total sample size, including all sites, was 1044 subjects, making the SCIP project the largest validity and reliability study of a diagnostic interview in psychiatry.

The SCIP project was conducted at 6 sites: Site 1: William R. Sharpe, Jr. Hospital, Weston, West Virginia; Site 2: Chestnut Ridge Center (inpatient and outpatient),

Morgantown, West Virginia; Site 3: Ain Shams University Hospital, Cairo, Egypt; Site 4: Mansoura University Hospital, Mansoura, Egypt; Site 5: Fairmont Physician Office, Fairmont, West Virginia; and Site 6: Rothbart Center, Toronto, Canada. The details of the design of the SCIP project were published in the previous articles [26–29].

The Main Outcomes of the SCIP Project

The Development of Reliable Psychopathology Items

Prior to the development of the SCIP, research on the reliability of individual psychopathology items was limited [30]. Renowned researchers such as Nancy Andreasen have stressed the importance of establishing reliability at the level of individual symptoms and signs. In the past, the absence of valid and reliable symptoms was the main limiting factor in creating dimensional measures [31]. The SCIP study removed this major obstacle by creating reliable symptoms and signs for 30 screening items and 200 psychopathology items, which paved the way for the creation of reliable and valid SCIP dimensions and scales. Table 2.1 shows interrater reliability (Kappa) and standard error for the SCIP 30 screening items and 200 psychopathology items in patients at William R. Sharpe Jr. Hospital, Chestnut Ridge Center (inpatient and outpatient), Ain Shams University Hospital, and Mansoura University Hospital.

The Development of Reliable and Valid SCIP Dimensions and Scales for Adult Psychiatric Disorders

Based upon reliable 230 psychopathology items, reliable dimensions of the main adult psychopathology were created and published in our previous manuscript [27]. The SCIP dimensions were used to create short and efficient SCIP scales. The initial items of the SCIP dimensions were formulated based upon the DSM and ICD criteria and experts' opinions. The sensitivity and specificity of the initial dimensions were calculated against the psychiatric diagnoses as determined by the psychiatrists who treated patients from admission to discharge at William R. Sharpe Jr. Hospital and Chestnut Ridge Center. Rules for shortening the lengthy initial dimensions and creating the final SCIP dimensions included removing items with low prevalence, low sensitivity, or low item rest correlation (<0.4). The reliability and validity of the remaining items were recalculated with repetitive iterations. The sensitivity and specificity of the final dimensions were approximately equal to the sensitivity and specificity of the initial dimensions. For example, the initial depression dimension included 19 symptoms and signs of depression. Three items not covered in the

Table 2.1 Interrater reliability kappa (*K*) and standard error (SE) for the SCIP 30 screening items and 200 psychopathology items in patients at William R. Sharpe Jr. Hospital, Chestnut Ridge Center (inpatient and outpatient), Ain Shams University Hospital, and Mansoura University Hospital

Item #	Item title/ subtitle	Item questions	# of cases	*K* ([a])	SE
Screening Items					
S1	**Generalized anxiety**	***Have you felt very anxious and afraid out of proportion to the situation (with or without physical symptoms) for a prolonged period almost every day?*** 0 Absent or non-significant 1 Symptom present . Not sure *or* not applicable *or* missing	**61**	**0.76**	**0.05**
S2	**Panic attacks**	***Did you have a panic attack, during which you suddenly felt anxious and frightened for a short time (up to 60 minutes) and developed physical symptoms*** **(e.g.,** ***fast heart beats, shaking, sweating)?*** 0 Absent or non-significant 1 Symptom present . Not sure *or* not applicable *or* missing	**54**	**0.81**	**0.05**
S3	**Agoraphobia**	***Have you been afraid of being alone (at home or outside of home), traveling in a car, train or plane, being in an open space*** **(e.g.,** ***park) or being in a closed space*** **(e.g.,** ***store), or being in crowds?*** 0 Absent or non-significant 1 Symptom present . Not sure *or* not applicable *or* missing	**26**	**0.52**	**0.05**
S4	**Social phobia**	***Have you been afraid and anxious when you do things in front of people, such as eating or speaking in public?*** 0 Absent or non-significant 1 Symptom present . Not sure *or* not applicable *or* missing	**22**	**0.51**	**0.05**
S5	**Screening for obsessions**	***Do you ever have an intrusive thought or image that does not make sense and keeps coming back to your mind even when you try not to have the thought or the image?*** 0 Absent or non-significant 1 Symptom present . Not sure *or* not applicable *or* missing	**38**	**0.70**	**0.04**

(continued)

Table 2.1 (continued)

S6	**Screening for compulsions**	***Do you find that you have to do things over and over, that is, checking things you have done (such as washing your hands even if they are clean, checking doors or repeating mental acts such as counting or praying)?*** 0 Absent or non-significant 1 Symptom present . Not sure *or* not applicable *or* missing	**31**	**0.58**	**0.05**
S7	**Witness or experience traumatic events**	***Have you ever witnessed or experienced a traumatic event that involved actual or threatened death or serious injury to you or someone else* (e.g., *physical or sexual abuse, terrorist attack, natural disaster, war…*)*?*** ***Did you feel intense fear and helplessness?*** 0 No traumatic events 1 One traumatic event 2 More than one traumatic event . Not sure *or* not applicable *or* missing	**69**	**0.75**	**0.05**
S8	**Re-experience traumatic events**	***Over the past month, have you re-experienced the event in a distressing way* (e.g., *flashbacks, nightmares, bad dreams*)*?*** 0 Absent or non-significant 1 Symptom present . Not sure *or* not applicable *or* missing	**34**	**0.89**	**0.05**
S9	**Depressed mood**	***Have you been feeling sad, depressed, or in low spirits?*** 0 Absent or non-significant 1 Symptom present . Not sure *or* not applicable *or* missing	**158**	**0.86**	**0.04**
S10	**Anhedonia**	***Have you been unable to experience pleasure and enjoy things that you used to enjoy like exercising, enjoying your hobbies or socializing with friends?*** 0 Absent or non-significant 1 Symptom present . Not sure *or* not applicable *or* missing	**125**	**0.87**	**0.04**
S11	**Suicidal ideation, intention, and plan**	***Have you had thoughts about harming yourself?*** ***Have you had the intention to carry out the suicidal thoughts?*** ***Have you had suicidal plans?*** ***Have you attempted to harm yourself during the past month?*** ***(multiple choices allowed)*** 0 Absent 1 Current suicidal ideation 2 Current suicidal intention 3 Current suicidal plans 4 Recent suicide attempts (past month) . Not sure *or* not applicable *or* missing.	**79**	**0.61**	**0.04**

(continued)

Table 2.1 (continued)

S12	**Self-mutilation behaviors**	***Have you attempted self-mutilation behaviors without intent to die (e.g., burning, cutting, scratching)?*** 0 Absent. 1 Current self-mutilation (past month). . Not sure *or* not applicable *or* missing.	**79**	**0.61**	**0.04**
S13	**Elated mood**	***Have you felt very happy, elated, on top of the world for no apparent reason?*** 0 Absent or non-significant 1 Symptom present . Not sure *or* not applicable *or* missing	**76**	**0.72**	**0.05**
S14	**Irritable mood**	***Have you felt easily irritated without reason? Have you found yourself so irritable that you shout at people or start arguments or actually become aggressive?*** 0 Absent or non-significant 1 Symptom present . Not sure *or* not applicable *or* missing	**65**	**0.75**	**0.05**
S15	**Mixed mood (same day mood changes)**	***Have you had mixed mood swings: periods of depression and elation or irritability on the same day?*** 0 Absent or non-significant 1 Symptom present . Not sure *or* not applicable *or* missing	**44**	**0.50**	**0.05**
S16	**Paranoid delusions**	***Have you felt that someone is spying on you or trying to harm you or has a plot or conspiracy against you?*** 0 Absent or non-significant 1 Symptom present . Not sure *or* not applicable *or* missing	**97**	**0.83**	**0.04**
S17	**Other delusions**	***Do you have strange thoughts such as that you are a prominent person in society, or you yourself are divine or you are God, or you receive special messages from TV or newspapers?*** 0 Absent or non-significant 1 Symptom present . Not sure *or* not applicable *or* missing	**39**	**0.77**	**0.04**
S18	**Auditory hallucinations**	***Have you had experiences of hearing voices or noises that other people cannot hear?*** 0 Absent or non-significant 1 Symptom present . Not sure *or* not applicable *or* missing	**92**	**0.76**	**0.04**
S19	**Visual hallucinations**	***Have you had experiences of seeing things (shadows, objects, people) that other people cannot see?*** 0 Absent or non-significant 1 Symptom present . Not sure *or* not applicable *or* missing	**51**	**0.68**	**0.05**

(continued)

Table 2.1 (continued)

S20	**Violence**	***Have you been violent (destructive to objects or violent towards people) in the past (with or without the influence of alcohol or drugs)?*** 0 No history of violence 1 Yes, due to alcohol and/or drugs 2 Yes, without use of alcohol or drugs 3 Both, with and without use of alcohol or drugs . Not sure *or* not applicable *or* missing	**74**	**0.64**	**0.04**
S21	**Disorganized behavior**	***There is evidence of disorganized behavior by observation during the interview (agitation, odd appearance, inappropriate social behavior, inappropriate affect).*** 0 Absent or non-significant 1 Symptom present . Not sure *or* not applicable *or* missing	**32**	**0.54**	**0.04**
S22	**Disorganized thoughts**	***Evidence of disorganized thoughts by observation during the interview (loose associations, tangentiality, incoherent speech)*** 0 Absent or non-significant 1 Symptom present . Not sure *or* not applicable *or* missing	**39**	**0.65**	**0.04**
S23	**Alcohol problems**	***During the past year, did alcohol cause problems for you at work or school, problems with family or friends, legal problems, or other problems such as getting in physical fights*?** 0 Absent or non-significant 1 Symptom present . Not sure *or* not applicable *or* missing	**53**	**0.89**	**0.06**
S24	**Drug problems**	***During the past year, did drug use (__________) cause problems for you at work or school, problems with family or friends, legal problems, or other problems such as getting in physical fights?*** 0 Absent or non-significant 1 Symptom present . Not sure *or* not applicable *or* missing	**17**	**0.78**	**0.06**
S25	**Somatic symptoms**	***Have you visited doctors due to physical illness and the doctors did the necessary work up and could not find a medical explanation (have patient give examples)?*** 0 Absent or non-significant 1 Symptom present . Not sure *or* not applicable *or* missing	**33**	**0.81**	**0.05**
S26	**Pain symptoms**	***Have you had pain and your doctor did the necessary work up and could not really explain why?*** 0 Absent or non-significant 1 Symptom present . Not sure *or* not applicable *or* missing	**24**	**0.93**	**0.05**

(continued)

Table 2.1 (continued)

S27	**Worry about weight gain**	***Have you worried about gaining weight to the point that you did things such as self-induced vomiting, using diet pills, laxatives, or heavy exercise?*** 0 Absent or non-significant 1 Symptom present . Not sure *or* not applicable *or* missing	**12**	**0.73**	**0.05**
S28	**Binge eating**	***Do you have episodes of binge eating (eating within 1 or 2-hour period what most people would consider an unusually large amount of food)?*** 0 Absent or non-significant 1 Symptom present . Not sure *or* not applicable *or* missing	**27**	**0.97**	**0.12**
S29	**Sustained attention impairment**	***Do you have difficulty concentrating on one thing for a long time* (e.g., *reading a book, writing a letter)?*** 0 Absent or non-significant 1 Patient has difficulty concentrating for a long period of time . Not sure *or* not applicable *or* missing	**39**	**0.95**	**0.12**
S30	**Fidgety**	***Do you have difficulty remaining seated (fidget with hands and feet, squirm or wiggle in seat) when expected to remain seated* (e.g., *in a meeting or a church service)?*** 0 Absent or non-significant 1 Patient fidgets with hands and feet, or wiggles in seat . Not sure *or* not applicable *or* missing	**41**	**0.81**	**0.12**

Psychopathology items:

Item #	Item Titles	Item Questions	# of Cases	*K*	SE
1	**Panic attacks**	***Did you have a panic attack, when you suddenly become anxious and frightened for a short period of time (up to 60 minutes)?*** ***During that time, did you feel that your heart was racing or pounding, or did you start shaking or sweating, or did you feel you were choking?*** 0 Patient had no panic attacks 1 Patient had panic attacks . Not sure *or* not applicable *or* missing	**30**	**0.92**	**0.06**

(continued)

Table 2.1 (continued)

Psychopathology items:

Item #	Item Titles	Item Questions	# of Cases	*K*	SE
2	**Worry about having another panic attack**	***After a panic attack, did you worry about having another attack?*** ***Did you worry about its effects* (e.g., *losing control, having a heart attack or going crazy)?*** 0 After a panic attack, patient did not worry about having another one 1 After a panic attack, patient worried about having another one or its effects . Not sure *or* not applicable *or* missing	**25**	**0.81**	**0.04**
3	**Action to end or prevent panic attacks**	***Did you have to do something to end the attack, like leaving a store, calling someone, taking deep breaths?*** ***Do you do anything to prevent attacks (like avoiding places that trigger the panic attacks)?*** 0 After a panic attack, patient does nothing to end or prevent another panic attack 1 After a panic attack, patient does something to end or prevent another panic attack . Not sure *or* not applicable *or* missing	**26**	**0.87**	**0.04**
4	**Social phobia**	***Have you been afraid and anxious when you do things in front of people, such as eating or speaking in public?*** ***Do you avoid social situations or endure them with intense fear?*** 0 Patient had no social phobia 1 Patient had social phobia . Not sure *or* not applicable o*r* missing	**22**	**0.51**	**0.05**
5	**Agoraphobia**	***Have you been afraid of being alone (at home or outside of home), traveling in a car, train or plane, being in an open space* (e.g., *park) or being in a closed space* (e.g., *store), or being in crowds?*** ***Do you avoid these situations, or require a companion, or endure with intense fear?*** 0 Patient had no agoraphobia 1 Patient had agoraphobia . Not sure *or* not applicable o*r* missing	**26**	**0.52**	**0.05**
6	**Generalized anxiety**	***Have you had excessive worry and anxiety for long periods (hours each day lasting several months), not just during panic attacks?*** ***Is it difficult to control the anxiety?*** 0 Patient has no generalized anxiety 1 Patient has generalized anxiety . Not sure *or* not applicable *or* missing	**25**	**0.84**	**0.04**

(continued)

Table 2.1 (continued)

7	**Restlessness with anxiety**	***Did you feel restless, keyed up, or on edge?*** 0 No 1 Yes . Not sure *or* not applicable *or* missing	**26**	**0.74**	**0.04**
8	**Tension with anxiety**	***Did you feel tense in your muscles?*** 0 No 1 Yes . Not sure *or* not applicable *or* missing	**22**	**0.77**	**0.04**
9	**Exhaustion with anxiety**	***Did you feel tired, or easily exhausted even without work?*** 0 No 1 Yes . Not sure *or* not applicable *or* missing	**22**	**0.79**	**0.05**
10	**Poor concentration with anxiety**	***Did you have difficulty concentrating when anxious?*** 0 No 1 Yes . Not sure *or* not applicable *or* missing	**27**	**0.76**	**0.05**
11	**Irritability with anxiety**	***Did you feel irritable when anxious?*** 0 No 1 Yes . Not sure *or* not applicable *or* missing	**28**	**0.83**	**0.04**
12	**Insomnia with anxiety**	***Did you have difficulty falling asleep or staying asleep when anxious?*** 0 No 1 Yes . Not sure *or* not applicable *or* missing	**25**	**0.82**	**0.05**
13	**Obsessions**	***Do you ever have an intrusive thought or image that does not make sense and keeps coming back to your mind even when you try to avoid the thought or the image?*** 0 Patient has no obsessions 1 Patient has obsessions less than 1 hour/day 2 Patient has obsessions 1–4 hours/day 3 Patient has obsessions more than 4 hours/day . Not sure *or* not applicable *or* missing	**26**	**0.85**	**0.04**
14	**Aggressive obsessions**	***Do you have obsessive thoughts related to aggression?*** 0 No 1 Yes . Not sure *or* not applicable *or* missing			
15	**Contamination obsessions**	***Do you have obsessive thoughts related to contamination?*** 0 No 1 Yes . Not sure *or* not applicable *or* missing			

(continued)

Table 2.1 (continued)

16	**Sexual obsessions**	***Do you have obsessive thoughts related to sex/ sexuality?*** 0 No 1 Yes . Not sure *or* not applicable *or* missing			
17	**Religious obsessions**	***Do you have obsessive thoughts related to religion?*** 0 No 1 Yes . Not sure *or* not applicable *or* missing			
18	**Somatic obsessions**	***Do you have obsessive thoughts related to your health?*** 0 No 1 Yes . Not sure *or* not applicable *or* missing			
19	**Appearance obsessions**	***Do you have obsessive thoughts about your physical appearance?*** 0 No 1 Yes . Not sure *or* not applicable *or* missing			
20	**Compulsions**	***Do you find that you have to do things over and over, that is, checking things you have done (such as washing your hands even if they are clean, checking doors or repeating mental acts such as counting or praying)?*** ***Do you get very anxious or tense if you do not repeat the act over and over?*** 0 Patient has no compulsions 1 Patient has compulsions less than 1 hour/day 2 Patient has compulsions 1–4 hours/day 3 Patient has compulsions more than 4 hours/ day . Not sure *or* not applicable *or* missing	**18**	**0.77**	**0.04**
21	**Checking compulsions**	***Do you feel the need to check things over and over again?*** 0 No 1 Yes . Not sure *or* not applicable *or* missing			
22	**Cleaning/ Washing Compulsions**	***Do you feel the need to clean/wash things over and over again?*** 0 No 1 Yes . Not sure *or* not applicable *or* missing			
23	**Repeating compulsions**	***Do you feel the need to repeat things many times?*** 0 No 1 Yes . Not sure *or* not applicable *or* missing			

(continued)

Table 2.1 (continued)

24	**Ordering/ arranging compulsions**	***Do you feel the need to arrange and rearrange things, order and reorder items over and over again?*** 0 No 1 Yes . Not sure *or* not applicable *or* missing			
25	**Hoarding/ collecting**	***Do you feel the need to collect and/or hoard things?*** 0 No 1 Yes . Not sure *or* not applicable *or* missing			
26	**Mental compulsions**	***Do you engage in any repetitive mental behaviors?*** 0 No 1 Yes . Not sure *or* not applicable *or* missing			
27	**Witness or experience traumatic events**	***Have you ever witnessed or experienced a traumatic event that involved actual or threatened death or serious injury to you or someone else (e.g., physical or sexual abuse, rape, terrorist attack, natural disaster, war...)? Did you feel intense fear and helplessness?*** 0 Patient had no traumatic events 1 Patient has experienced one traumatic event 2 Patient has experienced several traumatic events . Not sure *or* not applicable *or* missing	**69**	**0.75**	**0.05**
28	**Distressing recollection of events**	***Did you have recurrent upsetting memories (distressing recollection) of the event?*** 0 Patient had no significant symptom 1 Patient has recurrent upsetting memories (distressing recollection) of the event . Not sure *or* not applicable *or* missing	**30**	**0.88**	**0.05**
29	**Bad dreams or nightmares**	***Did you have recurrent upsetting dreams or nightmares of the event?*** 0 Patient had no significant symptom 1 Patient has recurrent upsetting dreams and nightmares of the event . Not sure *or* not applicable *or* missing	**26**	**0.94**	**0.05**
30	**Flashbacks**	***Did you have a sense or feeling that the event was happening again: the sense of reliving the event (flashbacks), auditory/visual hallucinations related to the event, or body/ somatosensory experiences of the event?*** 0 Patient had no significant symptom 1 Patient has a sense or feeling that the event is happening again, the sense of reliving the event (flashbacks) . Not sure *or* not applicable *or* missing	**23**	**0.87**	**0.05**

(continued)

Table 2.1 (continued)

31	**Avoidance of thoughts and feelings**	***Did you try to avoid thoughts and feelings associated with the event?*** 0 Patient had no significant symptom 1 Patient tries not to think about the event . Not sure *or* not applicable *or* missing	**27**	**0.94**	**0.05**
32	**Avoidance of people, places, and activities**	***Did you try to avoid things that reminded you of the event (such as certain people, certain places, or some activities)?*** 0 Patient had no significant symptom 1 Patient avoids things that are reminders of the event (such as certain people, certain places, or some activities) . Not sure *or* not applicable *or* missing	**27**	**0.94**	**0.05**
33	**Amnesia**	***Did you have difficulty remembering some or all important aspects of the event?*** 0 Patient had no significant symptom 1 Patient has difficulty remembering some or all important aspects of the event . Not sure *or* not applicable *or* missing	**15**	**0.70**	**0.06**
34	**Diminished social interest (asociality)**	***Did you spend less time or show less interest in activities with friends, family or hobbies that you used to enjoy due to the event?*** 0 Patient had no significant symptom 1 Patient spends less time or shows less interest in activities with friends/family or hobbies due to the event . Not sure *or* not applicable *or* missing	**17**	**0.83**	**0.05**
35	**Detachment and isolation**	***Did you feel distant, cut off, or isolated from other people due to the event?*** 0 Patient had no significant symptom 1 Patient feels distant, cut off, or isolated from other people due to the event . Not sure *or* not applicable *or* missing	**22**	**0.87**	**0.05**
36	**Diminished emotional feelings (Diminished experience of emotions)**	***Did you feel emotionally numb?*** ***Did you have trouble experiencing feelings (happiness, love feelings) due to the event?*** 0 Patient had no significant symptom 1 Patient feels emotionally numb. Patient has trouble experiencing feelings (such as happiness or love feelings) due to the event . Not sure *or* not applicable *or* missing	**24**	**0.88**	**0.05**
37	**Insomnia**	***Did you have difficulty falling or staying asleep due to the event?*** 0 Patient had no significant symptom. 1 Patient has difficulty falling or staying asleep due to the event . Not sure *or* not applicable *or* missing	**16**	**0.78**	**0.05**

(continued)

Table 2.1 (continued)

38	**Anger**	***Did you have periods of irritability or sudden outbursts of anger due to the event?*** 0 Patient had no significant symptom 1 Patient has periods of irritability or sudden outbursts of anger due to the event . Not sure *or* not applicable *or* missing	**19**	**0.80**	**0.05**
39	**Attention impairment (poor concentration)**	***Did you have difficulty concentrating due to the event?*** 0 Patient had no significant symptom. 1 Patient has difficulty concentrating due to the event. . Not sure *or* not applicable *or* missing.	**14**	**0.78**	**0.05**
40	**Hypervigilance**	***Did you feel very alert or watchful of things going on around you even when there was no need to be?*** 0 Patient had no significant symptom. 1 Patient feels very alert or watchful of things going on around even when there is no need to be . Not sure *or* not applicable *or* missing	**17**	**0.87**	**0.05**
41	**Startle response**	***Did you feel jumpy and easily startled? Were you easily scared or did you make a sudden movement or jump when you heard noises or if you were caught by surprise?*** 0 Patient had no significant symptom 1 Patient feels jumpy and has a startle response . Not sure *or* not applicable *or* missing	**20**	**0.86**	**0.05**
42	**Psychological distress due to events**	***Did you get emotionally upset* (e.g., *anxiety, agitation, shame, guilt) when something reminded you of the event?*** 0 Patient had no significant symptom 1 Patient gets emotionally upset (e.g., anxiety, agitation, shame, guilt) when reminded of the event . Not sure *or* not applicable *or* missing	**26**	**0.91**	**0.05**
43	**Physical reactions due to events**	***Did you have physical reactions* (e.g., *fast heart beats, fast breathing, sweating) when something reminded you of the event?*** 0 Patient had no significant symptom 1 Patient has physical reactions (e.g., fast heart beats, fast breathing, sweating) when reminded of the event . Not sure *or* not applicable *or* missing	**24**	**0.93**	**0.05**
44	**Daze (feeling out of touch with surroundings)**	***Did you feel out of touch with things going on around you* (e.g., *being in a daze or not aware of surroundings)?*** 0 Patient had no significant symptom 1 Patient feels out of touch with things going on around. . Not sure *or* not applicable *or* missing	**16**	**0.82**	**0.05**

(continued)

Table 2.1 (continued)

45	**Depressed mood**	***Have you been feeling sad, depressed or in low spirits?*** 0 Patient has no depressed mood 1 Patient has depressed mood less than half the time 2 Patient has depressed mood more than half the time . Not sure *or* not applicable *or* missing	**128**	**0.91**	**0.04**
46	**Anhedonia (loss of pleasure and interest)**	***Have you been unable to experience pleasure and enjoy things that you used to enjoy like exercising, enjoying your hobbies, or socializing with friends?*** 0 Patient has no anhedonia 1 Patient has anhedonia less than half the time 2 Patient has anhedonia more than half the time . Not sure *or* not applicable *or* missing	**121**	**0.87**	**0.04**
47	**Hopelessness**	***Have you felt hopeless about your future?*** 0 Patient is not hopeless 1 Patient feels hopeless less than half the time 2 Patient feels hopeless more than half the time . Not sure *or* not applicable *or* missing	**11**	**0.82**	**0.04**
48	**Attention impairment (poor concentration)**	***Have you found that your concentration has decreased and you are unable to complete a task (e.g., at work, reading an article, reading a book, or watching a movie), even though you were able to do that before?*** 0 Patient has no concentration problems 1 Patient has difficulty concentrating less than half the time 2 Patient has difficulty concentrating more than half the time . Not sure *or* not applicable *or* missing	**116**	**0.80**	**0.0**
49	**Psychomotor retardation/ slowing**	***Have you felt as though you were talking or moving more slowly than normal for you when depressed?*** 0 Patient has normal activity 1 Patient has psychomotor retardation less than half the time 2 Patient has psychomotor retardation more than half the time . Not sure *or* not applicable *or* missing	**97**	**0.72**	**0.04**
50	**Worthlessness (low self-esteem)**	***Have you felt that you are a worthless person in the society or a failure?*** 0 Patient has no feeling of worthlessness 1 Patient feels worthless less than half the time 2 Patient feels worthless more than half the time . Not sure *or* not applicable *or* missing	**97**	**0.78**	**0.04**
51	**Guilt**	***Have you felt guilty or ashamed of yourself for something you have done or thought?*** 0 Patient has no feeling of guilt 1 Patient feels guilty less than half the time 2 Patient feels guilty more than half the time . Not sure *or* not applicable *or* missing	**86**	**0.80**	**0.04**

(continued)

Table 2.1 (continued)

52	**Thoughts of suicide**	***Have you had thoughts, intention or plans to harm or kill yourself during the past month? Have you made a suicide attempt during the past month?*** 0 Patient had no suicidal thoughts or made a suicide attempt during the past month 1 Patient had thoughts, intention or plans to harm self 2 Patient made one recent suicide attempt during the past month 3 Patient made two or more recent suicide attempts during the past month . Not sure *or* not applicable *or* missing	**68**	**0.64**	**0.04**
53	**Crying when depressed**	***Have you cried when depressed?*** 0 Patient has no crying spells 1 Patient has crying spells due to sadness less than half the time 2 Patient has crying spells due to sadness more than half the time . Not sure *or* not applicable *or* missing	**11**	**0.76**	**0.04**
54	**Fatigue and loss of energy**	***Have you felt tired and exhausted during the day, even when you slept well and did not work very hard?*** 0 Patient has no fatigue or loss of energy 1 Patient feels tired and exhausted less than half the time 2 Patient feels tired and exhausted more than half the time . Not sure *or* not applicable *or* missing	**97**	**0.72**	**0.04**
55	**Loss of appetite when depressed**	***Have you lost your appetite when depressed?*** 0 Patient had no loss of appetite. 1 Patient had marked loss of appetite for 2 weeks or less. 2 Patient had marked loss of appetite for more than 2 weeks. . Not sure *or* not applicable *or* missing.	**93**	**0.79**	**0.04**
56	**Increased appetite when depressed**	***Has your appetite increased when depressed?*** 0 Patient had no increase of appetite 1 Patient had marked increase of appetite for 2 weeks or less 2 Patient had marked increase of appetite for more than 2 weeks . Not sure *or* not applicable *or* missing	**93**	**0.79**	**0.04**
57	**Weight loss**	***Did you lose weight when depressed?*** 0 Patient had no weight loss or minimal weight loss 1 Patient lost more than 5% of body weight in a month 2 Patient lost more than 15% of body weight in a year . Not sure *or* not applicable *or* missing	**62**	**0.71**	**0.04**

(continued)

Table 2.1 (continued)

58	**Weight gain**	***Did you gain weight when depressed?*** 0 Patient had no weight gain or minimal weight gain 1 Patient gained more than 5% of body weight in a month 2 Patient gained more than 15% of body weight in a year . Not sure *or* not applicable *or* missing	**15**	**0.76**	**0.05**
59	**Initial insomnia**	***Have you had difficulty falling asleep when depressed?*** 0 Patient has no sleeping problems 1 Patient has difficulty falling asleep (1 our or more) more than half the time when depressed . Not sure *or* not applicable *or* missing	**103**	**0.79**	**0.04**
60	**Middle insomnia**	***Have you had difficulty staying asleep when depressed?*** 0 Patient has no sleeping problems 1 Patient has difficulty staying asleep (awakens and stays awake 1 hour or more) more than half the time when depressed . Not sure *or* not applicable *or* missing	**79**	**0.65**	**0.04**
61	**Late insomnia**	***Have you been waking much earlier than your usual?*** 0 Patient has no sleeping problems 1 Patient has early waking (at least 2 hours) more than half the time when depressed . Not sure *or* not applicable *or* missing	**46**	**0.62**	**0.04**
62	**Hypersomnia**	***Have you been sleeping a lot more than usual when depressed?*** 0 Patient has no hypersomnia. 1 Patient has excessive sleep (sleeps longer than 12 hours in a 24-hour period including naps) more than half the time . Not sure *or* not applicable *or* missing	**26**	**0.68**	**0.05**
63	**Decreased libido**	***Has your interest in sex or your sexual activity been less than usual when depressed?*** 0 Patient has no change in sexual activities or interest in sex 1 Patient has much lower or no interest in sex or sexual activities . Not sure *or* not applicable *or* missing	**74**	**0.80**	**0.04**
64	**Elated (euphoric) mood (Expansive mood)**	***Have you sometimes felt very happy, elated, on top of the world without much reason?*** 0 Patient has no elated mood. 1 Patient has elated mood less than half the time 2 Patient has elated mood more than half the time . Not sure *or* not applicable *or* missing	**71**	**0.75**	**0.04**

(continued)

Table 2.1 (continued)

65	**Irritable mood**	***Have you sometimes felt that you were easily irritated without reason?*** ***Have you found yourself so irritable that you shout at people or start arguments or actually become aggressive?*** 0 Patient has no irritable mood 1 Patient has irritable mood less than half the time 2 Patient has irritable mood more than half the time . Not sure *or* not applicable *or* missing	**70**	**0.76**	**0.04**
66	**Mixed mood (mood lability) [same day mood changes]**	***Have you had mixed mood swings: periods of depression and elation or irritability on the same day?*** 0 Patient has no mixed mood swings 1 Patient has mixed mood less than half the time 2 Patient has mixed mood more than half the time . Not sure *or* not applicable *or* missing	**41**	**0.58**	**0.05**
67	**Racing thoughts**	***Have you felt that you had too many different thoughts racing through your mind compared with normal?*** 0 Patient has no racing thoughts 1 Patient has racing thoughts less than half the time 2 Patient has racing thoughts more than half the time . Not sure *or* not applicable *or* missing	**71**	**0.85**	**0.04**
68	**Pressured speech**	***Have you been talking faster than usual during this time (for example, people said that they were unable to understand you because you were speaking too fast or you felt a pressure to continue talking)?*** 0 Patient has normal speech 1 Patient has pressured speech less than half the time 2 Patient has pressured speech more than half the time . Not sure *or* not applicable *or* missing	**53**	**0.72**	**0.04**
69	**Flight of ideas**	***Flight of ideas (a combination of pressured speech and derailment):*** 0 Patient has no flight of ideas 1 Patient has flight of ideas . Not sure *or* not applicable *or* missing	**15**	**0.62**	**0.06**
70	**Increase in activities**	***Have you been more active and had more energy than usual?*** ***Did you do more things than usual at work or school?*** 0 Patient has no increased energy 1 Patient has too much energy less than half the time 2 Patient has too much energy more than half the time . Not sure *or* not applicable *or* missing	**68**	**0.83**	**0.04**

(continued)

Table 2.1 (continued)

71	**Decreased sleep**	***Have you needed less sleep than usual and without getting tired?*** 0 Patient has normal sleep 1 Patient sleeps 4 hours or less (in a 24-hour period including naps) and feels rested . Not sure *or* not applicable *or* missing	**56**	**0.78**	**0.04**
72	**Distraction (attention is distracted by environmental noises)**	***Do you find yourself easily distracted by unimportant activities or external noises happening around you?*** 0 Patient has no distraction 1 Patient has been easily distracted by external stimuli less than half the time 2 Patient has been easily distracted by external stimuli more than half the time . Not sure *or* not applicable *or* missing	**63**	**0.79**	**0.04**
73	**Grandiosity**	***Have you felt more self-confident than usual? Have you felt that you have special powers or special abilities?*** 0 Patient has no grandiosity 1 Patient has grandiose thoughts, but not of a delusional quality . Not sure *or* not applicable *or* missing	**40**	**0.81**	**0.04**
74	**Overspending (poor judgment in new activities)**	***Have you done something that you regretted later (e.g., spending a lot of money that you could not afford, writing bad checks, or investing money foolishly, sexual indiscretions)?*** 0 Patient did not go on a spending spree 1 Patient went on a spending spree during manic phase . Not sure *or* not applicable *or* missing	**49**	**0.74**	**0.04**
75	**Hypersexuality**	***Have you found that your interest in sex or your sexual activity has increased much compared with normal?*** 0 Patient has no change in sexual activities or interest in sex 1 Patient has been feeling hypersexual more than usual during manic phase . Not sure *or* not applicable *or* missing	**24**	**0.69**	**0.04**
76	**Clanging**	0 Normal speech 1 Clanging: association by sound 2 Punning: association by double meaning 3 Assonance: association by similar syllables 4 Mixed . Not sure *or* not applicable *or* missing	**12**	**0.49**	**0.04**

(continued)

Table 2.1 (continued)

77	**Auditory hallucinations (hallucination quality)**	**Do you hear noises (like music, whispering sounds) or voices talking to you when there is no one around?** **Are the voices like a real voice or just thoughts in your mind?** 0 Patient has no auditory hallucinations 1 Patient has auditory hallucinations 2 Patient has auditory hallucinations with command . Not sure *or* not applicable *or* missing	**54**	**0.90**	**0.04**
78	**Frequency of auditory hallucinations**	**How often do you hear noises (like music, whispering sounds) or voices talking to you when there is no one around?** 0 Patient has no auditory hallucinations 1 Patient has auditory hallucinations (1–4 days/month) 2 Patient has auditory hallucinations (5–15 days/month) 3 Patient has auditory hallucinations (>15 days/month) . Not sure *or* not applicable *or* missing	**54**	**0.93**	**0.05**
79	**Hallucination duration**	**On days when you hear noises or voices, how often do you hear them?** 0 Patient has no auditory hallucinations 1 Patient has auditory hallucinations (less than 1 hour / day) 2 Patient has auditory hallucinations (1–4 hours / day). 3 Patient has auditory hallucinations (more than 4 hours / day) . Not sure *or* not applicable *or* missing	**46**	**0.92**	**0.05**
80	**Audible thoughts**	***Do you think that your thoughts are so loud that someone close to you can hear what you are thinking?*** 0 Patient has no audible thoughts 1 Patient has audible thoughts . Not sure *or* not applicable *or* missing	**7**	**1.00**	**0.05**
81	**Voices arguing**	***Do you hear two or more voices that argue about what you are doing or thinking?*** 0 Voices do not argue with the patient 1 Voices argue about what the patient is doing or thinking . Not sure *or* not applicable *or* missing	**40**	**0.77**	**0.04**
82	**Voices commenting**	***Do you hear a voice or voices commenting on what you are doing or thinking?*** 0 Voices do not comment about the patient 1 Voices comment on what the patient is doing or thinking . Not sure *or* not applicable *or* missing	**40**	**0.77**	**0.04**

(continued)

Table 2.1 (continued)

83	**Internal hallucinations**	***Do you hear the voices or noises inside your head, or as though coming from outside?*** 0 No AH. 1 Mostly external hallucinations 2 Almost equal 3 Mstly internal hallucinations . Not sure *or* not applicable *or* missing	**50**	**0.84**	**0.04**
84	**Second/third hallucinations**	***Do you hear voices talking directly to you (second person) or talking to each other about you (third person)?*** 0 Voices do not talk to the patient or about the patient 1 Voices talk to the patient directly most of the time 2 Voices talk to the patient directly and talk to each other about the patient 3 Voices talk to each other about the patient most of the time . Not sure *or* not applicable *or* missing	**45**	**0.78**	**0.04**
85	**Observed hallucinations**	0 Patient has not been observed talking to self 1 Patient has been observed talking to self, talking to a mirror, or running a conversation with unseen person . Not sure *or* not applicable *or* missing	**12**	**0.55**	**0.04**
86	**Visual hallucinations**	***Do you see things other people cannot see*** **(e.g.,** ***shadows, objects or people)?*** 0 Patient has no visual hallucinations. 1 Patient has visual hallucinations . Not sure *or* not applicable *or* missing	**27**	**0.81**	**0.04**
87	**Olfactory hallucinations**	***Do you sometimes notice unusual smells that other people do not notice?*** 0 Patient has no olfactory hallucinations 1 Patient has olfactory hallucinations . Not sure *or* not applicable *or* missing	**8**	**0.78**	**0.05**
88	**Tactile hallucinations**	***Do you sometimes feel strange sensations on your body and you have no explanation for them?*** 0 Patient has no tactile hallucinations 1 Patient has tactile hallucinations . Not sure *or* not applicable *or* missing	**10**	**0.95**	**0.05**
89	**Somatic passivity**	***Do you feel or have bodily sensations*** **(e.g.,** ***something is crawling under your skin) and you think it is caused by an outside person or force?*** 0 Patient has no somatic passivity 1 Patient has somatic passivity . Not sure *or* not applicable *or* missing	**7**	**0.58**	**0.04**
90	**Thought insertion**	***Do you think that thoughts in your mind are not your own thoughts and that they were inserted into your mind by an outside person or force?*** 0 Patient has no delusions of thought insertion 1 Patient has delusions of thought insertion . Not sure *or* not applicable *or* missing	**16**	**0.76**	**0.04**

(continued)

Table 2.1 (continued)

91	**Thought withdrawal**	***Do you think that your thoughts were taken out of your mind by an outside person or force?*** 0 Patient has no delusions of thought withdrawal 1 Patient has delusions of thought withdrawal . Not sure *or* not applicable *or* missing	**6**	**0.80**	**0.04**
92	**Thought broadcasting**	***Do you think that your thoughts are broadcast so that people are able to know what you are thinking even if they are in different places?*** 0 Patient has no delusions of thought broadcast 1 Patient has delusions of thought broadcast . Not sure *or* not applicable *or* missing.	**16**	**0.71**	**0.04**
93	**Paranoid/ persecutory delusions**	***Have you felt that people are against you, or talking about you or laughing at you?*** ***Do you think someone is trying to harm you (e.g., trying to poison your food or trying to kill you)?*** 0 Patient has no paranoid/persecutory delusions 1 Patient has paranoid/persecutory delusions some of the time 2 Patient has paranoid/persecutory delusions most of the time . Not sure *or* not applicable *or* missing	**50**	**0.86**	**0.04**
94	**Conspiracy delusions**	***Do you think there is a plot or a conspiracy against you by anyone (e.g., a person, FBI, CIA)?*** 0 Patient has no delusions of conspiracy 1 Patient has delusions of conspiracy some of the time 2 Patient has delusions of conspiracy most of the time . Not sure *or* not applicable *or* missing	**49**	**0.84**	**0.04**
95	**Delusions of reference**	***When you are watching TV, listening to the radio, or reading the newspaper, do you think that special messages are intended specifically for you?*** 0 Patient has no delusions of reference 1 Patient has delusions of reference some of the time 2 Patient has delusions of reference most of the time . Not sure *or* not applicable *or* missing	**31**	**0.81**	**0.05**
96	**Delusions of reading thoughts**	***Do you think that you can read people's minds? Do you think that other people can read your thoughts?*** 0 Patient has no delusions of thought reading 1 Patient has delusions of thought reading . Not sure *or* not applicable *or* missing	**17**	**0.83**	**0.04**

(continued)

Table 2.1 (continued)

97	**Religious delusions**	***Do you have unusual religious thoughts, experiences, or practices that your friends or relatives consider very strange?*** ***Do you feel that you yourself are divine or that you are god?*** 0 Patient has no religious delusions 1 Patient has religious delusions some of the time 2 Patient has religious delusions most of the time . Not sure *or* not applicable *or* missing	**17**	**0.80**	**0.04**
98	**Grandiose delusions**	***Do you feel that you have special powers or great abilities that most people do not have?*** ***Do you think that you are a prominent person in society?*** 0 Patient has no grandiose delusions 1 Patient has grandiose delusions some of the time 2 Patient has grandiose delusions most of the time . Not sure *or* not applicable *or* missing	**16**	**0.77**	**0.05**
99	**Delusions of control**	***Do you think that some outside person or force is controlling your actions, impulses or emotions against your will?*** 0 Patient has no delusions of being controlled 1 Patient has delusions of being controlled . Not sure *or* not applicable *or* missing	**9**	**0.68**	**0.05**
100	**Other delusions**	***Do you have any other strange thoughts or beliefs that other people do not have?*** 0 Patient has no other delusions 1 Patient has other delusions . Not sure *or* not applicable *or* missing	**12**	**0.40**	**0.05**
101	**Bizarreness of delusions**	0 Patient has no bizarre delusions 1 Patient has bizarre delusions . Not sure *or* not applicable *or* missing	**14**	**0.43**	**0.05**
102	**Derailment (loose associations)**	0 Normal speech 1 Patient has derailment (loose associations): speech shifts to different topics, related or unrelated, but eventually comes back to the main topic 2 Patient has severe derailment (loose associations): speech shifts to different topics, mostly unrelated and never comes back to main topic . Not sure *or* not applicable *or* missing	**37**	**0.65**	**0.06**
103	**Tangentiality**	0 Normal speech 1 Patient has some tangentiality: replying to a question is related in some distant way 2 Patient has severe tangentiality: replying to a question is totally unrelated . Not sure *or* not applicable *or* missing	**28**	**0.57**	**0.06**

(continued)

Table 2.1 (continued)

104	**Incoherent speech**	0 Normal speech 1 Patient has incoherent speech: each sentence by itself makes sense. However, the first sentence is unrelated to the next sentence . Not sure *or* not applicable *or* missing	**18**	**0.41**	**0.06**
105	**Illogical speech**	0 Normal speech 1 Patient has illogical speech: taken together, speech is not logical . Not sure *or* not applicable *or* missing	**13**	**0.25**	**0.05**
106	**Other disorganized thoughts (e.g., word salad, clanging)**	0 Normal speech 1 Other disorganized thoughts . Not sure *or* not applicable *or* missing	**39**	**0.65**	**0.04**
107	**Agitation**	0 Patient has no verbal agitation. 1 Patient is **verbally agitated** causing people to **feel annoyed** (e.g., makes loud noises, shouts angrily, constant whining or constant attention seeking) 2 Patient is **verbally aggressive**, causing people to **feel insulted or scared** (e.g., cursing or using foul language, makes threats to others or self) 3 Patient is **physically agitated towards self** (e.g., pacing up and down or disrobing) 4 Patient is **destructive to objects** (e.g., slams doors, throws clothes or objects, kicks wall or furniture, breaks objects, smashes windows) . Not sure *or* not applicable *or* missing	**33**	**0.48**	**0.04**
108	**Violence toward others**	0 Patient is not violent towards people 1 Patient is **physically violent and threatening towards people without touching** (e.g., makes threatening gesture, swings at people) **2 Patient is physically violent and touches victims with or without resulting injury** (e.g., grabs at clothes, strikes, kicks, pulls hair, attacks) . Not sure *or* not applicable *or* missing	**25**	**0.64**	**0.04**
109	**Odd appearance and behavior**	0 Patient has appropriate appearance and behaviors 1 Patient has inappropriate appearance and behaviors . Not sure *or* not applicable *or* missing	**19**	**0.67**	**0.06**
110	**Inappropriate affect**	0 Patient has appropriate affect 1 Patient has inappropriate affect . Not sure *or* not applicable *or* missing	**14**	**0.77**	**0.06**
111	**Alogia**	0 Patient has normal speech 1 Patient has alogia less than half time 2 Patient has alogia more than half time . Not sure *or* not applicable *or* missing	**29**	**0.62**	**0.05**

(continued)

Table 2.1 (continued)

112	**Anhedonia (loss of pleasure and interest)**	***Have you been unable to experience pleasure and enjoy things that you used to enjoy like exercising, enjoying your hobbies, or socializing with friends?*** 0 Patient has no anhedonia 1 Patient has anhedonia less than half the time 2 Patient has anhedonia more than half the time . Not sure *or* not applicable *or* missing	**121**	**0.87**	**0.04**
113	**Blunted/flat affect (decrease in affective expression)** <u>**Other descriptors in Literature:**</u> **apathy, emotional apathy, emotional blunting, emotional indifference, blunting of emotional tone.**	0 Patient has broad affect 1 Patient has blunted affect 2 Patient has flat affect . Not sure *or* not applicable *or* missing	**42**	**0.68**	**0.05**
114	**Avolition (decrease in goal-directed activities)** <u>***(other descriptors in Literature:***</u> ***apathy, motor apathy, general apathy, lack of drive, lack of energy, lack of interest.***	0 Patient has normal activities 1 Patient has avolition less than half time 2 Patient has avolition more than half time . Not sure *or* not applicable *or* missing	**35**	**0.74**	**0.04**
115	**Diminished social interest (asociality)**	***Did you spend less time or show less interest in activities with friends, family or hobbies that you used to enjoy?*** 0 Patient had no significant symptom 1 Patient spends less time or shows less interest in activities with friends, family or hobbies . Not sure *or* not applicable *or* missing	**35**	**0.74**	**0.04**

(continued)

Table 2.1 (continued)

116	**Attention impairment (poor concentration)**	***Have you found that your concentration has decreased and you are unable to complete a task (e.g., at work, reading an article, reading a book, or watching a movie), even though you were able to do that before?*** 0 Patient has no concentration problems 1 Patient has difficulty concentrating less than half the time 2 Patient has difficulty concentrating more than half the time . Not sure *or* not applicable *or* missing	**41**	**0.92**	**0.12**
117	**Psychomotor retardation/ slowing**	***Have you felt as though you were talking or moving more slowly than normal for you?*** 0 Patient has normal activity 1 Patient has psychomotor retardation less than half the time 2 Patient has psychomotor retardation more than half the time . Not sure *or* not applicable *or* missing	**97**	**0.72**	**0.04**
118	**Poor self-care**	0 Patient has proper self-care 1 Patient has poor self-care less than half time 2 Patient has poor self-care more than half time . Not sure *or* not applicable *or* missing	**27**	**0.79**	**0.06**
119	**Alcohol tolerance**	***Did you use a lot more alcohol than you previously used to get the same effect (compared when you first started to drink)?*** ***Did you notice that the same amount of alcohol you take now has less effect than before (compared when you first started to drink)?*** 0 Patient had no tolerance to alcohol 1 Patient had tolerance to alcohol . Not sure *or* not applicable *or* missing	**39**	**0.99**	**0.06**
120	**Alcohol withdrawal**	***When you stopped or cut down on alcohol use, did you have withdrawal symptoms?*** ***(patient gives examples of alcohol withdrawal symptoms).*** 0 Patient had no withdrawal symptoms from alcohol 1 Patient had withdrawal symptoms from alcohol . Not sure *or* not applicable *or* missing	**33**	**0.93**	**0.06**
121	**Drinking alcohol to avoid withdrawal**	***Did you drink alcohol to avoid withdrawal symptoms?*** ***Did you use benzodiazepines (e.g., Ativan, Klonopin, Xanax) to avoid withdrawal symptoms?*** 0 Patient did not have to drink alcohol or use benzodiazepines to avoid withdrawal symptoms 1 Patient drank alcohol or used benzodiazepines to avoid withdrawal symptoms . Not sure *or* not applicable *or* missing	**29**	**0.96**	**0.06**

(continued)

Table 2.1 (continued)

122	**Unable to control alcohol**	***Did you drink more alcohol than you planned or intended?*** ***Did you drink alcohol for a longer period of time than you planned or intended?*** 0 Patient had control over alcohol drinking 1 Patient was unable to control alcohol drinking . Not sure *or* not applicable *or* missing	**51**	**0.96**	**0.06**
123	**Unable to reduce or stop alcohol**	***Did you try to reduce or stop alcohol use and not succeed?*** 0 Patient was able to stop or reduce alcohol drinking 1 Patient was unable to stop or reduce alcohol drinking . Not sure *or* not applicable *or* missing	**47**	**0.85**	**0.06**
124	**Time spent to drink alcohol**	***On days of alcohol use, did you spend substantial time obtaining, using or recovering from the effect of alcohol?*** ***Did alcohol drinking consume much of your time?*** 0 Patient did not lose substantial time due to alcohol 1 Patient lost substantial time due to alcohol . Not sure *or* not applicable *or* missing	**37**	**0.94**	**0.06**
125	**Failure to fulfil major obligations**	***Did alcohol use result in failure to fulfill major role obligations (work, school or home)?*** 0 Alcohol had no effect on work, school or social obligations 1 Alcohol had negative effect on work, school or social obligations . Not sure *or* not applicable *or* missing	**36**	**0.92**	**0.06**
126	**Giving up social or recreational activities**	***Did alcohol use result in giving up or reducing important social or recreational activities?*** 0 Alcohol use had no effect on social or recreational activities 1 Alcohol use had negative effect on social or recreational activities . Not sure *or* not applicable *or* missing	**36**	**0.92**	**0.06**
127	**Less time working due to alcohol use**	***Did alcohol use result in less time working?*** 0 Alcohol did not result in less time working 1 Alcohol resulted in missing one or more days of work . Not sure *or* not applicable *or* missing	**36**	**0.92**	**0.06**
128	**Alcohol-related work problems**	***Did alcohol cause any work-related problems?*** 0 Alcohol caused no work problems 1 Alcohol caused work problems . Not sure *or* not applicable *or* missing	**29**	**0.83**	**0.06**

(continued)

Table 2.1 (continued)

129	**Fighting when intoxicated**	***Did you get in physical fights when intoxicated?*** 0 Patient did not get in physical fights when intoxicated 1 Patient got in physical fights when intoxicated . Not sure *or* not applicable *or* missing	**31**	**0.90**	**0.06**
130	**Alcohol-related family problems**	***Did alcohol cause any family problems?*** 0 Alcohol caused no family problems 1 Alcohol caused family problems . Not sure *or* not applicable *or* missing	**51**	**0.82**	**0.06**
131	**Alcohol-related legal problems**	***Did alcohol cause any legal problems?*** 0 Alcohol caused no legal problems 1 Alcohol caused legal problems . Not sure *or* not applicable *or* missing	**29**	**0.92**	**0.06**
132	**Alcohol-induced medical problems**	***Did alcohol cause any medical problems* (e.g., *peptic ulcer disease, liver cirrhosis)?*** 0 Alcohol caused no medical problems 1 Alcohol caused medical problems . Not sure *or* not applicable *or* missing	**11**	**0.70**	**0.06**
133	**Alcohol-induced emotional problems**	***Did alcohol cause any emotional problems* (e.g., *depression, hallucinations)?*** 0 Alcohol caused no emotional problems 1 Alcohol caused emotional problems . Not sure *or* not applicable *or* missing	**24**	**0.90**	**0.06**
134	**Alcohol use in spite of problems**	***Did you continue to use alcohol even though you had problems?*** 0 Patient had no alcohol problems 1 Patient continued to use alcohol even though alcohol caused problems . Not sure *or* not applicable *or* missing	**57**	**0.87**	**0.06**
135	**Alcohol use in hazardous situations**	***Did you use alcohol in a situation, in which it was physically hazardous* (e.g., *driving a car or operating machinery)?*** 0 Patient did not use alcohol in hazardous situations 1 Patient used alcohol in hazardous situations . Not sure *or* not applicable *or* missing	**42**	**0.77**	**0.06**
136	**Alcohol binge**	***Did you go on binges when you kept drinking alcohol for a couple of days or more without sobering up?*** 0 Patient had no binge problem 1 Patient had binge problem . Not sure *or* not applicable *or* missing	**37**	**0.88**	**0.06**
137	**Alcohol blackout**	***Did you have a blackout after drinking so much alcohol that the next day you could not remember what you said or did?*** 0 Patient had no blackout 1 Patient had blackout . Not sure *or* not applicable *or* missing	**53**	**0.98**	**0.06**

(continued)

Table 2.1 (continued)

138	**Drug tolerance**	***Did you use a lot more of the drug than you previously used to get the same effect (compared when you first started to use the drug)?*** ***Did you notice that the same amount of the drug you take now has less effect than before (compared when you first started to use the drug)?*** 0 Patient had no tolerance to the drug 1 Patient had tolerance to the drug . Not sure *or* not applicable *or* missing	**49**	**0.95**	**0.06**
139	**Drug withdrawal**	***When you stopped or cut down on the drug use, did you have withdrawal symptoms?*** ***(patient gives examples of the drug withdrawal symptoms).*** 0 Patient had no withdrawal symptoms from the drug 1 Patient had withdrawal symptoms from the drug . Not sure *or* not applicable *or* missing	**46**	**0.97**	**0.06**
140	**Using drug to avoid withdrawal**	***Did you have to use the drug to avoid withdrawal symptoms?*** 0 Patient did not have to use the drug to avoid withdrawal symptoms 1 Patient had to use the drug to avoid withdrawal symptoms . Not sure *or* not applicable *or* missing	**40**	**0.94**	**0.06**
141	**Unable to control drug use**	***Did you use more of the drug than you planned or intended to use?*** ***Did you use the drug for a longer period of time than you had planned or intended?*** 0 Patient had control over the drug use 1 Patient used the drug more than what was planned or intended . Not sure *or* not applicable *or* missing	**55**	**0.97**	**0.06**
142	**Unable to reduce or stop drug use**	***Did you try to reduce or stop the drug use and not succeed?*** 0 Patient was able to stop or reduce the drug use 1 Patient was unable to stop or reduce the drug use . Not sure *or* not applicable *or* missing	**54**	**0.97**	**0.06**

(continued)

Table 2.1 (continued)

143	**Time spent to use drug**	***On days of drug use, did you spend substantial time obtaining, using or recovering from the effect of the drug?*** ***Did drug use consume much of your time?*** 0 Patient did not lose substantial time due to the drug use. 1 Patient lost substantial time due to the drug use. . Not sure *or* not applicable *or* missing.	**56**	**0.88**	**0.06**
144	**Failure to fulfil major obligations**	***Did the drug use result in failure to fulfill major role obligations at work, school or home?*** 0 Drug use had no effect on work, school or social obligations 1 Drug use had a negative effect on work, school or social obligations . Not sure *or* not applicable *or* missing	**50**	**0.95**	**0.06**
145	**Giving up social or recreational activities**	***Did the drug use result in giving up or reducing important social or recreational activities?*** 0 The drug had no effect on social or recreational activities 1 The drug had negative effect on social or recreational activities . Not sure *or* not applicable *or* missing	**50**	**0.95**	**0.06**
146	**Less time working due to drug use**	***Did drug use result in less time working?*** 0 Drug use did not result in less time working 1 Drug use resulted in missing one or more days of work . Not sure *or* not applicable *or* missing	**50**	**0.95**	**0.06**
147	**Drug-related work problems**	***Did drug use cause any work problems?*** 0 Drug use caused no work problems 1 Drug use caused work problems . Not sure *or* not applicable *or* missing	**34**	**0.83**	**0.06**
148	**Fighting when using drug**	***Did you get in physical fights when using the drug?*** 0 Patient did not get in physical fights when using the drug 1 Patient got in physical fights when using the drug . Not sure *or* not applicable *or* missing	**22**	**0.80**	**0.06**
149	**Drug-related family problems**	***Did drug use cause any family problems?*** 0 Drug use caused no family problems 1 Drug use caused family problems . Not sure *or* not applicable *or* missing	**58**	**0.80**	**0.06**
150	**Drug-related legal problems**	***Did drug use cause any legal problems?*** 0 Drug use caused no legal problems 1 Drug use caused legal problems . Not sure *or* not applicable *or* missing	**22**	**0.80**	**0.06**

(continued)

Table 2.1 (continued)

151	**Drug-induced mood problems**	***Did drug use cause any mood problems*** **(e.g.,** ***depression, mood swings)?*** 0 Drug use caused no mood problems 1 Drug use caused mood problems . Not sure *or* not applicable *or* missing	**19**	**0.76**	**0.06**
152	**Drug-induced psychosis**	***Did drug use cause any psychotic symptoms*** **(e.g.,** ***delusions, hallucinations)?*** 0 Drug use caused no psychotic symptoms 1 Drug use caused psychotic symptoms . Not sure *or* not applicable *or* missing	**16**	**0.59**	**0.06**
153	**Drug use in spite of problems**	***Did you continue to use the drug even though you had problems?*** 0 Patient had no problems from the drug use 1 Patient continued to use the drug even though the drug caused problems . Not sure *or* not applicable *or* missing	**64**	**0.91**	**0.06**
154	**Drug use in hazardous situations**	***Did you use the drug in a situation, in which it was physically hazardous*** **(e.g.,** ***driving a car or operating machinery)?*** 0 Patient did not use the drug in hazardous situations 1 Patient used the drug in hazardous situations . Not sure *or* not applicable *or* missing	**57**	**0.90**	**0.06**
155	**Being underweight**	***Have you ever been very thin and could not maintain a minimal normal weight?*** ***Have people ever said you weighed much less than normal?*** 0 Absent or non-significant 1 Symptoms present . Not sure *or* not applicable *or* missing	**32**	**0.83**	**0.11**
156	**Weight affects feelings**	***Do you feel that your weight and shape are very important and affect how you feel about yourself to the point that you do not worry about the health risks of being so little?*** 0 Absent or non-significant 1 Symptoms present . Not sure *or* not applicable *or* missing	**50**	**0.75**	**0.12**
157	**Fear of weight gain**	***Do you have an intense fear of gaining weight or becoming fat, even though you are underweight?*** 0 Absent or non-significant 1 Symptoms present . Not sure *or* not applicable *or* missing	**20**	**1.00**	**0.12**

(continued)

Table 2.1 (continued)

158	**Losing weight by fasting**	***Do you try to lose weight by fasting (not eating anything at all for at least 24 hours)?*** 0 Absent or non-significant 1 Symptoms present . Not sure *or* not applicable *or* missing	**32**	**0.95**	**0.12**
159	**Losing weight by exercise**	***Do you try to lose weight by exercising too much (more than 1 hour a day for at least 1 week)?*** 0 Absent or non-significant 1 Symptoms present . Not sure *or* not applicable *or* missing	**22**	**0.86**	**0.12**
160	**Losing weight by diet pills**	***Do you try to lose weight by using diet pills?*** 0 Absent or non-significant 1 Symptoms present . Not sure *or* not applicable *or* missing	**22**	**0.97**	**0.12**
161	**Losing weight by vomiting**	***Do you try to lose weight by inducing vomiting?*** 0 Absent or non-significant 1 Symptoms present . Not sure *or* not applicable *or* missing	**27**	**0.94**	**0.12**
162	**Losing weight by laxatives**	***Do you try to lose weight by taking laxatives or using enemas?*** 0 Absent or non-significant 1 Symptoms present . Not sure *or* not applicable *or* missing	**14**	**1.00**	**0.12**
163	**Losing weight by other methods**	***Do you try to lose weight by taking diuretics? Do you try to lose weight by other methods?*** 0 Absent or non-significant 1 Symptoms present . Not sure *or* not applicable *or* missing	**8**	**1.00**	**0.12**
164	**Binge eating**	***Do you have episodes of binge eating (eating within 1 or 2-hour period what most people would consider an unusually large amount of food)?*** 0 Absent or non-significant 1 Symptoms present . Not sure *or* not applicable *or* missing	**27**	**0.97**	**0.12**
165	**Binge eating frequency**	0 None 1 1–3 times per month 2 At least once a week for 3 months . Not sure *or* not applicable *or* missing	**27**	**0.85**	**0.09**
166	**Losing control with binge eating**	***During the episodes of binge eating, did you feel that you had lost control and could not stop eating?*** 0 Absent or non-significant 1 Symptoms present . Not sure *or* not applicable *or* missing	**17**	**0.96**	**0.12**

(continued)

Table 2.1 (continued)

167	**Eating fast during binge eating**	***During the episodes of binge eating, did you eat much more rapidly than usual?*** 0 Absent or non-significant 1 Symptoms present . Not sure *or* not applicable *or* missing	**16**	**1.00**	**0.12**
168	**Eating until uncomfortably full during binge eating**	***During the episodes of binge eating, did you eat until you felt uncomfortably full?*** 0 Absent or non-significant 1 Symptoms present . Not sure *or* not applicable *or* missing	**25**	**0.94**	**0.12**
169	**Eating when not hungry during binge eating**	***During the episodes of binge eating, did you eat a large amount of food when you did not feel physically hungry?*** 0 Absent or non-significant 1 Symptoms present . Not sure *or* not applicable *or* missing	**22**	**0.97**	**0.12**
170	**Eating alone during binge eating**	***During the episodes of binge eating, did you eat alone because you were embarrassed by how much you were eating?*** 0 Absent or non-significant 1 Symptoms present . Not sure *or* not applicable *or* missing	**16**	**0.96**	**0.12**
171	**Feeling disgusted and guilty during binge eating**	***During the episodes of binge eating, did you feel disgusted with yourself, depressed or guilty by your overeating***? 0 Absent or non-significant 1 Symptoms present . Not sure *or* not applicable *or* missing	**22**	**0.86**	**0.12**
172	**Distressed by overeating during binge eating**	***During the episodes of binge eating, did you feel quite upset or very distressed by your overeating?*** 0 Absent or non-significant 1 Symptoms present . Not sure *or* not applicable *or* missing	**24**	**0.77**	**0.11**
173	**Fasting after binge eating**	***After binge eating episodes, did you try to lose weight by fasting (not eating anything at all for at least 24 hours)?*** 0 Absent or non-significant. 1 Symptoms present. . Not sure *or* not applicable *or* missing.	**19**	**0.93**	**0.12**
174	**Exercise after binge eating**	***After binge eating episodes, did you try to lose weight by exercising too much (more than 1 hour a day for at least 1 week)?*** 0 Absent or non-significant. 1 Symptoms present. . Not sure *or* not applicable *or* missing.	**12**	**0.95**	**0.12**

(continued)

Table 2.1 (continued)

175	**Using diet pills after binge eating**	***After binge eating episodes, did you try to lose weight by using diet pills?*** 0 Absent or non-significant 1 Symptoms present . Not sure *or* not applicable *or* missing	**12**	**0.95**	**0.12**
176	**Vomiting after binge eating**	***After binge eating episodes, did you try to lose weight by inducing vomiting?*** 0 Absent or non-significant 1 Symptoms present . Not sure *or* not applicable *or* missing	**17**	**1.00**	**0.12**
177	**Taking laxatives after binge eating**	***After binge eating episodes, did you try to lose weight by taking laxatives or enemas?*** 0 Absent or non-significant 1 Symptoms present . Not sure *or* not applicable *or* missing	**14**	**1.00**	**0.12**
178	**Other losing weight methods after binge eating**	***After binge eating episodes, did you try to lose weight by taking diuretics?*** ***Do you try to lose weight by other methods?*** 0 Absent or non-significant 1 Symptoms present . Not sure *or* not applicable *or* missing	**9**	**1.00**	**0.12**
179	**Binge eating compensatory behavior frequency**	1 None. 2 1–3 times per month 3 at least once a week for 3 months . Not sure *or* not applicable *or* missing	**25**	**0.87**	**0.09**
180	**Other eating behaviors**	***Do you have any other eating behaviors?*** 0 Absent or non-significant 1 Symptoms present . Not sure *or* not applicable *or* missing	**4**	**0.39**	**0.09**
181	**Attention impairment (poor concentration)**	***Do you have difficulty paying attention and concentrating when reading an article, watching a TV show or a movie, or doing your work or school assignments?*** 0 Absent or non-significant 1 Patient has poor attention and concentration . Not sure *or* not applicable *or* missing	**41**	**0.92**	**0.12**
182	**Sustained attention impairment**	***Do you have difficulty concentrating on one thing for a long time*** (e.g., ***reading a book, writing a letter)?*** 0 Absent or non-significant 1 Patient has difficulty concentrating for a long period of time . Not sure *or* not applicable *or* missing	**39**	**0.95**	**0.12**

(continued)

Table 2.1 (continued)

183	**Avoiding sustained attention tasks**	***Do you avoid tasks that require a lot of concentration at work, school, or home* (e.g., *reading a book, writing a letter)?*** 0 Absent or non-significant 1 Patient avoids tasks that require sustained mental effort . Not sure *or* not applicable *or* missing	**34**	**0.97**	**0.12**
184	**Attention when spoken to**	***Do you have difficulty concentrating on what people say to you, even when they are speaking to you directly?*** 0 Absent or non-significant 1 Patient has difficulty concentrating on what people say . Not sure *or* not applicable *or* missing	**32**	**0.97**	**0.12**
185	**Organization and meeting deadlines**	***Do you have difficulty with tasks that require organization and keeping track of many things all at once* (e.g., *planning and organizing your work or household chores)?*** ***Do you have difficulty managing your time* (e.g., *usually fail to meet deadlines)?*** 0 Absent or non-significant 1 Patient has difficulty with tasks that require organization or meeting deadlines . Not sure *or* not applicable *or* missing	**30**	**0.82**	**0.12**
186	**Changing activities**	***Do you change from one activity to another without finishing the first?*** 0 Absent or non-significant 1 Patient changes from one activity to another without finishing the first . Not sure *or* not applicable *or* missing	**40**	**0.92**	**0.12**
187	**Distraction (attention is distracted by environmental noises)**	***Are you easily distracted from tasks by activity or noise around you?*** 0 Absent or non-significant 1 Patient is easily distracted from tasks by activity or noise around . Not sure *or* not applicable *or* missing	**43**	**0.97**	**0.12**
188	**Misplacing things**	***Do you lose or misplace things more often than others* (e.g., *wallets, keys, cell phones)?*** 0 Absent or non-significant 1 Patient loses or misplaces things more often than others . Not sure *or* not applicable *or* missing	**43**	**0.94**	**0.12**

(continued)

Table 2.1 (continued)

189	**Forgetting daily activities**	***Do you forget daily activities more often than others (*****e.g.*****, appointments, paying bills, returning phone calls)?*** 0 Absent or non-significant 1 Patient forgets daily activities more often than others . Not sure *or* not applicable *or* missing	**24**	**0.94**	**0.12**
190	**Losing track**	***Do you lose track of what you are doing (*****e.g.*****, forget why you went to get something)?*** 0 Absent or non-significant 1 Patient loses track of what he/she is doing . Not sure *or* not applicable *or* missing	**40**	**0.92**	**0.12**
191	**Fidgety**	***Do you have difficulty remaining seated (fidget with hands and feet, squirm or wiggle in seat) when expected to remain seated (*****e.g.*****, in a meeting or a church service)?*** 0 Absent or non-significant 1 Patient fidgets with hands and feet, or wiggles in seat . Not sure *or* not applicable *or* missing	**41**	**0.81**	**0.12**
192	**Leaving seats**	***Do you leave your seat in meetings or other situations (*****e.g.*****, during an appointment or a church service) where you are expected to remain seated?*** 0 Absent or non-significant 1 Patient leaves seat in meetings or other situations where expected to remain seated . Not sure *or* not applicable *or* missing	**30**	**0.88**	**0.12**
193	**Restlessness/ moving**	***Do you feel restless, fidgety and you must get up and move around?*** 0 Absent or non-significant 1 Patient feels restless, fidgety and must move around . Not sure *or* not applicable *or* missing	**49**	**0.61**	**0.12**
194	**Hyperactivity**	***Do you feel overly active and compelled to do things, like you are driven by a motor?*** 0 Absent or non-significant 1 Patient feels overly active and compelled to do things . Not sure *or* not applicable *or* missing	**22**	**0.97**	**0.12**
195	**Waiting in line**	***Is it difficult for you to wait in line for your turn when the situation calls for it?*** 0 Absent or non-significant 1 Patient has difficulty waiting in line . Not sure *or* not applicable *or* missing	**23**	**1.00**	**0.12**

(continued)

Table 2.1 (continued)

196	**Talking too much**	***Do you think you talk too much?*** ***Do others say that you talk too much?*** 0 Absent or non-significant 1 Patient talks too much . Not sure *or* not applicable *or* missing	**12**	**1.00**	**0.12**
197	**Loud and noisy**	***Do you think that you are a loud and noisy person?*** ***Do other people sometimes ask you to quiet down or lower your voice?*** 0 Absent or non-significant 1 Patient or others feel the patient is loud and noisy . Not sure *or* not applicable *or* missing	**22**	**0.58**	**0.11**
198	**Impulsivity**	***Are you impulsive (e.g., act before you think adequately about consequences of actions)?*** 0 Absent or non-significant 1 Patient is impulsive . Not sure *or* not applicable *or* missing	**41**	**0.92**	**0.12**
199	**Disturbing others**	***Do you disturb others or intrude on others (e.g., when people are talking or when people are involved in activities?)*** 0 Absent or non-significant 1 Patient disturbs others or intrudes on others . Not sure *or* not applicable *or* missing	**23**	**0.97**	**0.12**
200	**Blurt out answers**	***Do you have tendency to blurt out an answer before another person has finished asking the question?*** 0 Absent or non-significant 1 Patient blurts out the answers . Not sure *or* not applicable *or* missing	**32**	**0.89**	**0.12**

[a]Kappa values were calculated based upon interrater interviews of 322 patients at William R. Sharpe Jr. Hospital, Chestnut Ridge Center (inpatient and outpatient), Ain Shams University Hospital, and Mansoura University Hospital

DSM-5 (crying when depressed, feeling hopeless and reduced sexual desire) were included in the initial depression dimension because they have been recommended and used by experts and clinicians even before the existence of the DSM. The sensitivity and specificity of the initial depression scale were 93.24% and 74.15%, respectively. Following the rules of creating the SCIP scales, the final core depression scale has 10 items with sensitivity 93.24% and specificity 72.32% [29].

Based upon the reliable 230 psychopathology items and reliable SCIP dimensions, the SCIP is the only instrument that includes 18 clinician-administered scales to cover most adult symptom domains: anxiety, obsessions, compulsions, posttraumatic stress, depression, mania, delusions, hallucinations, disorganized thoughts, aggression, negative symptoms, alcohol use, drug use, attention deficit, hyperactivity, anorexia, binge-eating, and bulimia.

Table 2.2 The items of the SCIP generalized anxiety scale, item rest correlation, mean interitem correlation, and Cronbach's alpha with one-sided 95% confidence interval (CI), sensitivity, and specificity at the optimal cutpoint and receiver operating characteristic (ROC) area with standard error (SE)

Generalized anxiety scale items	Item rest correlation	Mean interitem correlation	Cronbach's alpha (one-sided 95% CI)	Validity at cutpoint	Sensitivity	Specificity	ROC Area (SE)
1. Anxiety	0.2854			≥2	77.78%	97.76%	0.9889 (0.0036)
2. Restlessness with anxiety	0.8957						
3. Tension with anxiety	0.9121						
4. Exhaustion with anxiety	0.867						
5. Poor concentration with anxiety	0.8926						
6. Irritability with anxiety	0.8485						
7. Insomnia with anxiety	0.9027						
		0.6774	0.9363 (≥0.9301)				

Data based upon 700 patients interviewed at Sharpe Hospital and Chestnut Ridge Center

Tables 2.2, 2.3, 2.4, 2.5, 2.6, 2.7, 2.8, 2.9, 2.10, 2.11, 2.12, 2.13, and 2.14 show the items included in the final SCIP scales, item rest correlation, mean interitem correlation, Cronbach's alpha with one-sided 95% confidence interval, sensitivity, and specificity at the optimal cutpoint and receiver operating characteristic (ROC) area with standard error. All of the SCIP scales have been validated with the exception of the obsessive-compulsive and eating disorders scales.

Self-administered versions of the SCIP scales were developed (15 self-administered scales to be completed by the patients) covering anxiety, obsessions, compulsions, posttraumatic stress, depression, mania, delusions, hallucinations, alcohol use, drug use, attention deficit, hyperactivity, anorexia, binge-eating, and bulimia. Chapter 4 includes the final version of the SCIP clinician-administered and self-administered scales.

Table 2.3 The items of the SCIP core PTSD scale, item rest correlation, mean interitem correlation, and Cronbach's alpha with one-sided 95% confidence interval (CI), sensitivity, and specificity at the optimal cutpoint and receiver operating characteristic (ROC) area with standard error (SE)

Core PTSD scale items	Item rest correlation	Mean interitem correlation	Cronbach's alpha (one-sided 95% CI)	Validity at cutpoint	Sensitivity	Specificity	ROC Area (SE)
1. Traumatic experience	0.6695			≥4	93.75%	98.42%	0.9868 (0.0082)
2. Distressing memories	0.8618						
3. Nightmares/ bad dreams	0.8354						
4. Flashback	0.8222						
5. Avoidance	0.8599						
6. Amnesia	0.608						
7. Diminished social interest	0.7384						
8. Detached/ distant	0.8118						
9. Diminished emotional feelings	0.8313						
10. Insomnia	0.8001						
11. Anger	0.7598						
12. Hypervigilance	0.7623						
13. Startle response	0.8162						
		0.6403	0.9586 (≥0.9547)				

Data based upon 700 patients interviewed at Sharpe Hospital and Chestnut Ridge Center

The Development of the SCIP Glossary of Psychiatric Symptoms and Signs

The SCIP glossary includes the definitions of 30 screening items and 200 psychopathology items and is the most consistent and comprehensive psychopathology vocabulary in psychiatric literature. The SCIP glossary is the only glossary that provides reliability estimates for each item. Interrater reliability was measured: among the 30 screening items, 19 items (63%) have good reliability (Kappa >0.7) and 11 items (37%) have fair reliability (Kappa ranges from 0.5 to 0.7). Among the

Table 2.4 The items of the SCIP core depression scale, item rest correlation, mean interitem correlation, and Cronbach's alpha with one-sided 95% confidence interval (CI), sensitivity, and specificity at the optimal cutpoint and receiver operating characteristic (ROC) area with standard error (SE)

Core scale items	Item rest correlation	Mean interitem correlation	Cronbach's alpha (one-sided 95% CI)	Validity at cutpoint	Sensitivity	Specificity	ROC Area (SE)
1. Depressed mood	0.84			≥6	93.24%	72.32%	0.8481 (0.0151)
2. Anhedonia	0.817						
3. Hopelessness	0.825						
4. Poor concentration	0.78						
5. Psychomotor retardation	0.693						
6. Worthlessness	0.786						
7. Guilt	0.668						
8. Suicide	0.325						
		0.563	0.912 (≥0.903)				

Data based upon 700 patients interviewed at Sharpe Hospital and Chestnut Ridge Center

200 psychopathology items, 7 items (3.5%) have poor reliability (Kappa <0.5), 24 items (12%) have fair reliability (Kappa ranges from 0.5 to 0.7), and 169 items (84.5%) have good reliability (Kappa >0.7). Chapter 5 will demonstrate the development of the SCIP glossary of symptoms and signs.

Measurement-Based Care (MBC) Training Curriculum for Mental Health Professionals and Psychiatry Residency Programs

The SCIP principles of rating symptoms and signs allow researchers and clinicians to use all the SCIP 18 clinician-administered scales covering most adult symptom domains: anxiety, obsessions, compulsions, posttraumatic stress, depression, mania, delusions, hallucinations, disorganized thoughts, aggression, negative symptoms, alcohol use, drug use, attention deficit, hyperactivity, anorexia, binge-eating, and bulimia. This unique property of the SCIP allowed the development of the first

Table 2.5 The items of the SCIP core mania scale, item rest correlation, mean interitem correlation, and Cronbach's alpha with one-sided 95% confidence interval (CI), sensitivity, and specificity at the optimal cutpoint and receiver operating characteristic (ROC) area with standard error (SE)

Core mania scale items	Item rest correlation	Mean interitem correlation	Cronbach's alpha (one-sided 95% CI)	Validity at cutpoint	Sensitivity	Specificity	ROC Area (SE)
1. Elated mood	0.6063			(≥4	95.12%	79.93%	0.9160 (0.0110)
2. Irritable mood	0.6301						
3. Mixed mood	0.3557						
4. Racing thoughts	0.7698						
5. Pressured speech	0.745						
6. Distraction	0.702						
7. Increase in activities	0.7982						
8. Grandiosity	0.5279						
9. Over spending	0.7661						
10. Decreased sleep	0.7125						
		0.4855	0.9042 (≥0.8951)				

Data based upon 700 patients interviewed at Sharpe Hospital and Chestnut Ridge Center

comprehensive training curriculum designed to teach psychiatrists and mental health professionals how to use rating scales in clinical practice. To ensure that future generations of psychiatrists have adequate training in using scales, a training curriculum for psychiatry residency programs was developed and published [32]. Measurement-Based Care (MBC) Training Curriculum for Mental Health Professionals and Psychiatry Residency Programs will be described in detail in Chap. 9.

Table 2.6 The items of the SCIP core schizophrenia scale, item rest correlation, mean interitem correlation, and Cronbach's alpha with one-sided 95% confidence interval (CI), sensitivity, and specificity at the optimal cutpoint and receiver operating characteristic (ROC) area with standard error (SE)

Core schizophrenia scale items	Item rest correlation	Mean interitem correlation	Cronbach's alpha (one-sided 95% CI)	Validity at cutpoint	Sensitivity	Specificity	ROC Area (SE)
1. Hallucination quality	0.6613			≥2	90.12	89.39	0.9265 (0.0150)
2. Hallucination frequency	0.6689						
3. Hallucination duration	0.6567						
4. Voices commenting	0.5977						
5. Visual hallucination	0.5415						
6. Other hallucinations	0.1696						
7. Thought insertion	0.5072						
8. Thought withdrawal	0.3182						
9. Thought broadcast	0.4717						
10. Paranoid delusions	0.5995						
11. Conspiracy delusion	0.4778						
12. Delusion of reference	0.3779						
13. Other delusion	0.1106						
14. Bizarreness of delusion	0.3817						
15. Derailment	0.2916						
16. Tangentiality	0.282						
17. Incoherent speech	0.1908						
18. Other disorganizations	0.2579						
		0.2154	0.8317 (≥0.8141)				

Data based upon 700 patients interviewed at Sharpe Hospital and Chestnut Ridge Center

Table 2.7 The items of the SCIP core alcohol scale, item rest correlation, mean interitem correlation, and Cronbach's alpha with one-sided 95% confidence interval (CI), sensitivity, and specificity at the optimal cutpoint and receiver operating characteristic (ROC) area with standard error (SE)

Core alcohol scale items	Item rest correlation	Mean interitem correlation	Cronbach's alpha (one-sided 95% CI)	Validity at cutpoint	Sensitivity	Specificity	ROC Area (SE)
1. Alcohol tolerance	0.6932			≥2	79.31%	97.10%	0.9391 (0.0111)
2. Alcohol withdrawal	0.7044						
3. Failure of obligations	0.775						
4. Alcohol-related social problems	0.5997						
5. Alcohol use in spite of problems	0.8431						
6. Alcohol use in hazardous situations	0.6499						
7. Blackout	0.7776						
		0.5828	0.9072 (≥0.8981)				

Data based upon 700 patients interviewed at Sharpe Hospital and Chestnut Ridge Center

Conclusions

The development of the SCIP suite with its four components (comprehensive and reliable 230 psychopathology items, a complete set of clinician-administered and self-administered scales, a comprehensive and consistent psychiatric glossary, and a measurement-based care curriculum) is compatible with the twenty-first century advances in neuroscience, measurement-based care, and personalized medicine in psychiatry. This will be explained in further detail in the next chapters of the manual.

Table 2.8 The items of the SCIP core drug scale, item rest correlation, mean interitem correlation, and Cronbach's alpha with one-sided 95% confidence interval (CI), sensitivity, and specificity at the optimal cutpoint and receiver operating characteristic (ROC) area with standard error (SE)

Core drug scale items	Item rest correlation	Mean interitem correlation	Cronbach's alpha (one-sided 95% CI)	Validity at cutpoint	Sensitivity	Specificity	ROC Area (SE)
1. Drug tolerance	0.7343			≥2	59.65%	91.54%	0.8514 (0.0168)
2. Drug withdrawal	0.7095						
3. Failure of obligations	0.7384						
4. Drug-related social problems	0.4353						
5. Drug use in spite of problems	0.803						
6. Drug use in hazardous situations	0.6279						
		0.5324	0.8723 (≥0.8596)				

Data based upon 700 patients interviewed at Sharpe Hospital and Chestnut Ridge Center

Table 2.9 The items of the SCIP core adult ADHD scale, item rest correlation, mean interitem correlation, and Cronbach's alpha with one-sided 95% confidence interval (CI), sensitivity, and specificity at the optimal cutpoint and receiver operating characteristic (ROC) area with standard error (SE)

Core adult ADHD	Item rest correlation scale items	Mean interitem correlation	Cronbach's alpha (one-sided 95% CI)	Validity at cutpoint	Sensitivity	Specificity	ROC Area (SE)
1. Attention impairment	0.367			≥5	94.74%	83.33%	0.9591 (0.0264)
2. Sustained attention impairment	0.4167						
3. Attention when spoken to	0.5383						
4. Changing activities	0.4024						
5. Distraction	0.5029						
6. Fidgety	0.4156						
7. Leaving seats	0.5507						
8. Restless and moving	0.4901						
9. Hyperactivity	0.3889						
10. Impulsivity	0.464						
		0.2666	0.7843 (≥0.6864)				

Data based upon 40 patients interviewed at Sharpe Hospital and Chestnut Ridge Center

Table 2.10 The items of the SCIP aggression scale, item rest correlation, mean interitem correlation, and Cronbach's alpha with one-sided 95% confidence interval (CI)

Aggression scale items	Item rest correlation	Mean interitem correlation	Cronbach's alpha (one-sided 95% CI)
Agitation	0.4046		
Violence	0.5073		
Violence a day	0.381		
Iolence a period	0.3818		
Odd behavior	0.5514		
Inappropriate affect	0.3251		
		0.2742	0.6939 (≥0.6635)

Data based upon 700 patients interviewed at Sharpe Hospital and Chestnut Ridge Center

Table 2.11 The items of the SCIP negativity scale, item rest correlation, mean interitem correlation, and Cronbach's alpha with one-sided 95% confidence interval (CI)

Negative symptom scale items	Item rest correlation	Mean interitem correlation	Cronbach's alpha (one-sided 95% CI)
1. Blunted affect	0.6847		
2. Avolition	0.5682		
3. Alogia	0.6744		
4. Psychomotor slowing	0.6096		
5. Poor self-care	0.5742		
		0.4877	0.8264 (≥0.8087)

Data based upon 700 patients interviewed at Sharpe Hospital and Chestnut Ridge Center

Table 2.12 The items of the SCIP anorexia scale, item rest correlation, mean interitem correlation, and Cronbach's alpha with one-sided 95% confidence interval (CI)

Anorexia scale items	Item rest correlation	Mean interitem correlation	Cronbach's alpha (one-sided 95% CI)
1. Being underweight	0.4009		
2. Weight affect feeling	0.3134		
3. Fear of weight gain	0.5464		
4 losing weight by fasting	0.6139		
5. Losing weight by exercise	0.2711		
6. Losing weight by diet pills	0.3373		
7. Losing weight by vomiting	0.5962		
8. Losing weight by laxatives	0.4392		
9. Other losing weight methods	0.3417		
		0.2496	0.7496 (≥0.6398)

Data based upon 40 patients interviewed at Sharpe Hospital and Chestnut Ridge Center

Table 2.13 The items of the SCIP binge-eating scale, item rest correlation, mean interitem correlation, and Cronbach's alpha with one-sided 95% confidence interval (CI)

Binge-eating scale items	Item rest correlation	Mean interitem correlation	Cronbach's alpha (one-sided 95% CI)
1. Binge-eating	0.9585		
2. Binge-eating frequency	0.9366		
3. Losing control	0.7628		
4. Binge-eating behavior	0.9585		
5. Eat fast	0.7743		
6. Eat until full	0.9315		
7. Eat when not hungry	0.8544		
8. Eat alone	0.6485		
9. Feel disgusted/guilty	0.7765		
10. Distressed by overeating	0.8714		
		0.7434	0.9666 (≥0.9521)

Data based upon 40 patients interviewed at Sharpe Hospital and Chestnut Ridge Center

Table 2.14 The items of the SCIP bulimia scale, item rest correlation, mean interitem correlation, and Cronbach's alpha with one-sided 95% confidence interval (CI)

Bulimia scale items	Item rest correlation	Mean interitem correlation	Cronbach's alpha (one-sided 95% CI)
1. Binge-eating	0.9187		
2. Binge-eating frequency	0.9437		
3. Losing control	0.7330		
4. Binge-eating behavior	0.9187		
5. Eat fast	0.7264		
6. Eat until full	0.9098		
7. Eat when not hungry	0.8223		
8. Eat alone	0.6721		
9. Feel disgusted/guilty	0.7574		
10. Distressed by overeating	0.8894		
11. Compensatory behavior	0.9190		
12. Losing weight by fasting	0.5864		
13. Losing weight by exercise	0.6744		
14. Losing weight by diet pills	0.6407		
15. Losing weight by vomiting	0.5884		
16. Losing weight by laxatives	0.5864		
17. Other losing weight methods	0.5817		
18. Compensatory behavior frequency	0.9418		
		0.6088	0.9655 (≥0.9511)

Data based upon 40 patients interviewed at Sharpe Hospital and Chestnut Ridge Center

References

1. Moore, T. (1933). In E. A. Pace (Ed.), *The essential psychoses and their fundamental syndromes: Studies in psychology and psychiatry from the Catholic University of America*. Williams and Wilkins.
2. Kay, S. R., Fiszbein, A., & Opler, L. A. (1987). The positive and negative syndrome scale (PANSS) for schizophrenia. *Schizophrenia Bulletin, 13*, 261–276.
3. Overall, J. E., & Gorham, D. R. (1988). The brief psychiatric rating scale (BPRS): Recent developments in ascertainment and scaling. *Psychopharmacology Bulletin, 24*, 97–99.
4. Goodman, W. K., Price, L. H., Rasmussen, S. A., Mazure, C., Delgado, P., Heninger, G. R., & Charney, D. S. (1989). The Yale-Brown obsessive compulsive scale. II. Validity. *Archives of General Psychiatry, 46*, 1012–1016.
5. Goodman, W. K., Price, L. H., Rasmussen, S. A., Mazure, C., Fleischmann, R. L., Hill, C. L., Heninger, G. R., & Charney, D. S. (1989). The Yale-Brown obsessive compulsive scale. I. Development, use, and reliability. *Archives of General Psychiatry, 46*, 1006–1011.
6. Hamilton, M. (1960). A rating scale for depression. *Journal of Neurology, Neurosurgery, and Psychiatry, 23*, 56–62.
7. Hamilton, M. (1959). The assessment of anxiety states by rating. *The British Journal of Medical Psychology, 32*, 50–55.
8. Wing, J. K., Birley, J. L., Cooper, J. E., Graham, P., & Isaacs, A. D. (1967). Reliability of a procedure for measuring and classifying "present psychiatric state". *The British Journal of Psychiatry: The Journal of Mental Science, 113*, 499–515.
9. Nasrallah, H. (2009). Long overdue: Measurement-based psychiatric practice. *Current Psychiatry, 8*, 14–16.
10. WHO. (1993). *The ICD-10 classification of mental and behavioral disorders: Diagnostic criteria for research* (10th ed.). World Health Organization.
11. American Psychiatric Association. (2013). *Diagnostic and statistical manual of mental disorders* (5th ed.). American Psychiatric Association.
12. Williams, J. B., Gibbon, M., First, M. B., Spitzer, R. L., Davies, M., Borus, J., Howes, M. J., Kane, J., Pope, H. G., Jr., Rounsaville, B., et al. (1992). The structured clinical interview for DSM-III-R (SCID). II. Multisite test-retest reliability. *Archives of General Psychiatry, 49*, 630–636.
13. Spitzer, R. L., Williams, J. B., Gibbon, M., & First, M. B. (1992). The structured clinical interview for DSM-III-R (SCID). I: History, rationale, and description. *Archives of General Psychiatry, 49*, 624–629.
14. Jk, W., Babor, T., Brugha, T., Burke, J., Cooper, J. E., Giel, R., Jablenski, A., Regier, D., & Sartorius, N. (1990). SCAN. Schedules for clinical assessment in neuropsychiatry. *Archives of General Psychiatry, 47*, 589–593.
15. Picardi, A., Adler, D. A., Rogers, W. H., Lega, I., Zerella, M. P., Matteucci, G., Tarsitani, L., Caredda, M., Gigantesco, A., & Biondi, M. (2013). Diagnostic accuracy of the primary care screener for affective disorder (PC-SAD) in primary care. *Clinical Practice and Epidemiology in Mental Health, 9*, 164–170.
16. Pinna, F., Deriu, L., Lepori, T., Maccioni, R., Milia, P., Sarritzu, E., Tusconi, M., & Carpiniello, B. (2013). Is it true remission? A study of remitted patients affected by schizophrenia and schizoaffective disorders. *Psychiatry Research, 210*, 739–744.
17. Sheehan, D. V., Lecrubier, Y., Sheehan, K. H., Amorim, P., Janavs, J., Weiller, E., Hergueta, T., Baker, R., & Dunbar, G. C. (1998). The Mini-International Neuropsychiatric Interview (M.I.N.I.): the development and validation of a structured diagnostic psychiatric interview for DSM-IV and ICD-10. *Journal of Clinical Psychiatry, 59*(Suppl 20), 22–33;quiz 34–57.
18. Aboraya, A. (2009). Use of structured interviews by psychiatrists in real clinical settings: Results of an open-question survey. *Psychiatry (Edgmont), 6*, 24–28.

19. Nienhuis, F. J., van de Willige, G., Rijnders, C. A., de Jonge, P., & Wiersma, D. (2010). Validity of a short clinical interview for psychiatric diagnosis: The mini-SCAN. *The British Journal of Psychiatry: The Journal of Mental Science, 196*, 64–68.
20. Gilbody, S. M., House AO, & Sheldon, T. A. (2002). Psychiatrists in the UK do not use outcomes measures. National survey. *The British Journal of Psychiatry: The Journal of Mental Science, 180*, 101–103.
21. Duffy, F. F., Chung, H., Trivedi, M., Rae, D. S., Regier, D. A., & Katzelnick, D. J. (2008). Systematic use of patient-rated depression severity monitoring: Is it helpful and feasible in clinical psychiatry? *Psychiatric Services, 59*, 1148–1154.
22. Morrison, J. (2008). *The first interview* (Third ed.). The Guilford Press.
23. Rettew, D. C., Lynch, A. D., Achenbach, T. M., Dumenci, L., & Ivanova, M. Y. (2009). Meta-analyses of agreement between diagnoses made from clinical evaluations and standardized diagnostic interviews. *International Journal of Methods in Psychiatric Research, 18*, 169–184.
24. Bastiaens, L. (2011). Poor practice, managed care, and magic pills: Have we created a mental health monster? *Psychiatric Times, 28*, 1–4.
25. Busner, J., Kaplan, S. L., Greco, N., & Sheehan, D. V. (2011). The use of research measures in adult clinical practice. *Innovations of Clinical Neuroscience, 8*, 19–23.
26. Aboraya, A. (2015). The validity results of the standard for clinicians' interview in psychiatry (SCIP). *Schizophrenia Bulletin, 41*, S103–S104.
27. Aboraya, A., El-Missiry, A., Barlowe, J., John, C., Ebrahimian, A., Muvvala, S., Brandish, J., Mansour, H., Zheng, W., Chumber, P., Berry, J., Elswick, D., Hill, C., Swager, L., Abo Elez, W., Ashour, H., Haikal, A., Eissa, A., Rabie, M., … Price, E. (2014). The reliability of the standard for clinicians' interview in psychiatry (SCIP): a clinician-administered tool with categorical, dimensional and numeric output. *Schizophrenia Research, 156*, 174–183.
28. Aboraya, A., Nasrallah, H., Muvvala, S., El-Missiry, A., Mansour, H., Hill, C., Elswick, D., & Price, E. C. (2016). The standard for clinicians' interview in psychiatry (SCIP): A clinician-administered tool with categorical, dimensional, and numeric output-conceptual development, design, and description of the SCIP. *Innovations of Clinical Neuroscience, 13*, 31–77.
29. Aboraya, A., Nasrallah, H. A., Elswick, D. E., Ahmed, E., Estephan, N., Aboraya, D., Berzingi, S., Chumbers, J., Berzingi, S., Justice, J., Zafar, J., & Dohar, S. (2018). Measurement-based care in psychiatry-past, present, and future. *Innovations of Clinical Neuroscience, 15*, 13–26.
30. Rodgers, B., & Mann, S. A. (1986). The reliability and validity of PSE assessments by lay interviewers: A national population survey. *Psychological Medicine, 16*, 689–700.
31. Andreasen, N. C., Flaum, M., & Arndt, S. (1992). The comprehensive assessment of symptoms and history (CASH). An instrument for assessing diagnosis and psychopathology. *Archives of General Psychiatry, 49*, 615–623.
32. Aboraya, A., et al. (2021). Measurement-based care training curriculum in psychiatry residency programs: I: Description of the curriculum and demonstration of implementation. *Annals of Clinical Psychiatry, 33*, 168–179.

Chapter 3
The SCIP Principles of Rating Symptoms, Signs, and Creating Reliable Questions and Dimensions

In essence, the Standard for Clinicians' Interview in Psychiatry (SCIP) is a state-of-art process of psychopathology assessment which is compatible with the twenty-first century advances in neuroscience and personalized medicine in psychiatry. Chapter 3 describes the SCIP process of assessment of symptoms and signs and creating reliable questions and dimensions. Evaluation of episodes and assessment of causes of mental disorders are reviewed.

Principles of Designing the SCIP Questions

As in the case of medicine, modern psychiatric diagnosis depends on the assessment of psychopathological symptoms and signs. The SCIP interview reflects a state-of-the-art approach to assessment and includes questions designed to evaluate symptoms and signs of mental illness. **The SCIP questions were designed with four principles:**

(a) Questions are worded to be simple and easily understood by patients regardless of their intellectual level.
(b) Questions simulate what seasoned psychiatrists usually ask.
(c) The meaning of the questions and examples are embedded in the questions so that each question and the response reflect the criterion being examined.
(d) Responses to questions have the fewest possible subcategories to reflect the clinical significance of the symptom, **following the principle of least subcategories of symptom severity (LSSS).** The fewer the subcategories reflecting symptom severity, the more efficient the interview and the more likely that clinicians will use the questions.

A. S. Aboraya, *Manual for the Standard for Clinicians' Interview in Psychiatry (SCIP)*, Advances in Mental Health and Addiction,
https://doi.org/10.1007/978-3-030-94930-3_3

For example, one criterion for a major depressive episode is “diminished ability to think or concentrate.” Here is the SCIP question and possible responses:

Attention impairment (poor concentration)	***Have you found that your concentration has decreased and you are unable to complete a task* (e.g., *at work, reading an article, reading a book, or watching a movie), even though you were able to do that before?*** 0 Patient has no concentration problems 1 Patient has difficulty concentrating less than half the time 2 Patient has difficulty concentrating more than half the time . Not sure *or* Not applicable *or* Missing	**Kappa 0.80**

The question and responses explain the criterion, give examples of impaired concentration, and measure the severity of the problem (less than half the time or more than half the time).

Coding Symptoms of Psychopathology

First, questions are asked regarding a specific period (past week, past month, past year, etc.). The interviewer decides on the specific time frame for the questions. The interviewer may choose the past month when evaluating mood, the past year when evaluating alcohol use, and so on. The general principle is to code 0 for absent or subclinical symptoms. Many questions have ratings of 0 (absent or subclinical symptom) and 1 (clinical symptom).

Panic attacks	**Did you have a panic attack, when you suddenly become anxious and frightened for a short period of time (up to 60 minutes)?** **During that time, did you feel that your heart was racing or pounding, or did you start shaking or sweating, or did you feel you were choking?** 0 Patient had no panic attacks 1 Patient had panic attacks . Not sure *or* Not applicable *or* Missing	**Kappa** 0.92

Some questions have the following codes:

0 Absent or non-significant
1 A symptom is present for less than 50% of the time or less than 50% of times.
The mere presence of a symptom does not qualify for a rating of one. To receive a rating of one, a symptom must be more than what a normal person would experience, or cause at least some distress, or force the patient to seek professional help.
2 The same as a rating of one. In addition, the symptom is present for more than 50% of the time or more than 50% of times.

Hopelessness	***Have you felt hopeless about your future?*** 0 Patient is not hopeless 1 Patient feels hopeless less than half the time 2 Patient feels hopeless more than half the time . Not sure *or* Not applicable *or* Missing	**Kappa 0.82**

Some questions have possible responses of 0 (absent or subclinical), 1, 2, and 3 to allow for severity measurement and to generate a dimensional score when added to responses from other questions.

Hallucination duration	**On days when you hear noises or voices, how often do you hear them?**	**Kappa**
	0 Patient has no auditory hallucinations 1 Patient has auditory hallucinations (less than 1 hour/day) 2 Patient has auditory hallucinations (1–4 hours/day) 3 Patient has auditory hallucinations (more than 4 hours/day) . Not sure *or* Not applicable *or* Missing	**0.92**

Coding Signs of Psychopathology

The SCIP interview includes observational items to assess for signs of mental illness. The interviewer listens to the patient, asks him/her questions, examines the patient, and rates the observational items.

Some observational items have questions. For example, the interviewer observes the patient's speech and can ask about symptom of pressured speech over a specific period of time.

Pressured speech	***Have you been talking faster than usual during this time (for example, people said that they were unable to understand you because you were speaking too fast or you felt a pressure to continue talking)?*** 0 Patient has normal speech 1 Patient has pressured speech less than half the time 2 Patient has pressured speech more than half the time . Not sure *or* Not applicable *or* Missing	**Kappa 0.72**

Some observational items require active interviewer's observation and examination, as in catatonia. The interviewer observes the patient; tests for mobility, rigidity, catalepsy, and waxy flexibility; and rates catatonia items.

Catalepsy: Patients maintain any odd or unusual posture the interviewer places them in. 0 Patient has no catalepsy 1 Patient has catalepsy

Waxy flexibility: Patient maintains a limb in a certain position. When the interviewer moves the limb, the limb feels as if it were made of wax. 0 Patient has no waxy flexibility 1 Patient has waxy flexibility

Some observational items are described and observed.

Flight of ideas	***Flight of Ideas (a combination of pressured speech and derailment):*** 0 Patient has no flight of ideas 1 Patient has flight of ideas . Not sure *or* Not applicable *or* Missing	**Kappa 0.62**

Observed hallucinations	0 Patient has not been observed talking to self 1 Patient has been observed talking to self, talking to a mirror, or running a conversation with unseen person . Not sure *or* Not applicable *or* Missing	**Kappa 0.55**

Derailment (loose associations)	0 Normal speech 1 Patient has derailment (loose associations): speech shifts to different topics, related or unrelated, but eventually comes back to the main topic 2 Patient has severe derailment (loose associations): speech shifts to different topics, mostly unrelated and never comes back to main topic . Not sure *or* Not applicable *or* Missing	**Kappa 0.65**

Tangentiality	0 Normal speech. 1 Patient has some tangentiality: replying to a question is related in some distant way 2 Patient has severe tangentiality: replying to a question is totally unrelated . Not sure *or* Not applicable *or* Missing	**Kappa 0.57**

Incoherent speech	0 Normal speech 1 Patient has incoherent speech: each sentence by itself makes sense. However, the first sentence is unrelated to the next sentence . Not sure *or* Not applicable *or* Missing	**Kappa 0.41**

General Notes on Ratings

(a) Do not overrate symptoms. If the symptom is present and the clinician is not sure whether to rate 1 or 2, the code should be 1. If the clinician decides that the patient has a concentration problem, but he/she forgot to ask about the duration of the problem, the code should be 1 and not 2.
(b) A symptom rated 1 will qualify for diagnostic criteria.
(c) If the clinician is not sure whether the symptom is present after a thorough questioning, the clinician can make a judgment call about whether the symptom is present or absent. If the clinician does not feel comfortable making a decision, he/she can choose the rating of "." for "Not Sure."

Special Notes on Delusions

Delusions are ideas with the following criteria:

(a) The idea is false based on what most people of the same culture know (false idea).
(b) The patient is convinced that the idea is true (firm idea).
(c) If the patient is provided with evidence that contradicts the idea, the patient is still convinced that the idea is true (fixed idea).

If the patient has paranoid delusions less than half the time, the rating is one. If the patient has paranoid delusions more than half the time, the rating is two. Typically, a patient with delusions goes through three phases:

(a) **Initial partial delusions:** The initial transition from normal thoughts to delusional thoughts. The delusional thoughts gradually occupy some of the patient's time. As time goes on without treatment, the delusional thoughts occupy more of the patient's time.
(b) **Full delusions:** The delusions occupy most or the entirety of a patient's time. Typically, when patients are admitted to hospitals, they have full delusions.
(c) **Residual partial delusions:** As the patient receives antipsychotic medications and improves, the patient starts to question his/her delusional thoughts. The delusional thoughts occupy less and less of the patient's time. Eventually, the delusional thoughts disappear.

Principles of Designing Clinically Useful Psychological Dimensions

The SCIP study measured Kappa for 200 psychological symptoms and signs and 30 screening questions. Based upon reliable SCIP items, the SCIP dimensions were created. The SCIP questions were designed so that dimensional measures can be generated easily whether the interviewer is using the paper version or the SCIP software. ***The SCIP method of creating reliable and clinically relevant dimensions was based upon the following nine principles:***

1. **Reliable dimensions require reliable symptoms and signs.** Psychological symptoms and signs are the building blocks of psychological dimensions. The SCIP study confirmed the hypothesis that reliable psychological dimensions require reliable symptoms and signs. The absence of valid and reliable symptoms was the main limiting factor in prior attempts to create dimensional models [1]. The SCIP reliable symptoms and signs removed this major obstacle. Based upon reliable SCIP items, the SCIP dimensions were created and have evidenced reliability [2].
2. **Each item is given one score, regardless of the number of questions exploring the item.** Typically, a SCIP item is assessed with one question. The question has embedded examples, if needed, so that each question and the response reflect the criterion being examined. Sometimes, one criterion needs to be assessed using several questions. In that case, even if the patient responds yes to several questions evaluating the criterion, the score is the same as if the criterion was measured with one question.

   For example, the symptom of suicidal ideation can be assessed by the following eight questions:

   Have you had thoughts of suicide?
   Have you had thoughts of ending your life?
   Have you had thoughts about killing yourself?
   Have you had thoughts of wishing to be dead?
   Have you had thoughts that life is not worth living?
   Have you had thoughts that you would not care if you did not wake in the morning?
   Have you had thoughts the world is better off without you?
   Have you had thoughts you would be better off dead?

   If the patient responds yes to the first four questions, these questions still only reflect one criterion: suicidal ideation.
3. **Dimensions are built upon significant symptoms and signs.** Absent or mild symptoms are coded "0" in the SCIP.
4. **The principle of least subcategories of symptom severity (LSSS):** Symptom severity subcategories should be used sparingly and reflect the symptom's clinical significance. The symptom of panic attacks can be assessed as absent or

present (0, 1). The symptom of poor concentration in a patient with depression can be assessed as absent, less than half the time and more than half the time (0, 1, 2). It is important to know how much of the time the concentration problem is present because it may affect the patient's functioning at work or in school. The fewer the subcategories reflecting symptom severity, the more efficient the interview and the more likely that clinicians will use the questions. If there are too many unnecessary subcategories of symptoms severity, clinically useful dimensions cannot be created. For example, the Positive and Negative Syndrome Scale (PANSS) has seven subcategories: absent, minimal, mild, moderate, moderate severe, severe, and extreme [3]. For clinicians, the differences between minimal and mild, moderate and moderate severe, and severe and extreme are not useful or relevant. Not surprisingly, psychiatrists do not use the PANSS in clinical settings [4].

5. **The frequency of symptoms:** The more frequent the symptom, the higher the score on the item. A good example is the frequency of auditory hallucinations:

Frequency of auditory hallucinations	**How often do you hear noises (like music, whispering sounds) or voices talking to you when there is no one around?** 0 Patient has no auditory hallucinations 1 Patient has auditory hallucinations (1–4 days/month) 2 Patient has auditory hallucinations (5–15 days/month) 3 Patient has auditory hallucinations (>15 days/month) . Not sure *or* Not applicable *or* Missing	**Kappa 0.93**

6. **The duration of symptoms:** The longer the duration of a symptom, the higher the score on the item.

Obsessions	**Do you ever have an intrusive thought or image that does not make sense and keeps coming back to your mind even when you try to avoid the thought or the image?** 0 Patient has no obsessions 1 Patient has obsessions less than 1 hour/day 2 Patient has obsessions 1–4 hours/day 3 Patient has obsessions more than 4 hours/day . Not sure *or* Not applicable *or* Missing	**Kappa 0.85**

7. **The recency of a symptom:** More recent behavior has a higher score than temporally distant behavior. For example, in response to the timing of the suicidal ideation question:

Have you ever had thoughts of suicide?	
0	Patient has never had suicidal ideation
1	Patient had suicidal ideation in past, but not in the past 3 months
2	Patient had suicidal ideation during the past 3 months (excluding past week)
3	Patient had suicidal ideation during the past week

Suicidal thoughts during the past week receive a score of 3, past 3 months receive a score of 2, and if the patient has had suicidal thoughts before the past 3 months, this receives a score of 1. A patient with suicidal thoughts during the past week, past 3 months, and past year receives a score of 6.

8. **The quality of symptoms:** Certain qualities of some symptoms increase the score on the item. For example, auditory hallucination with and without commands.

Auditory hallucinations (hallucination quality)	**Do you hear noises (like music, whispering sounds) or voices talking to you when there is no one around?** **Are the voices like a real voice or just thoughts in your mind?** 0 Patient has no auditory hallucinations 1 Patient has auditory hallucinations 2 Patient has auditory hallucinations with command . Not sure *or* Not applicable *or* Missing	**Kappa 0.90**

9. **Summation principle:** The total score of a dimension is the summation of symptom presence, recency, frequency, duration, and quality.

Evaluation of Episodes

In psychiatry, an episode is a significant symptom or a cluster of symptoms occurring during a specific period of time during the course of a mental disorder. For example, a patient may have an episode of auditory hallucinations that lasted 3 months until the patient responded to clozapine. Another patient may have an episode of binge-eating that lasted for 5 months. More often, patients have episodes of a group of symptoms occurring together during a specific period of time. A patient may have an episode of depression (depressed mood with anhedonia, psychomotor retardation, hopelessness, poor concentration, and suicidal thoughts) that lasted for 2 months until the antidepressant medication took effect to alleviate the depression. To delineate one episode from another, a 2-month or longer interval without significant symptoms has been recommended [5]. The DSM-5 followed the 2-month interval of absence of significant symptoms as demonstrated in dysthymia diagnostic criteria ("the individual has never been without the symptoms in Criteria A and B for more than 2 months at a time") [6]. Depending on the timing of the episode, the following main episodes have been described:

1. **Present episode (PE):** The present episode is measured from the onset of significant symptom(s) to the present time. The present episode may vary from 1 day or a few days to several months or years, as long as no symptom-free intervals have lasted for 2 months or more. A patient may have had a recent

depressive episode that started 2 weeks ago until now. Another patient may have had a depressive episode for the last 3 years.

2. **Representative episode (RE):** A patient may have had several depressive or manic episodes in the past, and the interviewer may choose to evaluate one representative episode. The clinician decides on the type of episode to serve diagnostic and clinical purposes. If a patient is presenting with a recent depressive episode, the clinician may choose another depressive episode in the past as a representative episode to use when comparing the severity of depression between the two periods. For another patient presenting with a recent depressive episode, the clinician may choose a manic episode in the past as representative episode to confirm the diagnosis of bipolar disorder. The clinician can decide on the duration of the RE (e.g., a week if evaluating a manic episode, a 2-week period if evaluating a depressive episode, or a month if evaluating a psychotic episode).
3. **Present state (PS):** The present state describes the psychopathology during the month before the interview and has been an essential part of the Present State Examination (PSE) developed by Professor John Wing [7–11]. If the present episode is longer than a month, the present state is the most recent part of the present episode [5]. The clinician makes a clinical judgment whether to use the PS or the PE for a particular patient, depending on the goals of the interview.

Finally, the diagnostic criteria of mental disorders may define the length of the period evaluated as follows:

Manic episode: The usual period is 1 week or longer.
Major depressive episode: The usual period is 2 weeks or longer.
Eating disorders: The usual period is 3 months or longer.
Schizophrenia: The usual period is 6 months or longer.
Alcohol and drug disorders: The usual period is 12 months or longer.
Dysthymia: The usual period is 2 years or longer.

Etiological Assessment of Mental Disorders

The psychiatrist explores potential causes of psychopathology and uses medical knowledge and clinical skills to decide if any specific medical condition has caused or exacerbated psychiatric symptoms. The SCIP method of psychiatric assessment does not exclude any particular school of thought. A clinician is welcome to use any theory or theories to elucidate the causes of mental disorders, as long as the clinician has scientific data to support those theories. Causal specifiers include definite etiopathies and factors contributing to manifestations of the mental disorders (contributing factors) as shown in Appendix I [12, 13].

Definite Etiopathy (DE) Definite etiopathy is a factor that is determined to be the cause of a mental disorder. For example, a 45-year-old lawyer with no psychiatric problems sustains a head trauma in a car accident. The MRI after the car accident shows a subdural hematoma. A mental status evaluation and neuropsychological testing show significant memory deficits. The final diagnosis is amnestic disorder due to head trauma. The head trauma or the subsequent subdural hematoma is a definite etiopathy (DE) in this case. ***Remember, definite etiopathies are rare in medicine and psychiatry.*** Most of the causal specifiers are Factors Contributing to Manifestations of Mental Disorders (FCM_MD). These contributing factors (biological, environmental, social, developmental, or others) play a part in contributing to the manifestations of the illness, but they stop short of being definite etiopathies. These contributing factors are very important in case formulation, differential diagnosis, and treatment decisions. As our understanding of these contributing factors improves, some contributing factors may be upgraded to definite etiopathies. Appendix II (causal specifiers of mental disorders) covers a wide range of factors that may cause or contribute to manifestations of mental disorders.

Conclusions

The SCIP includes simple and unified principles of psychopathology assessment which allowed the development of a complete set of 18 clinician-administered and 15 self-administered scales (Chap. 4) and the first comprehensive training curriculum designed to teach psychiatrists and mental health professionals how to use rating scales in clinical practice (Chap. 9).

Appendix I: Degree of Certainty of Causal Specifiers

0 No cause
1 Some evidence exists: Factors Contributing to Manifestations of Mental Disorders
(FCM_MD)
2 Strong evidence exists: Definite etiopathy (DE)

Appendix II: Causal Specifiers of Mental Disorders

A. ***Biological***

1. Drug abuse

   A. Alcohol
   B. Illicit drugs (e.g., THC, cocaine...etc.)
   C. Toxins (e.g., heavy metals)

2. Effects of prescribed medications (e.g., antidepressants, neuroleptics)
3. Effects of somatic treatment (e.g., ECT)
4. Discontinuing psychotropic medications
5. Biological Diseases

    A. Cerebral diseases:

        1. Trauma
        2. Infection (e.g., HIV, meningitis, cerebritis)
        3. Tumors
        4. Vascular (e.g., stroke)
        5. Seizure
        6. Hereditary (e.g., Huntington's disease)
        7. Age related (e.g., dementia)
        8. Brain imaging changes
        9. Neurological diseases
        10. Others

    B. Systematic diseases:

        1. Trauma
        2. Infections
        3. Tumors
        4. Cardiovascular diseases
        5. Hematologic diseases
        6. Respiratory diseases
        7. Nutritional diseases
        8. Autoimmune disease (e.g., SLE)
        9. Endocrine diseases
        10. Encephalopathies (e.g., hepatic)
        11. Gastrointestinal diseases
        12. Renal diseases
        13. Hypoxia
        14. Electrolyte's imbalances
        15. Metabolic disease
        16. Others

    C. Specific conditions:

        1. Peri-menstrual
        2. Postpartum
        3. Peri-menopausal
        4. Others

6. Other biological factors

B. ***Genetic/familial profile***
C. ***Neuroscience profile***

1. Neurobiological profile
2. Neurotransmitter's profile
3. Molecular biology profile
4. Biomarkers
5. Others

D. ***Environmental***

1. Life events (e.g., death of a parent when the child was very young)
2. Adverse events in childhood
   A. Poverty
   B. Neglect of a child
   C. Removal of a child from home
   D. Migration
   E. Other
3. Childhood abuse
   A. Emotional
   B. Physical
   C. Sexual
   D. Other abuse
4. Traumatic events (catastrophes, wars...etc.)
5. Other environmental factors

E. ***Developmental***

1. Developmental milestones (age of walking and talking, puberty changes)
2. Developmental problems:
   A. Intellectual developmental disorder
   B. Learning disabilities
   C. Others
3. History of serious illnesses in childhood
4. Family factors
5. Religious upbringing
6. Cultural factors
7. Other developmental factors

F. ***Social***

1. Relationship factors
   A. Marriage
   B. Separation
   C. Divorce
   D. Children
   E. Problem with significant other

   F. Living alone
   G. Others

2. Change in support system

   A. Family
   B. Friends
   C. Doctors, therapists
   D. Others

3. Social stressors

   A. Jobs:

      1. Unemployment
      2. Underemployment
      3. Stressful work
      4. Stressful schedule
      5. Job change
      6. Discord with boss or co-workers

   B. Financial
   C. Educational:

      1. Illiteracy
      2. Problems in school
      3. Discord with teachers or classmates
      4. Other problems

   D. Housing:

      1. Homeless
      2. Inadequate housing
      3. Moving to a new area
      4. Unsafe neighborhood
      5. Discord with neighbors
      6. Other

   E. Physical illness of the patient, family member, or others
   F. Death of family members or friends
   G. Access to healthcare services:

      1. No health insurance
      2. Inadequate health insurance
      3. Transportation problem

   H. Others

4. Legal
5. Other social factors

G. ***Psychodynamic factors***
H. ***Behavioral factors***
I. ***Cognitive factors***
J. ***Personality characteristics factors***
K. ***Other Categories***

References

1. Andreasen, N. C., Flaum, M., & Arndt, S. (1992). The Comprehensive Assessment of Symptoms and History (CASH). An instrument for assessing diagnosis and psychopathology. *Archives of General Psychiatry, 49*, 615–623.
2. Aboraya, A., El-Missiry, A., Barlowe, J., John, C., Ebrahimian, A., Muvvala, S., Brandish, J., Mansour, H., Zheng, W., Chumber, P., Berry, J., Elswick, D., Hill, C., Swager, L., Abo Elez, W., Ashour, H., Haikal, A., Eissa, A., Rabie, M., … Price, E. (2014). The reliability of the standard for clinicians' interview in psychiatry (SCIP): A clinician-administered tool with categorical, dimensional and numeric output. *Schizophrenia Research, 156*, 174–183.
3. Kay, S. R., Fiszbein, A., & Opler, L. A. (1987). The positive and negative syndrome scale (PANSS) for schizophrenia. *Schizophrenia Bulletin, 13*, 261–276.
4. Nasrallah, H. (2009). Long overdue: Measurement-based psychiatric practice. *Current Psychiatry., 8*, 14–16.
5. WHO. (1998). *Schedules for clinical assessment in neuropsychiatry glossary*. World Health Organization.
6. American Psychiatric Association. (2013). *Diagnostic and statistical manual of mental disorders* (Fifth ed.). American Psychiatric Association.
7. Wing, J., Nixon, J., von Cranach, M., & Strauss, A. (1977). Further developments of the 'present state examination' and CATEGO system. *Archiv für Psychiatrie und Nervenkrankheiten, 224*, 151–160.
8. Wing, J., Babor, T., Brugha, T., Burke, J., Cooper, J. E., Giel, R., Jablenski, A., Regier, D., & Sartorius, N. (1990). SCAN. Schedules for clinical assessment in neuropsychiatry. *Archives of General Psychiatry, 47*, 589–593.
9. Wing, J. K., Birley, J. L., Cooper, J. E., Graham, P., & Isaacs, A. D. (1967). Reliability of a procedure for measuring and classifying "present psychiatric state". *The British Journal of Psychiatry: The Journal of Mental Science, 113*, 499–515.
10. Wing, J. K., Cooper, J. E., & Sartorius, N. (1974). *The measurement and classification of psychiatric symptoms: An Instruction Manual for the PSE and Catego Program*. Cambridge University Press.
11. Wing, J. K., Nixon, J. M., Mann, S. A., & Leff, J. P. (1977). Reliability of the PSE (ninth edition) used in a population study. *Psychological Medicine, 7*, 505–516.
12. Aboraya, A. (2010). Scientific forum on the diagnostic and statistical manual of mental disorders, fifth edition (DSM-V)-an invitation. *Psychiatry (Edgmont), 7*, 32–36.
13. Aboraya, A. (2010). Recommendation for DSM-V: A proposal for adding causal specifiers to axis I diagnoses. *Psychiatry (Edgmont), 7*, 24–28.

Chapter 4
The Standard for Clinicians' Interview in Psychiatry (SCIP) Screening Questionnaire and Scales

This chapter discusses the development of the SCIP screening questionnaire, the SCIP clinician-administered (CA) scales, and self-administered (SA) scales.

The SCIP Screening Questionnaire

Screening for mental disorders may be performed at the individual or population level. At the individual level, an important part of the clinical interview is to screen for mental disorders, in addition to the chief complaint that brought the patient to the clinic. The term "psychiatric review of symptoms" is used to describe this process of psychiatric evaluation [1]. For example, if a patient is evaluated and found to meet the diagnostic criteria for a major depressive episode, the clinician needs to screen for past manic or hypomanic episodes, as well as for alcohol and drug use, to rule out comorbid diagnoses of bipolar disorder or alcohol or drug use disorders. Psychiatrists and clinical psychologists usually have adequate training to screen for mental disorders before making provisional differential diagnoses and final psychiatric diagnosis(es). At the population level, screening is "the examination of a group of usually asymptomatic individuals to detect those with a high probability of having a given disease, typically by means of an inexpensive diagnostic test" [2]. Screening may take place within a general population or a specific population. Individuals who screen positive for a diagnosis are targeted for more detailed evaluation and medical work-up to diagnose and treat the specific disorder(s) [3–6].

Recently, two self-report questionnaires were published that screen for a wide range of DSM-IV Axis I disorders: the Composite International Diagnostic – Screener (CID-S) and the Psychiatric Diagnostic Screening Questionnaire (PDSQ) [7, 8]. The Composite International Diagnostic – Screener (CID-S) is a 12-item self-report questionnaire based on core diagnostic questions from the Composite

A. S. Aboraya, *Manual for the Standard for Clinicians' Interview in Psychiatry (SCIP)*, Advances in Mental Health and Addiction,
https://doi.org/10.1007/978-3-030-94930-3_4

International Diagnostic Interview (CIDI) and covers a wide range of DSM-IV diagnoses: somatoform, anxiety, depressive, other affective, and substance-use disorders. The composite International Diagnostic – Screener (CID-S) was found to be an efficient diagnostic screening tool for most mental disorders (except for somatoform and substance use disorders) [7]. Another advantage of the CID-S is that test-retest reliability (kappa) for the core (stem) questions of the CID-S items was found to be satisfactory [9]. The Psychiatric Diagnostic Screening Questionnaire (PDSQ) is a 90-item self-administered questionnaire that screens for 13 DSM-IV disorders [8]. The final version of the PDSQ consists of 126 questions assessing the symptoms of 13 DSM-IV disorders: major depressive disorder, eating disorder, PTSD, panic disorder, agoraphobia, social phobia, GAD, OCD, alcohol abuse/dependence, drug abuse/dependence, somatization, hypochondriasis, and psychosis [10].

More recently, the development of the Standard for Clinicians' Interview in Psychiatry (SCIP) as a new valid and reliable semi-structured diagnostic interview provided a comprehensive screening section (the SCIP screening questionnaire). The SCIP screening questions were designed to be administered by clinicians and consist of 30 questions covering most of the adult psychiatric disorders: generalized anxiety, panic, agoraphobia, social phobia, obsessive-compulsive, posttraumatic, major depressive, dysthymic, bipolar, schizoaffective, schizophrenia, attention deficit/hyperactivity, anorexia nervosa, bulimia nervosa, binge-eating, alcohol use, drug use, and somatic symptom disorders. The time needed to administer the SCIP screening questions ranges from 10 to 20 minutes. The screening questions were shown to have high interrater reliability (kappa), as shown in Chap. 2.

The SCIP screening questions were chosen to include all the "gate," "core," or "stem" criterion or criteria of the disorders [7, 11]. For example, a major depressive episode has two core criteria: depressed mood and anhedonia, and both of these were included in the screening section. For a schizophrenia diagnosis, at least one of the three core criteria (delusions, hallucinations, and disorganized thoughts) is required, and thus the three core criteria are included in the SCIP screening questionnaire. On the other hand, attention-deficit hyperactivity disorder (ADHD) diagnosis is based on the presence of a minimum number of criteria and no gate criterion or criteria required for the diagnosis [11]. Recent research by M. Zimmerman (2017) showed that difficulty sustaining attention and fidgetiness have been found to have the highest sensitivity and negative predictive value and were recommended for use as a 2-item screening for ADHD [11]. Consequently, the author of the SCIP added both items to the SCIP screening section. The final SCIP screening section includes 30 questions. Table 2.1 in Chap. 2 shows the 30-item SCIP screening questions, interrater reliability (kappa), and the standard error, based upon 322 patients interviewed at William R. Sharpe Jr. Hospital, Chestnut Ridge Center (inpatient and outpatient), Ain Shams University Hospital, and Mansoura University Hospital. Out of 30 screening items, 19 items (63%) had good agreement (kappa values >0.7), and 11 items (37%) had fair agreement (kappa values ranging from 0.5 to 0.7).

Finally, the SCIP screening section was tested and found to have high sensitivity as a screening tool with a primary-care population in India [12] and has the potential to be useful in screening for mental disorders in general populations. Appendix I includes the final version of the SCIP screening questionnaire.

The SCIP Clinician-Administered (CA) Scales

As described in Chap. 2, one of the main outcomes of the SCIP study is the creation of reliable dimensions to measure the main psychopathology domains. The initial items of the SCIP dimensions were formulated based upon the DSM and ICD criteria and experts' opinions. The sensitivity and specificity of the initial dimensions were calculated against the psychiatric diagnoses as determined by the psychiatrists who treated patients from admission to discharge. To create short and valid scales that are practical to use in clinical settings, the following principles were used to create the SCIP scales:

Principles of including items in the final SCIP scales:

1. All the "gate," "core," or "stem" criterion or criteria of the disorders are included in the scales. For example, depressed mood and anhedonia items are included in the SCIP depression scale.
2. Items with relatively high prevalence, high sensitivity (≥75%), and high item rest correlations (≥0.4) are included in the final scales.
3. Clinicians' input was considered in the final version of the scales. For example, the somatic passivity item was not one of the initial Schneiderian dimension. However, somatic passivity was included in the final SCIP delusions scale due to its clinical and historical significance [13].
4. Items that were not included in the final SCIP scale are considered in the last item of each scale as "other symptoms."

Principles of excluding items in the final SCIP scales:

1. Items with relatively low prevalence, low sensitivity (<75%), and low item rest correlations (<0.4).
2. Items that did not affect the sensitivity and specificity of the scales, regardless of whether they are included in the model or not.

Process of identifying items of the final SCIP scales:

1. The sensitivity and specificity of the initial dimensions were calculated against the psychiatric diagnoses as determined by the psychiatrists who treated patients from admission to discharge.
2. Following the rules of excluding items as described above, the sensitivity and specificity of the remaining items were recalculated with repetitive iterations.
3. After adequate iterations, the sensitivity and specificity of the final dimensions were approximately equal to the sensitivity and specificity of the initial dimensions.
4. Clinicians' input was considered in the final version of the scales.

Appendix II includes the final version of the 18 SCIP clinician-administered scales:

1. SCIP anxiety scale.
2. SCIP panic scale.
3. SCIP phobia scale.
4. SCIP obsessive-compulsive (OCD) scale.
5. SCIP posttraumatic stress (PTSD) scale.
6. SCIP depression scale.
7. SCIP mania scale.
8. SCIP hallucinations scale.
9. SCIP delusions scale.
10. SCIP disorganized thoughts scale.
11. SCIP aggression scale.
12. SCIP negative symptoms scale.
13. Core schizophrenia scale.
14. SCIP alcohol use scale.
15. SCIP drug use scale.
16. SCIP attention deficit/hyperactivity (ADHD) scale.
17. SCIP anorexia nervosa scale.
18. SCIP binge/bulimia scale.

The SCIP Self-Administered (SA) Scales

The SCIP self-administered scales were developed based upon the reliable and validated clinician-administered scales.

Principles of creating the SCIP self-administered scales:

1. The SCIP study resulted in creating reliable and validated SCIP clinician-administered scales. The logic is to use the SCIP reliable questions and modify them to be in a self-administered format so that patients read the questions and answer them on their own.
2. Most of the SCIP SA questions were kept the same as the CA questions. A few SCIP SA questions were modified to be even simpler than the SCIP CA questions.
   An example is the following anhedonia question:
   Anhedonia (clinician-administered version).

2. Anhedonia (loss of pleasure and interest)	
Have you been unable to experience pleasure and enjoy things that you used to enjoy like exercising, enjoying your hobbies, or socializing with friends?	
0	Patient has no anhedonia
1	Patient has anhedonia less than half the time
2	Patient has anhedonia more than half the time
	Not sure *or* Not applicable *or* Missing

Anhedonia (self-administered version).

2. Did you lose interest in things, or not enjoy things you normally would?

0 No.
1 Yes, some of the time.
2 Yes, most of the time.
Not sure *or* Not applicable *or* Missing

3. The questions' sequence and numbers were kept the same in the CA version and SA version. The anhedonia question above was # 2 in both CA and SA versions. That was done to create coherence between the two versions of the SCIP scales and facilitate data entry and analyses.
4. Some items require two questions to elicit the criterion evaluated. For example, a panic attack requires both fear and somatic symptoms. Clinicians know this and therefore ask about fear and somatic symptoms. For patients who do not necessarily know this, two questions were written separately for the patient to read and make a choice.

   Panic attacks (clinician-administered version).

PAN1. Panic attacks (without phobias)

Did you have a panic attack, when you suddenly become anxious and frightened for a short period of time (up to 60 minutes)?
During that time, did you feel that your heart was racing or pounding, or did you start shaking or sweating, or did you feel you were choking?

0 Patient had no panic attacks.
1 Patient had panic attacks.
. Not sure *or* Not applicable *or* Missing

Panic attacks (self-administered version).

1a. Did you have a panic attack, when you suddenly become anxious and frightened for a short period of time (up to 60 minutes)?

0 *No.*
1 *Yes.*
. Not sure or Not applicable or Missing.

1b. During that time, did you feel that your heart was racing or pounding, or did you start shaking or sweating, or did you feel you were choking?

0 *No.*
1 *Yes*
. Not sure or Not applicable or Missing

5. One important principle of the SCIP assessment is that a rating of 0 means the symptom is absent or non-significant. For the patient, a rating of 0 was described as "No, *or* Sometimes, but it does not bother me."

Attention impairment (clinician-administered version).

1. Attention impairment/poor concentration	
Do you have difficulty paying attention and concentrating when reading an article, watching a TV show or a movie, or doing your work or school assignments?	
0	Absent or non-significant
1	Patient has poor attention and concentration
	. = Not sure *or* Not applicable *or* Missing

Attention impairment (self-administered version).

1. Do you have difficulty paying attention and concentrating when reading an article, watching a TV show or a movie, or doing your work or school assignments?	
0	No, *or* Sometimes, but it does not bother me
1	Yes
	. Not sure *or* Not applicable *or* Missing

Appendix III includes the final version of the 15 SCIP self-administered scales:

1. SCIP anxiety scale.
2. SCIP panic scale.
3. SCIP phobia scale.
4. SCIP obsessive-compulsive (OCD) scale.
5. SCIP posttraumatic stress (PTSD) scale.
6. SCIP depression scale.
7. SCIP mania scale.
8. SCIP hallucinations scale.
9. SCIP delusions scale.
10. SCIP alcohol use scale.
11. SCIP drug use scale.
12. SCIP attention deficit/hyperactivity (ADHD) scale.
13. SCIP anorexia nervosa scale.
14. SCIP binge/bulimia scale.
15. Intake self-administered scale.

Psychometric Properties of the SCIP Self-Administered (SA) Scales

To measure the psychometric properties of the SCIP self-administered (SA) scales, 120 patients were recruited from the following sites: Chestnut Ridge Center (52 patients), United Hospital Center (11 patients), W.R. Sharpe Jr. Hospital (9 patients), and Chestnut Ridge Clinic (48 patients). Patients completed the SA scales pertaining to their presenting symptoms in the hospital or in the outpatient clinic. The mean patient age was 37 years old. Fifty-four percent of the sample were identified as female, 93% identified as White, and 63% reported that they had 12 years of education or less.

Of the 120 patients recruited, 52 patients completed only the SA scales. Sixty-eight patients completed the SA scales and were interviewed by one or more of the clinicians who administered the corresponding clinician-administered (CA) scales on the same day. Some patients were interviewed by one clinician, which generated a comparison between the SA scale and corresponding CA scales. Some patients were interviewed by two or more clinicians. For example, if a patient was interviewed by three clinicians (i.e., A, B, C), a comparison was made between the SA scale and Clinician A, the same SA scale and Clinician B, and the same SA scale and Clinician C. A total of 135 comparisons between the SA scales and CA scales allowed the calculation of kappa for 103 SA SCIP questions versus the same CA SCIP questions.

Internal Consistency Reliability of the SCIP SA Scales

Cronbach's alpha measured internal consistency reliability of the SCIP SA scales [14–16]. Cronbach's alpha considers the mean interitem correlation; its value increases as the average interitem correlation and the number of items increase. The reliability of a dimension is considered "substantial" if Cronbach's alpha is > 0.7, "moderate" if alpha ranges from 0.5 to 0.7, and "poor" if alpha is < 0.5.

Tables 4.1, 4.2, 4.3, 4.4, 4.5, 4.6, 4.7, 4.8, 4.9, and 4.10 present item-rest correlations, interitem correlations, mean interitem correlations, and mean alphas for the SCIP SA scales. Cronbach's alpha values ranged from 0.7720 to 0.9873. Cronbach's alpha for the hallucinations scale was 0.7777 and included only 5 main questions (hallucinations quality, hallucination frequency, hallucination duration, visual hallucinations, and other hallucinations). Cronbach's alpha for the delusions scale was 0.7720 and did not include the somatic passivity item due to insufficient data. Overall, the internal consistency reliability measures of the SCIP SA scales are good.

Table 4.1 Anxiety scale

	Item-rest	Interitem	Alpha	Label
	Correlation		Correlation	
SA_anxiety1	0.9148	0.8737	0.9765	Anxiety
SA_anxiety2	0.9237	0.8700	0.9757	Restlessness
SA_anxiety3	0.8905	0.8807	0.9779	Tense
SA_anxiety4	0.9081	0.8773	0.9772	Exhausion
SA_anxiety5	0.9534	0.8622	0.9740	Poor concentration
SA_anxiety6	0.9436	0.8660	0.9749	Irritability
SA_anxiety7	0.9166	0.8737	0.9765	Insomnia
Mean		0.8719	0.9795	

Table 4.2 Panic scale

	Item-rest	Interitem	Alpha	Label
	Correlation		Correlation	
SA_panic1	0.9550	0.8967	0.9630	Panic
SA_panic2	0.9327	0.9130	0.9692	Panic apprehension
SA_panic3	0.9504	0.9000	0.9643	Panic prevention
SA_panic4	0.9141	0.9267	0.9743	Panic physical symptoms
Mean		0.9091	0.9756	

Table 4.3 PTSD scale

	Item-rest	Interitem	Alpha	Label
	Correlation		Correlation	
SA_PTSD1	0.9173	0.6994	0.9721	Trauma
SA_PTSD2	0.9345	0.6972	0.9719	Recollection
SA_PTSD3	0.6929	0.7234	0.9751	Dreams/nightmares
SA_PTSD4	0.8495	0.7080	0.9732	Flashback
SA_PTSD5	0.9098	0.7005	0.9723	Avoid thoughts
SA_PTSD6	0.8537	0.7095	0.9734	Avoid people
SA_PTSD7	0.6830	0.7281	0.9757	Amnesia
SA_PTSD8	0.7196	0.7188	0.9746	Dimished social interest
SA_PTSD9	0.8453	0.7078	0.9732	Detachment/isolation
SA_PTSD10	0.9345	0.6972	0.9719	Dimished emotional feeling
SA_PTSD11	0.7767	0.7164	0.9743	Insomnia
SA_PTSD12	0.8708	0.7045	0.9728	Anger
SA_PTSD13	0.8403	0.7105	0.9736	Poor concentration
SA_PTSD14	0.9441	0.6988	0.9721	Hypervigilance
SA_PTSD15	0.9442	0.6960	0.9717	Startle response
SA_PTSD16	0.6402	0.7298	0.9759	Other
Mean		0.7091	0.9750	

Table 4.4 Depression scale

	Item-rest	Interitem	Alpha	Label
	Correlation		Correlation	
SA_depres ~ n1	0.8648	0.5717	0.9362	Depressed mood
SA_depres ~ n2	0.8991	0.5664	0.9349	Anhedonia
SA_depress ~ 3	0.9005	0.5666	0.9350	Hopelessness
SA_depress ~ 4	0.8875	0.5685	0.9354	Poor concentration
SA_depress ~ 5	0.7764	0.5846	0.9393	Psychom. Retardation
SA_depress ~ 6	0.8788	0.5697	0.9358	Worthlessness
SA_depress ~ 7	0.8359	0.5749	0.9370	Guilt
SA_depress ~ 8	0.6629	0.6002	0.9429	Other
SA_depress ~ 9	0.7950	0.5811	0.9385	Suicidal ideation
SA_depres ~ 10	0.6944	0.5960	0.9420	Suicidal intention
SA_depres ~ 11	0.4844	0.6282	0.9489	Suicidal plan
SA_depres ~ 12	0.2844	0.6593	0.9551	Suicidal attempt
Mean		0.5889	0.9450	

Table 4.5 Mania scale

	Item-rest Correlation	Interitem	Alpha Correlation	Label
SA_mania1	0.7928	0.6315	0.9449	Elated mood
SA_mania2	0.7849	0.6325	0.9451	Irritable mood
SA_mania3	0.8020	0.6291	0.9443	Mixed mood
SA_mania4	0.9255	0.6092	0.9397	Racing thoughts
SA_mania5	0.8214	0.6267	0.9438	Pressured speech
SA_mania6	0.8901	0.6151	0.9411	Distraction
SA_mania7	0.7424	0.6415	0.9471	Overactivity
SA_mania8	0.5855	0.6648	0.9520	Grandiosity
SA_mania9	0.7278	0.6429	0.9474	Over spending
SA_mania10	0.8246	0.6265	0.9437	Decreased sleep
SA_mania11	0.6264	0.6574	0.9505	Risky behaviors
Mean		0.6343	0.9502	

Table 4.6 Hallucinations scale

	Item-rest Correlation	Interitem	Alpha Correlation	Label
SA_hal1	0.7369	0.3429	0.6761	Hallucination quality
SA_hal2	0.7811	0.3193	0.6523	Hallucination frequency
SA_hal3	0.6634	0.3653	0.6972	Hallucination duration
SA_hal7	0.2865	0.5278	0.8172	Visual hallucinations
SA_hal9	0.3541	0.5031	0.8020	Other hallucinations
Mean		0.4116	0.7777	

Table 4.7 Delusions scale

	Item-rest Correlation	Interitem	Alpha Correlation	Label
SA_del2	0.2565	0.3395	0.7825	Thought insertion
SA_del3	0.2565	0.3395	0.7825	Thought withdrawal
SA_del4	0.5587	0.2826	0.7339	Thought broadcast
SA_del5	0.5020	0.2888	0.7398	Paranoid delusions
SA_del6	0.5902	0.2724	0.7238	Conspiracy delusions
SA_del7	0.2689	0.3445	0.7862	Delusion of reference
SA_del8	0.7614	0.2435	0.6926	Other delusions
SA_del9	0.6325	0.2686	0.7199	Bizarre delusions
Mean		0.2974	0.7720	

Table 4.8 Alcohol scale

	Item-rest Correlation	Interitem	Alpha Correlation	Label
SA_alc1	0.7429	0.6786	0.9366	Tolerance
SA_alc2	0.8391	0.6547	0.9299	Withdrawal
SA_alc3	0.8849	0.6435	0.9267	Obligations failure
SA_alc4	0.9367	0.6311	0.9229	Social problems
SA_alc5	0.9302	0.6327	0.9234	Alcohol despite problems
SA_alc6	0.5550	0.7274	0.9492	Alcohol with hazard
SA_alc7	0.8086	0.6621	0.9321	Alcohol blackout
SA_alc8	0.6362	0.7059	0.9438	Other problems
Mean		0.6670	0.9413	

Table 4.9 Drug scale

	Item-rest Correlation	Interitem	Alpha Correlation	Label
SA_drug1	0.9839	0.9072	0.9832	Tolerance
SA_drug2	0.8833	0.9404	0.9895	Withdrawal
SA_drug3	0.9864	0.9042	0.9826	Obligations failure
SA_drug4	0.9862	0.9054	0.9829	Social problems
SA_drug5	0.9862	0.9054	0.9829	Drug despite problems
SA_drug6	0.8985	0.9329	0.9881	Drug with hazard
SA_drug7	0.9288	0.9248	0.9866	Other problems
Mean		0.9172	0.9873	

Table 4.10 ADHD scale

	Item-rest Correlation	Interitem	Alpha Correlation	Label
SA_ADHD1	0.8966	0.5393	0.9570	Attention
SA_ADHD2	0.9372	0.5361	0.9564	Long attention
SA_ADHD3	0.7999	0.5470	0.9582	Avoid tasks
SA_ADHD4	0.8466	0.5432	0.9576	Attention when speaking to
SA_ADHD5	0.8453	0.5434	0.9576	Organization
SA_ADHD6	0.8827	0.5400	0.9571	Changing activities
SA_ADHD7	0.8435	0.5436	0.9577	Distraction
SA_ADHD8	0.8220	0.5453	0.9580	Misplace things
SA_ADHD9	0.8022	0.5469	0.9582	Forgetting activities
SA_ADHD10	0.8163	0.5457	0.9580	Losing track
SA_ADHD11	0.7123	0.5534	0.9593	Fidgety
SA_ADHD12	0.4097	0.5786	0.9631	Leaving seats
SA_ADHD13	0.7022	0.5548	0.9595	Restless and moving
SA_ADHD14	0.5958	0.5633	0.9608	Over activities
SA_ADHD15	0.5835	0.5640	0.9609	Waiting in line
SA_ADHD16	0.5271	0.5686	0.9616	Talking too much
SA_ADHD17	0.4467	0.5753	0.9626	Loud and noisy
SA_ADHD18	0.8167	0.5457	0.9580	Impulsivity
SA_ADHD19	0.6253	0.5609	0.9604	Disturb others
SA_ADHD20	0.6715	0.5575	0.9599	Blurt out answers
Mean		0.5526	0.9611	

Validation of the SCIP SA Scales

The 135 comparisons between the SA scales and CA scales allowed for evaluation of the validity of the SA scales using criterion validity and convergent and discriminant validity.

Criterion Validity of the SCIP SA Scales

Considering that the CA scales were administered by clinicians with expertise in mental health and who can clarify patients' responses when there is a contradiction, the CA scales can be viewed as the "criterion" or "gold standard" by which to validate the patients' SA scale responses. The index of agreement kappa (K), which measures the proportion of agreement corrected for chance agreement [17–19], compared the agreement between patient responses of the SA scales and the clinicians' CA scale assessment. In general, kappa values greater than 0.7 indicate good agreement, kappa values ranging from 0.5 to 0.7 indicate fair agreement, and kappa values less than 0.5 indicate poor agreement [20]. Table 4.11 shows kappa and the standard error of 103 psychopathology items.

Excluding the hallucinations and delusions scales, 85 psychopathology items remain. Among these 85 psychopathology items, kappa was poor for only 5 items (items # 27, 47, 50, 76, and 93 in Table 4.11). This indicates good criterion validity for the SCIP SA scales, with the exception of the hallucinations and delusions scales. Among the nine items of hallucinations scale, one item (other hallucinations) evidenced good reliability, four items produced fair reliability (frequency of hallucinations, voices arguing, voices commenting, and visual hallucinations), and four items demonstrated poor reliability (hallucinations quality, hallucinations duration, audible thoughts, and observed hallucinations). Of the nine items of the delusions

Table 4.11 Index of agreement kappa (K) between the items of self-administered scales and clinician-administered scales

Scale	Item number	Scale items	Item titles	Kappa (standard error)
Anxiety	1	1	Generalized anxiety	0.9359 (0.0861)
	2	2	Restlessness with anxiety	0.9327 (0.0862)
	3	3	Tension with anxiety	0.8964 (0.0860)
	4	4	Exhaustion with anxiety	1.0000 (0.0861)
	5	5	Poor concentration with anxiety	0.9687 (0.0860)
	6	6	Irritability with anxiety	0.7759 (0.0842)
	7	7	Insomnia with anxiety	0.9700 (0.0860)

(continued)

Table 4.11 (continued)

Scale	Item number	Scale items	Item titles	Kappa (standard error)
Panic	8	1	Panic attacks	1.0000 (0.0861)
	9	2	Worry about having another panic attack	0.8820 (0.0874)
	10	3	Action to end or prevent panic attacks	0.9252 (0.0860)
	11	4	Panic physical symptoms	1.0000 (0.0861)
PTSD	12	1	Witness or experience traumatic events	0.8312 (0.0762)
	13	2	Distressing recollection of events	0.9712 (0.0860)
	14	3	Bad dreams or nightmares	0.6494 (0.0806)
	15	4	Flashbacks	0.8679 (0.0856)
	16	5	Avoidance of thoughts and feelings	0.8439 (0.0850)
	17	6	Avoidance of people, places, and activities	0.6915 (0.0856)
	18	7	Amnesia	0.7421 (0.0877)
	19	8	Diminished social interest (asociality)	0.5380 (0.0822)
	20	9	Detachment and isolation	0.7789 (0.0873)
	21	10	Diminished emotional feelings (diminished experience of emotions)	0.6301 (0.0800)
	22	11	Insomnia	0.9189 (0.0888)
	23	12	Anger	0.6486 (0.0821)
	24	13	Attention impairment (poor concentration)	0.8767 (0.0854)
	25	14	Hypervigilance	0.8179 (0.0856)
	26	15	Startle response	0.8362 (0.0852)
	27	16	Other symptoms	−0.0102 (0.0820)
Depression	28	1	Depressed mood	0.9005 (0.0728)
	29	2	Anhedonia (loss of pleasure and interest)	0.7933 (0.0735)
	30	3	Hopelessness	0.8411 (0.0675)
	31	4	Attention impairment (poor concentration)	0.7675 (0.0653)
	32	5	Psychomotor retardation/slowing	0.6535 (0.0683)
	33	6	Worthlessness (low self-esteem)	0.6835 (0.0653)
	34	7	Guilt	0.7928 (0.0695)
	35	8	Other symptoms	0.5048 (0.0863)
	36	9	Thoughts of suicide	0.9015 (0.0860)
	37	10	Suicidal intention	0.8920 (0.0861)
	38	11	Suicidal plan	0.7166 (0.0825)
	39	12	Suicidal attempt	0.8717 (0.0774)

(continued)

Table 4.11 (continued)

Scale	Item number	Scale items	Item titles	Kappa (standard error)
Mania	40	1	Elated (euphoric) mood (expansive mood)	0.6967 (0.0672)
	41	2	Irritable mood	0.6594 (0.0669)
	42	3	Mixed mood (same day mood changes)	0.7597 (0.0660)
	43	4	Racing thoughts	0.8234 (0.0704)
	44	5	Pressured speech	0.6543 (0.0670)
	45	6	Distraction	0.6499 (0.0657)
	46	7	Increase in activities	0.6299 (0.0669)
	47	8	Grandiosity	0.3117 (0.0822)
	48	9	Overspending (poor judgment in new activities)	0.7755 (0.0851)
	49	10	Decreased sleep	0.7069 (0.0858)
	50	11	Other risky behaviors	0.4810 (0.0818)
Hallucinations	51	1	Auditory hallucinations (hallucination quality)	0.4127 (0.0557)
	52	2	Frequency of auditory hallucinations	0.6475 (0.0627)
	53	3	Hallucination duration	0.4972 (0.0606)
	54	4	Audible thoughts	−0.0331 (0.0796)
	55	5	Voices arguing	0.6563 (0.0817)
	56	6	Voices commenting	0.5869 (0.0793)
	57	7	Visual hallucinations	0.6396 (0.0841)
	58	8	Observed hallucinations	−0.0370 (0.0701)
	59	9	Other hallucinations	0.7158 (0.0857)
Delusions	60	1	Somatic passivity	Too few categories
	61	2	Thought insertion	0.7166 (0.0825)
	62	3	Thought withdrawal	−0.0261 (0.0851)
	63	4	Thought broadcasting	0.7162 (0.0841)
	64	5	Paranoid/persecutory delusions	0.6860 (0.0716)
	65	6	Conspiracy delusions	0.2130 (0.0517)
	66	7	Delusions of reference	0.4867 (0.0676)
	67	8	Other delusions	0.0690 (0.0775)
	68	9	Bizarreness of delusions	−0.0135 (0.0504)

(continued)

Table 4.11 (continued)

Scale	Item number	Scale items	Item titles	Kappa (standard error)
Alcohol	69	1	Alcohol tolerance	0.9588 (0.0863)
	70	2	Alcohol withdrawal	0.9636 (0.0860)
	71	3	Failure to fulfil major obligations	1.0000 (0.0861)
	72	4	Social or interpersonal problems	1.0000 (0.0861)
	73	5	Alcohol use in spite of problems	0.9016 (0.0856)
	74	6	Alcohol use in hazardous situations	1.0000 (0.0861)
	75	7	Alcohol blackout	1.0000 (0.0861)
	76	8	Other problems	0.0997 (0.0824)
Drug	77	1	Drug tolerance	1.0000 (0.0867)
	78	2	Drug withdrawal	0.9560 (0.0863)
	79	3	Failure to fulfil major obligations	1.0000 (0.0867)
	80	4	Social or interpersonal problems	1.0000 (0.0867)
	81	5	Drug use in spite of problems	1.0000 (0.0864)
	82	6	Drug use in hazardous situations	0.7627 (0.0848)
	83	7	Other problems	0.7373 (0.0853)
ADHD	84	1	Attention impairment (poor concentration)	0.8908 (0.0856)
	85	2	Sustained attention impairment	0.9654 (0.0863)
	86	3	Avoiding sustained attention tasks	0.9483 (0.0863)
	87	4	Attention when spoken to	0.8304 (0.0851)
	88	5	Organization and meeting deadlines	0.8679 (0.0853)
	89	6	Changing activities	0.8920 (0.0862)
	90	7	Distraction	0.9655 (0.0860)
	91	8	Misplacing things	0.8410 (0.0850)
	92	9	Forgetting daily activities	0.8921 (0.0856)
	93	10	Losing track	0.4101 (0.0822)
	94	11	Fidgety	0.7050 (0.0822)
	95	12	Leaving seats	1.0000 (0.0864)
	96	13	Restlessness/moving	0.8302 (0.0848)
	97	14	Hyperactivity	0.7886 (0.0844)
	98	15	Waiting in line	0.8851 (0.0855)
	99	16	Talking too much	0.5622 (0.0774)
	100	17	Loud and noisy	0.7964 (0.0843)
	101	18	Impulsivity	0.8921 (0.0856)
	102	19	Disturbing others	Too few categories
	103	20	Blurt out answers	0.3927 (0.0686)

scale, two items evidenced good reliability (thought insertion and thought broadcast), one item produced average reliability (paranoid/persecutory delusions), five items revealed poor reliability (thought withdrawal, conspiracy delusions, delusions of references, other delusions, and bizarreness of delusions), and one item (somatic passivity) had too few categories to assess. Therefore, the hallucinations and delusions scales evidenced poor criterion validity overall. In sum, the SCIP SA scales are valid, with the exception of the hallucinations and delusions scales.

Convergent and Discriminant Validity

Convergent validity (expected high positive correlations among scales that measure the same construct) and discriminant validity (expected low correlations among scales that measure different constructs) analyses were performed using the 135 comparisons between the SCIP SA scales and the SCIP CA scales. The scale scores of ADHD, panic, anxiety, PTSD, depression, mania, hallucinations, delusions, alcohol use, and drug use were calculated by summing the positive items of each scale for both the SCIP SA and the SCIP CA scales. Correlations among the scores of SCIP SA and the SCIP CA scales are shown in Table 4.12. The correlations between the scales of the same construct (SA versus CA) were high (>0.90) for all scales, except the hallucinations and delusions scales (0.5626 and 0.6353, respectively), which provides fair evidence of convergent validity. The correlations between the scales of different constructs were low or even negatively correlated, which provides evidence of discriminant validity. Relatively low correlations were found between the hallucinations SA and hallucinations CA scales (0.5626) and delusions SA and delusions CA scales (0.6353). This finding confirms that the hallucinations SA scale and delusions SA scale are not valid for assessing hallucinations and delusions. This conclusion was further confirmed by criterion validity analyses evidencing that 9 items of the hallucinations and delusions scales had poor agreement with corresponding items of the CA scales (Table 4.11). One limitation of this study is that the analyses were limited to the SCIP scales and did not compare the SCIP scales against other published scales.

In sum, the SCIP SA scales are reliable. The SCIP SA scales are also valid, with the exception of hallucinations and delusions scales. The clinical implication of these findings is that administration of CA scales is required in order to produce valid diagnoses for severe mood disorders with psychotic features, schizoaffective disorder, and schizophrenia.

Table 4.12 Correlations among the self-administered (SA) and clinician-administered (CA) scales scores

	ADHD _SA	Panic SA	Anxiety SA	PTSD SA	Dep[a] SA	Mania SA	Hal[b] SA	Del[c] SA	Alcohol SA	Drug SA
ADHD_CA	***0.9615***	0.0187	0.0221	−0.0912	−0.1175	0.2327	−0.1042	−0.1478	0.2099	−0.0593
Panic_CA	0.0294	***0.9846***	0.2096	0.2802	−0.0254	−0.2149	−0.1411	−0.2001	−0.0325	0.0167
Anxiety_CA	0.0812	0.2441	***0.9736***	−0.1130	0.4873	−0.1743	−0.1146	−0.1627	0.2160	−0.1818
PTSD_CA	−0.1047	0.3101	−0.1195	***0.9481***	−0.1455	−0.0390	−0.0818	−0.1162	0.0094	−0.1753
Dep[a]_CA	−0.1184	−0.0805	0.4591	−0.1387	***0.9724***	−0.2075	−0.1406	−0.1995	0.0900	−0.2870
Mania_CA	0.0604	−0.2528	−0.2018	0.0536	−0.2380	***0.9372***	0.3746	0.1320	−0.1070	−0.2957
Hal[b]_CA	−0.1093	−0.1565	−0.1247	−0.0842	−0.1519	0.2371	***0.5626***	0.2225	−0.0843	−0.1830
Del[c]_CA	−0.1431	−0.2049	−0.1634	−0.1104	−0.1990	0.0545	0.4636	***0.6353***	0.0694	−0.2396
Alcohol_CA	0.2757	−0.0399	0.2396	0.0608	0.0463	−0.1140	−0.0254	0.0630	***0.9896***	−0.1425
Drug_CA	−0.0835	0.0490	−0.1711	−0.1624	−0.2605	−0.2514	−0.1647	−0.2336	−0.1446	***0.9813***

[a]*Dep* depression
[b]*Hal* hallucinations
[c]*Del* delusions

References

1. Carlat, D. J. (1999). *The psychiatric interview*. Lippincott Williams & Wilkins.
2. Spraycar, M., & Randolph, E. (Eds.). (1995). *Stedman: Stedman's medical dictionary*. Williams&Wilkins.
3. Wittchen, H. U., Nelson, C. B., & Lachner, G. (1998). Prevalence of mental disorders and psychosocial impairments in adolescents and young adults. *Psychological Medicine, 28*, 109–126.
4. Cherpitel, C. J. (1999). Screening for alcohol problems in the U.S. general population: A comparison of the CAGE and TWEAK by gender, ethnicity, and services utilization. *Journal of Studies on Alcohol., 60*, 705–711.
5. Cherpitel, C. J. (1998). Performance of screening instruments for identifying alcohol dependence in the general population, compared with clinical populations. *Alcoholism, Clinical and Experimental Research, 22*, 1399–1404.
6. Grut, M., Fratiglioni, L., Viitanen, M., & Winblad, B. (1993). Accuracy of the mini-mental status examination as a screening test for dementia in a Swedish elderly population. *Acta Neurologica Scandinavica, 87*, 312–317.
7. Hea, W. (1999). Screening for mental disorders: Performance of the Composite International Diagnostic – Screener (CID–S). *International Journal of Methods in Psychiatric Research., 8*, 59–70.
8. Zimmerman, M., & Mattia, J. I. (1999). The reliability and validity of a screening questionnaire for 13 DSM-IV Axis I disorders (the psychiatric diagnostic screening questionnaire) in psychiatric outpatients. *The Journal of Clinical Psychiatry, 60*, 677–683.
9. Wittchen, H. U., Lachner, G., Wunderlich, U., & Pfister, H. (1998). Test-retest reliability of the computerized DSM-IV version of the Munich-Composite International Diagnostic Interview (M-CIDI). *Social Psychiatry and Psychiatric Epidemiology, 33*, 568–578.
10. Zimmerman, M., & Mattia, J. I. (2001). A self-report scale to help make psychiatric diagnoses: The psychiatric diagnostic screening questionnaire. *Archives of General Psychiatry, 58*, 787–794.
11. Zimmerman, M., Gorlin, E., Dalrymple, K., & Chelminiski, I. (2017). A clinically useful screen for attention-deficit/hyperactivity disorder in adult psychiatric outpatients. *Annals of Clinical Psychiatry, 29*, 160–166.
12. Raghuraman, P., Balasundaram, S., Sarkar, S., & Subramaniam, E. (2019). A cross-sectional study of psychiatric morbidity and quality of life among participants utilizing the preventive health-care services of a tertiary hospital. *Indian Journal of Psychiatry, 61*, 192–197.
13. Kendler, K. S., & Mishara, A. (2019). The prehistory of Schneider's First-rank symptoms: Texts from 1810 to 1932. *Schizophrenia Bulletin, 45*, 971–990.
14. Cronbach, L. J. (1951). Coefficient alpha and the internal structure of tests. *Psychometrika., 16*, 297–334.
15. Carmines, E. G., & Zeller, R. A. (1979). *Reliability and validity assessment*. SAGE.
16. Schene, A. H., Koeter, M., van Wijngaarden, B., Knudsen, H. C., Leese, M., Ruggeri, M., White, I. R., & Vazquez-Barquero, J. L. (2000). Methodology of a multi-site reliability study. EPSILON study 3. European psychiatric services: Inputs linked to outcome domains and needs. *The British journal of psychiatry. Supplement, 39*, s15–s20.
17. Cohen, J. (1960). A coefficient of agreement for nominal scales. *Educational and Psychological Measurement., 20*, 37–46.
18. Fleiss, J. (1981). *Statistical methods for rates and proportions* (2nd ed.). Wiley.
19. Kraemer, H. C., Periyakoil, V. S., & Noda, A. (2002). Tutorial in biostatistics: Kappa coefficient in medical research. *Statistics in Medicine., 21*, 2109–2129.
20. Williams, J. B., Gibbon, M., First, M. B., Spitzer, R. L., Davies, M., Borus, J., Howes, M. J., Kane, J., Pope, H. G., Jr., Rounsaville, B., et al. (1992). The Structured Clinical Interview for DSM-III-R (SCID). II. Multisite test-retest reliability. *Archives of General Psychiatry, 49*, 630–636.

Chapter 5
The Standard for Clinicians' Interview in Psychiatry (SCIP) as a Consistent and Comprehensive Glossary of Psychiatric Symptoms and Signs

The science of descriptive psychopathology (mental symptoms and signs) was developed in Europe in the nineteenth century, prompted by the nineteenth century practice of building asylums where patients with mental disorders were confined in the asylums for years. This allowed the nineteenth century alienists to be in direct contact with patients of mental illness; examine and describe their behaviors, symptoms, and signs; and observe the changes of behaviors and actions over time. The science of descriptive psychopathology continued to develop in the twentieth century, prompted by the development of rating scales which correlated with more detailed descriptions of symptoms and signs and rating their severity (e.g., mild, moderate, severe). Father Thomas Verner Moore (1877–1969), a psychologist and psychiatrist, created modern psychiatric rating scales. As described in Chap. 1, the book "The Essential Psychoses and Their Fundamental Syndromes: Studies in Psychology and Psychiatry from the Catholic University of America" (Moore, T) outlined the details of the rating scales. The following is an example of the definition of hypochondriacal delusions: "This symptom was termed positive if the patient's delusions had to do with ideas about impossible pathological conditions, e.g., that his heart was gone, that his brain had wasted away to nothing, etc." [1].

There are now hundreds of scales that exist to measure many aspects of human behaviors, symptoms, and signs. However, with many scales developed by different authors across several generations and covering the same disorder (e.g., major depression), the consistency of definitions of psychopathology items has been a challenge. A systematic review of historical textbooks in psychiatry published between 1899 and 1956 by Kendler showed that the same psychopathology item was defined differently by various authors with different titles and labels. Even different psychopathology items like emotional blunting and avolition were given the same label "apathy" [2, 3].

With the development of many scales and definitions of psychopathology, the need to develop consistent and comprehensive definitions of psychiatric symptoms and signs has emerged. The Association for Methodology and Documentation in

A. S. Aboraya, *Manual for the Standard for Clinicians' Interview in Psychiatry (SCIP)*, Advances in Mental Health and Addiction,
https://doi.org/10.1007/978-3-030-94930-3_5

Psychiatry (AMDP) was founded in 1965 by a group of European psychiatrists (from Germany, France, Spain, Switzerland, Belgium, and Austria) to develop uniform definitions of psychiatric symptoms and signs which would be useful in both clinical practice and psychopharmacological research. The system could serve as the basis for the development of international standards in psychiatric diagnosis and research [4]. The final version is the AMDP-III that consists of five parts: Part 1: Demographic data, Part 2: Life events, Part 3: Psychiatric history, Part 4: Psychopathological symptoms (100), and Part 5: Somatic signs (40 signs). The AMDP contains a glossary of definitions for 100 symptoms (covering mainly anxiety, phobia, affect, mood, obsessions, compulsions, delusions, hallucinations, and formal thought disorders) and a glossary of definitions for 40 signs (covering sleep, appetite, gastrointestinal, cardiac, respiratory, autonomic, neurological, and other somatic symptoms). The final AMDP version was translated into 12 languages, including English, in 1982 [5]. **The AMDP manual was published by Springer-Verlag and is 121 pages (4.5 × 7 inches).** AMDP symptoms glossary covers 24 pages and AMDP signs glossary covers 7 pages. The raters of the AMDP were trained by experienced supervisors to make ratings based upon objective data from observation by the staff and subjective data obtained directly from the patient. The raters used a logical model to decide on the presence of the symptom and its severity (mild, moderate, severe, or extreme). The definitions are provided in the glossary, but no specific questions that reflect specific glossary items. Interest in AMDP disappeared in 1980s due to the development of DSM-III [5] and the Present State Examination (PSE) by Professor John Wing and his colleagues at the Institute of Psychiatry, London University. The PSE is a structured clinical interview designed to assess the presence or absence of psychiatric symptoms and signs and make psychiatric diagnoses using the clinical experience of the interviewer. The PSE has passed through several editions (PSE 7, 8, 9 and 10) and has been used in research worldwide [6–14]. The PSE-9 sections cover anxiety, panic, depression, mania, obsessions, compulsions, delusions, hallucinations, behaviors, affect, and speech. A major advantage of the PSE-9 version is the glossary of definitions of 140 items of psychopathology (46 pages). Compared to the AMDP glossary, the definitions in the PSE are more detailed and the PSE 9 provided specific questions to elicit the items.

Comparison

AMDP: 10. Concentration: The inability to focus on a topic and remain focused. Failure to keep one's attention on a specific matter or objective for a reasonable period of time. In everyday language, the inability "to stick to a task."

PSE-9: 20. Poor concentration: The subject complains that he cannot give his full attention to matters which require it or not for as long as they require. The experience is unpleasant, it is beyond the subject's power to correct except for very brief intervals, and it is out of proportion to the difficulty of the problems being considered. At its most intense, the subject cannot even read a few sentences in a newspaper, cannot watch television, and cannot take in a conversation. Severity is rated on the basis of frequency and intensity during the past month.

The PSE-9 questions regarding poor concentration:

Q.1 What has your concentration been like recently?
Q.2 Can you read an article in the paper or watch a TV program right through?
Q.3 Do your thoughts drift off so that you do not take things in?

Drawbacks of PSE-9:

1. Multiple questions are usually required to assess a single item, which is time-intensive and often less feasible in busy clinical settings.
2. The reliability of individual items is limited. Rodgers 1986 article measured the reliability of 48 questions on anxiety and depression [15].

The PSE-10 was built on the PSE-9 and added new sections to cover somatoform disorders, dissociative and eating disorders, alcohol and drug use disorders, and cognitive impairment. The Schedules for Clinical Assessment in Neuropsychiatry (SCAN) glossary were developed from the PSE-9 glossary and added definitions for the newly added sections [16]. The PSE-9 glossary and the SCAN glossary of definitions provided important contributions to the science of psychopathology definitions.

The publication of the DSM-III in 1982 and its widespread use all over the world added a new spin on the concept of glossary of definitions. The DSM-III and its subsequent editions included diagnostic criteria, which are brief definitions that provide no guidelines or specific questions for eliciting the criteria. Moreover, the number of psychiatric diagnoses has increased from 106 diagnoses in the DSM-I to 297 diagnoses in the DSM-IV [17]. The hierarchy of psychiatric diagnoses (diagnoses that are higher on the hierarchy subsume diagnoses that are lower on the hierarchy) has been present and dominant in virtually all systems of psychiatric nosology [18, 19]. The fourth revision of the Diagnostic and Statistical Manual (DSM-IV) relaxed the hierarchical constraint and allowed more than one diagnosis to be assigned on axis I [20]. The DSM-IV excluded lower diagnoses only if they were "better accounted for" by a higher diagnosis. The result of this important change is that one patient could be diagnosed with several psychiatric disorders (comorbidity) and one symptom could be used as a diagnostic criterion for several psychiatric disorders. For example, poor concentration is a symptom of generalized anxiety disorder (GAD), posttraumatic stress disorder, major depression, negative symptom of schizophrenia, and attention-deficit hyperactivity disorder (ADHD). Here are the DSM-5 definitions of poor concentration as they pertain to different psychiatric disorders:

GAD: "Difficulty concentrating or mind going blank".

Major depressive episode: "Diminished ability to think or concentrate, or indecisiveness, nearly every day (either by subjective account or as observed by others)".

Posttraumatic stress disorder: "Problems with concentration".

ADHD: "Often fails to give close attention to details or makes careless mistakes in schoolwork, at work, or during other activities (e.g., overlooks or misses details, work is inaccurate)".

The DSM-5 included a 15-page glossary of technical terms (179 technical terms) which is considered a step backward in the science of descriptive psychopathology.

Despite the aforementioned progress in the glossary of definitions of psychopathology, three problems still exist. **First, research on the reliability of individual symptoms and signs is limited.** The mental health system exists because patients come to doctors with symptoms and signs; it is therefore a starting point [21]. Mental health professionals ask patients questions to inquire more about the details of symptoms and signs (e.g., symptom severity, duration, history, etc.). Although researchers realized the importance of reliability at the level of individual symptoms and signs [22], this line of research is limited [15]. This gap in the literature was one of the important goals addressed by the SCIP project. Specifically, the SCIP sought to develop reliable questions to measure symptoms and signs of mental disorders. **Second, no guidelines exist for the titles and labels of psychopathology items.** Many labels like apathy, asociality, and alogia are defined inconsistently and can be misleading for clinicians [23]. **Third, the same psychopathology item can have different labels based on the diagnosis.** For example, the DSM-5 criteria of "loss of interest or pleasure" is explained as "Markedly diminished interest or pleasure in all, or almost all, activities most of the day, nearly every day (as indicated by either subjective account or observation)." The DSM-5 has a similar definition for anhedonia: "Lack of enjoyment from, engagement in, or energy for life's experiences; deficits in the capacity to feel pleasure and take interest in things." So, for a patient diagnosed with schizophrenia, the loss of pleasure is labeled as "anhedonia." However, for another patient diagnosed with a major depressive episode, this loss of pleasure would be labeled as "loss of interest or pleasure."

The SCIP glossary of psychiatric symptoms and signs (GPSS) is a continuation of decades of research that has aimed to develop a uniform system of definitions of psychopathology and to correct the shortcomings of existing glossaries. One of the main objectives of the SCIP project was to develop reliable questions for psychopathology. **By the end of the SCIP project, kappa coefficients for 30 screening and 200 psychopathology questions/items covering most adult psychiatric disorders were measured.** The definitions of psychopathology items were written to reflect the questions.

Each SCIP psychopathology item had a single title; some SCIP items have a title and subtitle that are commonly described and used in literature. **The rule is that the title or the subtitle should be descriptive of the psychopathology item.** Whether the SCIP item has one title or a title/subtitle, each SCIP item has the same definition. For example, the inability to experience pleasure and enjoyments in the SCIP has one title and a subtitle: anhedonia (loss of pleasure and interest). The item also has one definition: The patient has been unable to experience pleasure and enjoy things that he/she used to enjoy like exercising, enjoying hobbies, or socializing with friends. Table 5.1 shows the 30 SCIP screening items and 200 adult psychopathology items. Each item has two codes: a measurement-based care (MBC) code and a personalized medicine in psychiatry (PMP) code, a title/subtitle, item definition, item question(s), a kappa, and the standard error of kappa. Inter-rater reliability kappa was measured: among the 30 screening items, 19 items (63%) have good reliability (kappa >0.7) and 11 items (37%) have fair reliability (kappa ranges from 0.5 to 0.7). Among the 200 psychopathology items, 7 items (3.5%) have poor reliability (kappa <0.5), 24 items (12%) have fair reliability (kappa ranges from 0.5 to 0.7), and 169 items (84.5%) have good reliability (kappa >0.7).

Table 5.1 The Standard for Clinicians' Interview in Psychiatry (SCIP) glossary of psychiatric symptoms and signs (GPSS)

Screening items

MBC Code[a] (PMP Code)[b]	Item title/ subtitle	Item definitions	Item questions	# of cases	K	SE
PS1_ANX (PS1)	**Generalized anxiety**	**Patient feels very anxious and afraid out of proportion to the situation (with or without physical symptoms) for a prolonged period almost every day**	***Have you felt very anxious and afraid out of proportion to the situation (with or without physical symptoms) for a prolonged period almost every day?*** 0 Absent or non-significant 1 present . Not sure *or* Not applicable *or* Missing	**61**	**0.76**	**0.05**
PS2_PANIC (PS2)	**Panic attacks**	**Panic attack: Patient suddenly feels anxious and frightened for a short time (up to 60 minutes) and develops physical symptoms such as fast heart beats, shaking, sweating, difficulty breathing**	***Did you have a panic attack, during which you suddenly felt anxious and frightened for a short time (up to 60 minutes) and developed physical symptoms (e.g., fast heart beats, shaking, sweating)?*** 0 Absent or non-significant 1 Symptom present . Not sure *or* Not applicable *or* Missing	**54**	**0.81**	**0.05**
PS3_ AGORAPHOB (PS3)	**Agoraphobia**	**Patient is afraid of being alone (at home or outside of home), traveling in a car, train or plane, being in an open space (e.g., park) or being in a closed space (e.g., store), or being in crowds**	***Have you been afraid of being alone (at home or outside of home), traveling in a car, train or plane, being in an open space (e.g., park) or being in a closed space (e.g., store), or being in crowds?*** 0 Absent or non-significant 1 Symptom present . Not sure *or* Not applicable *or* Missing	**26**	**0.52**	**0.05**

(continued)

PS4_SOC_ PHOB (PS4)	**Social Phobia**	**Patient is afraid and anxious when he/she does things in front of people, such as eating or speaking in public**	***Have you been afraid and anxious when you do things in front of people, such as eating or speaking in public?*** 0 Absent or non-significant 1 Symptom present . Not sure *or* Not applicable *or* Missing	**22**	**0.51**	**0.05**
PS5_OBS (PS5)	**Screening for obsessions**	**The patient has an intrusive thought or image that does not make sense and keeps coming back to his/her mind even when the patient tries not to have the thought or the image**	***Do you ever have an intrusive thought or image that does not make sense and keeps coming back to your mind even when you try not to have the thought or the image?*** 0 Absent or non-significant 1 Symptom present . Not sure *or* Not applicable *or* Missing	**38**	**0.70**	**0.04**
PS6_COMP (PS6)	**Screening for compulsions**	**The patient has to do things over and over, that is, checking things he/she has done (such as washing hands even if they are clean, checking doors or repeating mental acts such as counting or praying)**	***Do you find that you have to do things over and over, that is, checking things you have done (such as washing your hands even if they are clean, checking doors, or repeating mental acts such as counting or praying)?*** 0 Absent or non-significant 1 Symptom present . Not sure *or* Not applicable *or* Missing	**31**	**0.58**	**0.05**
PS7_TRAUM (PS7)	**Witness or experience traumatic events**	**The patient witnessed or experienced a traumatic event that involved actual or threatened death or serious injury to the patient or someone else (e.g. physical or sexual abuse, terrorist attack, natural disaster, war…). The patient felt intense fear and helplessness**	***Have you ever witnessed or experienced a traumatic event that involved actual or threatened death or serious injury to you or someone else*** **(e.g.,** ***physical or sexual abuse, terrorist attack, natural disaster, war…)?*** ***Did you feel intense fear and helplessness?*** 0 No traumatic events 1 One traumatic event 2 More than one traumatic event . Not sure *or* Not applicable *or* Missing	**69**	**0.75**	**0.05**

PS8_RE_EXP (PS8)	**Re-experience traumatic events**	**The patient has re-experienced the event in a distressing way (e.g., flashbacks, nightmares, bad dreams)**	***Over the past month, have you re-experienced the event in a distressing way (e.g., flashbacks, nightmares, bad dreams)?*** 0 Absent or non-significant 1 Symptom present . Not sure *or* Not applicable *or* Missing	**34**	**0.89**	**0.05**
PS9_DEP (PS9)	**Depressed mood**	**The patient has been feeling sad, depressed or in low spirits**	***Have you been feeling sad, depressed or in low spirits?*** 0 Absent or non-significant 1 Symptom present . Not sure *or* Not applicable *or* Missing.	**158**	**0.86**	**0.04**
PS10_ ANHED (PS10)	**Anhedonia**	**The patient has been unable to experience pleasure and enjoy things that he/she used to enjoy like exercising, enjoying hobbies or socializing with friends**	***Have you been unable to experience pleasure and enjoy things that you used to enjoy like exercising, enjoying your hobbies, or socializing with friends?*** 0 Absent or non-significant 1 Symptom present . Not sure *or* Not applicable *or* Missing.	**125**	**0.87**	**0.04**
PS11_SUICID (PS11)	**Suicidal ideation, intention and plan**	**The patient had thoughts about harming self.** **The patient had the intention to carryout the suicidal thoughts.** **The patient had specific suicidal plans.** **The patient had one or more suicide attempts during the past month**	***Have you had thoughts about harming yourself?*** ***Have you had the intention to carry out the suicidal thoughts?*** ***Have you had suicidal plans?*** ***Have you attempted to harm yourself during the past month? (multiple choices allowed)*** 0 Absent 1 Current suicidal ideations 2 Current suicidal intention 3 Current suicidal plans 4 Recent suicide attempts (past month) . Not sure *or* Not applicable *or* Missing	**79**	**0.61**	**0.04**
PS12_MUTIL (PS12)	**Self-mutilation behaviors**	**The patient engages in self-mutilation behaviors without intending to die (e.g., burning, cutting, scratching)**	***Have you attempted self-mutilation behaviors without intent to die (e.g., burning, cutting, scratching)?*** 0 Absent 1 Current self-mutilation (past month) . Not sure *or* Not applicable *or* Missing	**79**	**0.61**	**0.04**

PS13_ ELATED (PS13)	**Elated mood**	**The patient feels very happy, elated, on top of the world for no apparent reason**	***Have you felt very happy, elated, on top of the world for no apparent reason?*** 0 Absent or non-significant 1 Symptom present . Not sure *or* Not applicable *or* Missing	**76**	**0.72**	**0.05**
PS14_ IRRITAB (PS14)	**Irritable mood**	**The patient feels easily irritated without reason.** **The patient feels so irritable that he/she shouts at people or starts arguments or actually becomes aggressive**	***Have you felt easily irritated without reason?*** ***Have you found yourself so irritable that you shout at people or start arguments or actually become aggressive?*** 0 Absent or non-significant 1 Symptom present . Not sure *or* Not applicable *or* Missing	**65**	**0.75**	**0.05**
PS15_MIXED (PS15)	**Mixed mood (same day mood changes)**	**The patient has mixed mood swings: Periods of depression and elation or irritability on the same day.**	***Have you had mixed mood swings: Periods of depression and elation or irritability on the same day?*** 0 Absent or non-significant 1 Symptom present . Not sure *or* Not applicable *or* Missing	**44**	**0.50**	**0.05**
PS16_ PARANOID (PS16)	**Paranoid delusions**	**The patient feels that someone is spying on him/her or trying to harm the patient or has a plot or conspiracy against the patient**	***Have you felt that someone is spying on you or trying to harm you or has a plot or conspiracy against you?*** 0 Absent or non-significant. 1 Symptom present . Sure *or* Not applicable *or* Missing	**97**	**0.83**	**0.04**
PS17_DEL (PS17)	**Other delusions**	**The patient has strange thoughts such as that he/she is a prominent person in society, or he/she is divine or God, or he/she receives special messages from TV or newspapers**	***Do you have strange thoughts such as that you are a prominent person in society, or you yourself are divine or you are God, or you receive special messages from TV or newspapers?*** 0 Absent or non-significant 1 Symptom present . Not sure *or* Not applicable *or* Missing	**39**	**0.77**	**0.04**
PS18_AUDH (PS18)	**Auditory hallucinations**	**The patient has experiences of hearing voices or noises that other people cannot hear**	***Have you had experiences of hearing voices or noises that other people cannot hear?*** 0 Absent or non-significant. 1 Symptom present. . Not sure *or* Not applicable *or* Missing	**92**	**0.76**	**0.04**

PS19_VISH (PS19)	**Visual hallucinations**	**The patient has experiences of seeing things (shadows, objects, people) that other people cannot see**	***Have you had experiences of seeing things (shadows, objects, people) that other people cannot see?*** 0 Absent or non-significant. 1 Symptom present. . Not sure *or* Not applicable *or* Missing	**51**	**0.68**	**0.05**
PS20_VIOL (PS20)	**Violence**	**The patient has been violent (destructive to objects or violent towards people) in the past (with or without the influence of alcohol or drugs)**	***Have you been violent (destructive to objects or violent towards people) in the past (with or without the influence of alcohol or drugs)?*** 0 No history of violence. 1 Yes, due to alcohol and/or drugs. 2 Yes, without use of alcohol or drugs. 3 Both, with and without use of alcohol or drugs. . Not sure *or* Not applicable *or* Missing	**74**	**0.64**	**0.04**
PS21_ DISBHV (PS21)	**Disorganized behavior**	**There is evidence of disorganized behavior by observation during the interview (agitation, odd appearance, inappropriate social behavior, inappropriate affect)**	***There is evidence of disorganized behavior by observation during the interview (agitation, odd appearance, inappropriate social behavior, inappropriate affect)*** 0 Absent or non-significant 1 Symptom present . Not sure *or* Not applicable *or* Missing	**32**	**0.54**	**0.04**
PS22_ DISTHOT (PS22)	**Disorganized thoughts**	**Evidence of disorganized thoughts by observation during the interview (loose associations, tangentiality, incoherent speech)**	***Evidence of disorganized thoughts by observation during the interview (loose associations, tangentiality, incoherent speech)*** 0 Absent or non-significant. 1 Symptom present. . Not sure *or* Not applicable *or* Missing	**39**	**0.65**	**0.04**
PS23_ALCP (PS23)	**Alcohol problems**	**Alcohol causes problems for the patient at work or school, problems with family or friends, legal problems, or other problems such as physical fights**	***During the past year, did alcohol cause problems for you at work or school, problems with family or friends, legal problems, or other problems such as getting in physical fights?*** 0 Absent or non-significant. 1 Symptom present. . Not sure *or* Not applicable *or* Missing	**53**	**0.89**	**0.06**

PS24_DRGP (PS24)	**Drug problems**	**Drug use (__________) causes problems for the patient at work or school, problems with family or friends, legal problems, or other problems such as getting in physical fights**	***During the past year, did drug use (__________) cause problems for you at work or school, problems with family or friends, legal problems, or other problems such as getting in physical fights?*** 0 Absent or non-significant. 1 Symptom present. . Not sure *or* Not applicable *or* Missing	**17**	**0.78**	**0.06**
PS25_SOMS (PS25)	**Somatic symptoms**	**The patient had visited doctors due to physical illness and the doctors did the necessary work up and could not find a medical explanation for the symptoms**	***Have you visited doctors due to physical illness and the doctors did the necessary work up and could not find a medical explanation (have patient give examples)?*** 0 Absent or non-significant 1 Symptom present . Not sure *or* Not applicable *or* Missing	**33**	**0.81**	**0.05**
PS26_PAINS (PS26)	**Pain symptoms**	**The patient had pain and the doctor did the necessary work up and could not really explain why**	***Have you had pain and your doctor did the necessary work up and could not really explain why?*** 0 Absent or non-significant. 1 Symptom present. . Not sure *or* Not applicable *or* Missing	**24**	**0.93**	**0.05**
PS27_ **WTGAIN (PS27)**	**Worry about weight gain**	**The patient worried about gaining weight to the point that he/she engaged in self-induced vomiting, using diet pills, laxatives, or heavy exercise**	***Have you worried about gaining weight to the point that you did things such as self-induced vomiting, using diet pills, laxatives, or heavy exercise?*** 0 Absent or non-significant. 1 Symptom present. . Not sure *or* Not applicable *or* Missing.	**12**	**0.73**	**0.05**
PS28_BINGE (PS28)	**Binge-eating**	**The patient had episodes of binge -eating (eating within 1- or 2- hour period what most people would consider an unusually large amount of food)**	***Do you have episodes of binge-eating (eating within 1- or 2-hour period what most people would consider an unusually large amount of food)?*** 0 Absent or non-significant. 1 Symptom present. . Not sure *or* Not applicable *or* Missing	**27**	**0.97**	**0.12**

PS29_SUST_ ATTN (PS29)	**Sustained attention impairment**	**The patient has difficulty concentrating on one thing for a long time (e.g., reading a book, writing a letter)**	***Do you have difficulty concentrating on one thing for a long time* (e.g., *reading a book, writing a letter*)?** 0 Absent or non-significant 1 Patient has difficulty concentrating for a long period of time . = Not sure *or* Not applicable *or* Missing	**39**	**0.95**	**0.12**
PS30_ FIDGETY (PS30)	**Fidgety**	**The patient has difficulty remaining seated (fidgets with hands and feet, squirms or wiggles in seat) when he/she is expected to remain seated (e.g., in a meeting or a church service)**	***Do you have difficulty remaining seated (fidget with hands and feet, squirm or wiggle in seat) when expected to remain seated* (e.g., *in a meeting or a church service*)?** 0 = Absent or non-significant. 1 = Patient fidgets with hands and feet, or wiggles in seat. . = Not sure *or* Not applicable *or* Missing	**41**	**0.81**	**0.12**

Psychopathology items

MBC Code[a] (PMP Code)[b]	Item titles	Item definitions	Item questions	# of Cases	K	SE
1_PAN (P_A1)	**Panic attacks**	**The patient suddenly becomes anxious and frightened for a short period of time (up to 60 minutes). During that time, the patient feels that the heart is racing or pounding, or he/she is shaking or sweating, or choking**	***Did you have a panic attack, when you suddenly become anxious and frightened for a short period of time (up to 60 minutes)?*** ***During that time, did you feel that your heart was racing or pounding, or did you start shaking or sweating, or did you feel you were choking?*** 0 Patient had no panic attacks. 1 Patient had panic attacks. . Not sure *or* Not applicable *or* Missing.	**30**	**0.92**	**0.06**
2_PAN_ WORRY (P_A2)	**Worry about having another panic attack**	**After a panic attack, the patient worries about having another attack.** **The patient worries about its effects (e.g., losing control, having a heart attack or going crazy)**	***After a panic attack, did you worry about having another attack?*** ***Did you worry about its effects* (e.g., *losing control, having a heart attack or going crazy*)?** 0 After a panic attack, patient did not worry about having another one. 1 After a panic attack, patient worried about having another one or its effects. . Not sure *or* Not applicable *or* Missing	**25**	**0.81**	**0.04**

Psychopathology items

MBC Code[a] (PMP Code)[b]	Item titles	Item definitions	Item questions	# of Cases	K	SE
3_PAN_END (P_A3)	**Action to end or prevent panic attacks**	**The patient does something to end the attack, like leaving a store, calling someone, taking deep breaths.** **The patient does something to prevent attacks (like avoiding places that trigger the panic attacks)**	***Did you have to do something to end the attack, like leaving a store, calling someone, taking deep breaths?*** ***Do you do anything to prevent attacks (like avoiding places that trigger the panic attacks)?*** 0 After a panic attack, patient does nothing to end or prevent another panic attack. 1 After a panic attack, patient does something to end or prevent another panic attack. . Not sure *or* Not applicable *or* Missing	**26**	**0.87**	**0.04**
4_SOC_PHOB (P_A4)	**Social phobia**	**The patient becomes afraid and anxious when he/she does things in front of people, such as eating or speaking in public.** **The patient avoids social situations or endures them with intense fear**	***Have you been afraid and anxious when you do things in front of people, such as eating or speaking in public?*** ***Do you avoid social situations or endure them with intense fear?*** 0 Patient had no social phobia 1 Patient had social phobia . Not sure *or* Not applicable *or* Missing	**22**	**0.51**	**0.05**
5_ AGORAPHOB (P_A5)	**Agoraphobia**	**The patient is afraid of being alone (at home or outside of home), traveling in a car, train or plane, being in an open space (e.g., park) or being in a closed space (e.g., store), or being in crowds.** **The patient avoids these situations, or requires a companion, or endures with intense fear**	***Have you been afraid of being alone (at home or outside of home), traveling in a car, train or plane, being in an open space (e.g., park) or being in a closed space (e.g., store), or being in crowds?*** ***Do you avoid these situations, or require a companion, or endure with intense fear?*** 0 Patient had no agoraphobia. 1 Patient had agoraphobia. . Not sure *or* Not applicable *or* Missing	**26**	**0.52**	**0.05**

6_GEN_ANX (P_A6)	**Generalized anxiety**	**The patient has excessive worry and anxiety for long periods (hours each day lasting several months), not just during panic attacks.** **The patient has difficulty controlling the anxiety**	***Have you had excessive worry and anxiety for long periods (hours each day lasting several months), not just during panic attacks?*** ***Is it difficult to control the anxiety?*** 0 Patient has no generalized anxiety 1 Patient has generalized anxiety . Not sure *or* Not applicable *or* Missing	**25**	**0.84**	**0.04**
7_RESTLESS (P_A7)	**Restlessness with anxiety**	**The patient feels restless, keyed up or on edge**	***Did you feel restless, keyed up or on edge?*** 0 No. 1 Yes . Not sure *or* Not applicable *or* Missing.	**26**	**0.74**	**0.04**
8_TENSION (P_A8)	**Tension with anxiety**	**The patient feels tense in muscles**	***Did you feel tense in your muscles?*** 0 No. 1 Yes. . Not sure *or* Not applicable *or* Missing.	**22**	**0.77**	**0.04**
9_ EXHAUSION (P_A9)	**Exhaustion with anxiety**	**The patient feels tired, or easily exhausted even without work**	***Did you feel tired, or easily exhausted even without work?*** 0 No. 1 Yes. . Not sure *or* Not applicable *or* Missing.	**22**	**0.79**	**0.05**
10_POOR_ CONC (P_A10)[a]	**Poor concentration with anxiety**	**The patient has difficulty paying attention and concentrating when reading an article, watching a TV show or a movie, or doing work or school assignments due to anxiety**	***Did you have difficulty concentrating when anxious?*** 0 No 1 Yes . Not sure *or* Not applicable *or* Missing	**27**	**0.76**	**0.05**
11_IRRITAB (P_A11)	**Irritability with anxiety**	**The patient feels irritable when anxious**	***Did you feel irritable when anxious?*** 0 No. 1 Yes. . Not sure *or* Not applicable *or* Missing	**28**	**0.83**	**0.04**
12_ INSOMNIA (P_A12)	**Insomnia with anxiety**	**The patient has difficulty falling asleep or staying asleep when anxious**	***Did you have difficulty falling asleep or staying asleep when anxious?*** 0 No. 1 Yes. . Not sure *or* Not applicable *or* Missing.	**25**	**0.82**	**0.05**

[a]The item is repeated again in different contexts (PTSD item # 39, depression item # 48, negative symptom item # 116, ADHD item # 181)

13_OBS (P_OBS13)	**Obsessions**	**The patient has an intrusive thought or image that does not make sense and keeps coming back to the patient's mind even when he/she tries to avoid the thought or the image**	***Do you ever have an intrusive thought or image that does not make sense and keeps coming back to your mind even when you try to avoid the thought or the image?*** 0 Patient has no obsessions 1 Patient has obsessions less than 1 hour/day 2 Patient has obsessions 1–4 hours/day 3 Patient has obsessions more than 4 hours/day . Not sure *or* Not applicable *or* Missing	**26**	**0.85**	**0.04**
14_OBS_ AGGRESS (P_OBS14)	**Aggressive obsessions**	**Potential examples: Fears of harming oneself, fears of unintentionally hurting someone, urges to stab someone, thoughts of "losing control" and hurting a partner or significant other**	***Do you have obsessive thoughts related to aggression?*** 0 No. 1 Yes. . Not sure *or* Not applicable *or* Missing			
15_OBS_ CONTAM (P_OBS15)	**Contamination obsessions**	**Potential examples: Fear of contamination in public bathrooms, outdoors, or public places, fear of what might happen after touching one's own bodily secretions, fear of getting germs or viruses from others**	***Do you have obsessive thoughts related to contamination?*** 0 No. 1 Yes. . Not sure *or* Not applicable *or* Missing.			
16_OBS_SEX (P_OBS16)	**Sexual obsessions**	**Potential examples: Disturbing thoughts about sex, unwanted images of sexual acts toward strangers, family members or children, fear of being found with pornography**	***Do you have obsessive thoughts related to sex/sexuality?*** 0 No. 1 Yes. . Not sure *or* Not applicable *or* Missing.			

17_OBS_ RELIG (P_OBS17)	**Religious obsessions**	**<u>Potential examples</u>: fear of having blasphemous or "sinful" thoughts, concerns for engaging in sinful or forbidden behavior, feeling the need to complete a certain number of prayers or "good deeds"**	***Do you have obsessive thoughts related to religion?*** 0 No 1 Yes . Not sure *or* Not applicable *or* Missing			
18_OBS_ SOMAT (P_OBS18)	**Somatic obsessions**	**<u>Potential examples:</u> Worries about having an undiagnosed illness like cancer or heart disease, fear of contracting a deadly disease, images of your own death**	***Do you have obsessive thoughts related to your health?*** 0 No. 1 Yes. . Not sure *or* Not applicable *or* Missing.			
19_OBS_ APPEAR (P_OBS19)	**Appearance obsessions**	**<u>Potential examples:</u> Worries about the size of certain body parts (ears, nose, mouth), fears of certain body parts being disgusting to others**	***Do you have obsessive thoughts about your physical appearance?*** 0 No. 1 Yes. . Not sure *or* Not applicable *or* Missing			
20_COMP (P_COM20)	**Compulsions**	**The patient has to do things over and over, that is, checking things he/she has done (such as washing hands even if they are clean, checking doors or repeating mental acts such as counting or praying). The patient gets very anxious or tense if he/she does not repeat the act over and over**	***Do you find that you have to do things over and over, that is, checking things you have done (such as washing your hands even if they are clean, checking doors or repeating mental acts such as counting or praying)?*** ***Do you get very anxious or tense if you do not repeat the act over and over?*** 0 Patient has no compulsions 1 Patient has compulsions less than 1 hour/day 2 Patient has compulsions 1–4 hours/day 3 Patient has compulsions more than 4 hours/day . Not sure *or* Not applicable *or* Missing	**18**	**0.77**	**0.04**
21_COMP_ CHECK (P_COM21)	**Checking compulsions**	**Potential examples: Checking door locks, switches, or appliances many times before leaving the house, checking one's appearance for an excessive amount of time before leaving the house**	***Do you feel the need to check things over and over again?*** 0 No 1 Yes . Not sure *or* Not applicable *or* Missing			

22_COMP_ CLEAN (P_COM22)	**Cleaning/ washing compulsions**	**Potential examples: Excessively changing your clothes, excessive handwashin, tooth brushing, showering, scrubbing surfaces**	***Do you feel the need to clean/wash things over and over again?*** 0 No 1 Yes . Not sure *or* Not applicable *or* Missing
23_COMP_REPEAT (P_COM23)	**Repeating compulsions**	**Potential examples: re-reading text out of concerns that one "missed something," re-writing or re-tracing words, re-entering buildings or living spaces, re-tying one's shoes**	***Do you feel the need to repeat things many times?*** 0 No 1 Yes . Not sure *or* Not applicable *or* Missing
24_COMP_ORDER (P_COM24)	**Ordering/ arranging compulsions**	**Potential examples: Re-arranging one's pantry or refrigerator, spending excessive amounts of time organizing one's desk or workspace**	***Do you feel the need to arrange and rearrange things, order and reorder items over and over again?*** 0 No 1 Yes . Not sure *or* Not applicable *or* Missing
25_COMP_HOARD (P_COM25)	**Hoarding/ collecting**	**Potential examples: Picking up, collecting or buying useless things, owning an excessive amount of items and being unable to donate or get rid of them.**	***Do you feel the need to collect and/or hoard things?*** 0 No 1 Yes . Not sure *or* Not applicable *or* Missing.
26_COMP_MENTAL (P_COM26)	**Mental compulsions**	**Potential examples: Repetitively counting certain numbers or avoiding certain "bad" numbers, repeating certain words, counting senseless things (e.g., ceiling tiles), reciting prayers or statements.**	***Do you engage in any repetitive mental behaviors?*** 0 No 1 Yes . Not sure *or* Not applicable *or* Missing

27_TRAUMA (P_PTSD27)	**Witness or experience traumatic events**	**The patient witnessed or experienced a traumatic event that involved actual or threatened death or serious injury to the patient or someone else (e.g., physical or sexual abuse, rape, terrorist attack, natural disaster, war…)**	***Have you ever witnessed or experienced a traumatic event that involved actual or threatened death or serious injury to you or someone else* (e.g., *physical or sexual abuse, rape, terrorist attack, natural disaster, war…)?*** ***Did you feel intense fear and helplessness?*** 0 Patient had no traumatic events 1 Patient has experienced one traumatic event 2 Patient has experienced several traumatic events . Not sure *or* Not applicable *or* Missing	**69**	**0.75**	**0.05**
28_TRAUMA_ DISTRESS (P_PTSD28)	**Distressing recollection of events**	**The patient had recurrent upsetting memories (distressing recollection) of the event**	***Did you have recurrent upsetting memories (distressing recollection) of the event?*** 0 Patient had no significant symptom 1 Patient has recurrent upsetting memories (distressing recollection) of the event . Not sure *or* Not applicable *or* Missing	**30**	**0.88**	**0.05**
29_TRAUMA_ NGTMARE (P_PTSD29)	**Bad dreams or nightmares**	**The patient had recurrent upsetting dreams or nightmares of the event**	***Did you have recurrent upsetting dreams or nightmares of the event?*** 0 Patient had no significant symptom 1 Patient has recurrent upsetting dreams and nightmares of the event . Not sure *or* Not applicable *or* Missing	**26**	**0.94**	**0.05**
30_TRAUMA_ FLASH (P_PTSD30)	**Flashbacks**	**The patient had a sense or feeling that the event was happening again: the sense of reliving the event (flashbacks), auditory/visual hallucinations related to the event, or body/somatosensory experiences of the event**	***Did you have a sense or feeling that the event was happening again: the sense of reliving the event (flashbacks), auditory/ visual hallucinations related to the event, or body/ somatosensory experiences of the event?*** 0 Patient had no significant symptom 1 Patient has a sense or feeling that the event is happening again, the sense of reliving the event (flashbacks) . Not sure *or* Not applicable *or* Missing	**23**	**0.87**	**0.05**

31_TRAUMA_ AVOIDTH (P_PTSD31)	**Avoidance of thoughts and feelings**	**The patient tries to avoid thoughts and feelings associated with the event**	***Did you try to avoid thoughts and feelings associated with the event?*** 0 Patient had no significant symptom. 1 Patient tries not to think about the event . Not sure *or* Not applicable *or* Missing	**27**	**0.94**	**0.05**
32_TAUMA_ AVOIDPLE (P_PTSD32)	**Avoidance of people, places, and activities**	**The patient tries to avoid things that reminded him/her of the event (such as certain people, certain places, or some activities)**	***Did you try to avoid things that reminded you of the event (such as certain people, certain places, or some activities)?*** 0 Patient had no significant symptom 1 Patient avoids things that are reminders of the event (such as certain people, certain places, or some activities) . Not sure *or* Not applicable *or* Missing	**27**	**0.94**	**0.05**
33_TRAUMA_ AMNESIA (P_PTSD33)	**Amnesia**	**The patient has difficulty remembering some or all important aspects of the event**	***Did you have difficulty remembering some or all important aspects of the event?*** 0 Patient had no significant symptom 1 Patient has difficulty remembering some or all important aspects of the event . Not sure *or* Not applicable *or* Missing	**15**	**0.70**	**0.06**
34_TRAUMA_ ASOCIAL (P_PTSD34)[a]	**Diminished social interest (asociality)**	**The patient spends less time or shows less interest in activities with friends, family or hobbies that he/she used to enjoy due to the even**	***Did you spend less time or show less interest in activities with friends, family or hobbies that you used to enjoy due to the event?*** 0 Patient had no significant symptom 1 Patient spends less time or shows less interest in activities with friends/family or hobbies due to the event . Not sure *or* Not applicable *or* Missing	**17**	**0.83**	**0.05**
35_Tauma_ Detach (P_PTSD35)	**Detachment and isolation**	**The patient feels distant, cut off, or isolated from other people due to the event**	***Did you feel distant, cut off, or isolated from other people due to the event?*** 0 Patient had no significant symptom 1 Patient feels distant, cut off, or isolated from other people due to the event . Not sure *or* Not applicable *or* Missing	**22**	**0.87**	**0.05**

[a]The item is repeated again in a different context (negative symptoms, item # 115)

36_TRAUMA_ NUMB (P_PTSD36)[a]	**Diminished emotional feelings (diminished experience of emotions)**	**The patient feels emotionally numb. The patient has trouble experiencing feelings (happiness, love feelings) due to the event**	***Did you feel emotionally numb? Did you have trouble experiencing feelings (happiness, love feelings) due to the event?*** 0 Patient had no significant symptom 1 Patient feels emotionally numb. Patient has trouble experiencing feelings (such as happiness or love feelings) due to the event . Not sure *or* Not applicable *or* Missing	**24**	**0.88**	**0.05**
37_TRAUMA_ INSOMNIA (P_PTSD37)	**Insomnia**	**The patient has difficulty falling or staying asleep due to the event**	***Did you have difficulty falling or staying asleep due to the event?*** 0 Patient had no significant symptom 1 Patient has difficulty falling or staying asleep due to the event . Not sure *or* Not applicable *or* Missing	**16**	**0.78**	**0.05**
38_TAUMA_ ANGER (P_PTSD38)	**Anger**	**The patient has periods of irritability or sudden outbursts of anger due to the event**	***Did you have periods of irritability or sudden outbursts of anger due to the event?*** 0 Patient had no significant symptom 1 Patient has periods of irritability or sudden outbursts of anger due to the event . Not sure *or* Not applicable *or* Missing	**19**	**0.80**	**0.05**

[a]Note that item #36 is ***different*** from item # 113

39_TRAUMA_ POOR_CONC (P_PTSD39)[a]	**Attention impairment (poor concentration)**	**The patient has difficulty concentrating due to the event. The patient has decreased concentration and he/she is unable to complete a task (e.g., at work, reading an article, reading a book, or watching a movie), even though the patient was able to do that before**	***Did you have difficulty concentrating due to the event?*** 0 Patient had no significant symptom 1 Patient has difficulty concentrating due to the event . Not sure *or* Not applicable *or* Missing	**14**	**0.78**	**0.05**

40_TRAUMA_ VIGIL (P_PTSD40)	**Hypervigilance**	**The patient feels very alert or watchful of things going on around even when there is no need to be**	***Did you feel very alert or watchful of things going on around you even when there was no need to be?*** 0 Patient had no significant symptom 1 Patient feels very alert or watchful of things going on around even when there is no need to be . Not sure *or* Not applicable *or* Missing.	**17**	**0.87**	**0.05**
41_TRAUMA_ STARTLE (P_PTSD41)	**Startle response**	**The patient feels jumpy and easily startled.** **The patient is easily scared or makes a sudden movement or jump when he/she hears noises or caught by surprise**	***Did you feel jumpy and easily startled?*** ***Were you easily scared or did you make a sudden movement or jump when you heard noises or if you were caught by surprise?*** 0 Patient had no significant symptom 1 Patient feels jumpy and has a startle response . Not sure *or* Not applicable *or* Missing	**20**	**0.86**	**0.05**

[a]The item is repeated again in different contexts (anxiety item # 10, depression item # 48, negative symptom item # 116, ADHD item # 181)

42_TRAUMA_ EMOTION (P_PTSD42)	**Psychological distress due to events**	**The patient gets emotionally upset (e.g., anxiety, agitation, shame, guilt) when something reminded him/her of the event**	***Did you get emotionally upset* (e.g., *anxiety, agitation, shame, guilt) when something reminded you of the event?*** 0 Patient had no significant symptom 1 Patient gets emotionally upset (e.g., anxiety, agitation, shame, guilt) when reminded of the event . Not sure *or* Not applicable *or* Missing	**26**	**0.91**	**0.05**
43_TRAUMA_ PHYSICAL (P_PTSD43)	**Physical reactions due to events**	**The patient has physical reactions (e.g., fast heart beats, fast breathing, sweating) when something reminded him/her of the event**	***Did you have physical reactions* (e.g., *fast heart beats, fast breathing, sweating) when something reminded you of the event?*** 0 Patient had no significant symptom 0 Patient has physical reactions (e.g., fast heart beats, fast breathing, sweating) when reminded of the event . Not sure *or* Not applicable *or* Missing	**24**	**0.93**	**0.05**
44_TRAUMA_ DAZE (P_PTSD44)	**Daze (feeling out of touch with surroundings)**	**The patient feels out of touch with things going on around (e.g., being in a daze or not aware of surroundings)**	***Did you feel out of touch with things going on around you* (e.g., *being in a daze or not aware of surroundings)?*** 0 Patient had no significant symptom 1 Patient feels out of touch with things going on around . Not sure *or* Not applicable *or* Missing.	**16**	**0.82**	**0.05**

45_DEP (P_DEP45)	**Depressed mood**	**The patient feels sad, depressed or in low spirits**	***Have you been feeling sad, depressed or in low spirits?*** 0 Patient has no depressed mood 1 Patient has depressed mood less than half the time 2 Patient has depressed mood more than half the time . Not sure *or* Not applicable *or* Missing	**128**	**0.91**	**0.04**
46_ANHED ONIA (P_DEP46)[a]	**Anhedonia (loss of pleasure and interest)**	**The patient has been unable to experience pleasure and enjoy things that he/she used to enjoy like exercising, enjoying hobbies, or socializing with friends**	***Have you been unable to experience pleasure and enjoy things that you used to enjoy like exercising, enjoying your hobbies, or socializing with friends?*** 0 Patient has no anhedonia 1 Patient has anhedonia less than half the time 2 Patient has anhedonia more than half the time . Not sure *or* Not applicable *or* Missing	**121**	**0.87**	**0.04**
47_HOPE LESSNESS (P_DEP47)	**Hopelessness**	**The patient feels hopeless about his/her future**	***Have you felt hopeless about your future?*** 0 Patient is not hopeless 1 Patient feels hopeless less than half the time 2 Patient feels hopeless more than half the time . Not sure *or* Not applicable *or* Missing	**11**	**0.82**	**0.04**

[a]The item is repeated again in a different context (negative symptom item # 112)

48_POOR_ CONC (P_DEP48)[a]	**Attention impairment (poor concentration)**	**The patient has decreased concentration and he/she is unable to complete a task (e.g., at work, reading an article, reading a book, or watching a movie), even though the patient was able to do that before**	***Have you found that your concentration has decreased and you are unable to complete a task (*****e.g.*****, at work, reading an article, reading a book, or watching a movie), even though you were able to do that before?*** 0 Patient has no concentration problems 1 Patient has difficulty concentrating less than half the time 2 Patient has difficulty concentrating more than half the time. . Not sure *or* Not applicable *or* Missing	**116**	**0.80**	**0.04**
49_ PSYCHOM_ SLOW (P_DEP49)[b]	**Psychomotor retardation/ slowing**	**The patient is talking or moving more slowly than normal when depressed**	***Have you felt as though you were talking or moving more slowly than normal for you when depressed?*** 0 Patient has normal activity 1 Patient has psychomotor retardation less than half the time 2 Patient has psychomotor retardation more than half the time . Not sure *or* Not applicable *or* Missing	**97**	**0.72**	**0.04**

50_ WORTHLESS (P_DEP50)	**Worthlessness (low self-esteem)**	**The patient has low self-esteem and feels that he/she is a worthless person in the society or a failure**	***Have you felt that you are a worthless person in the society or a failure?*** 0 Patient has no feeling of worthlessness 1 Patient feels worthless less than half the time 2 Patient feels worthless more than half the time . Not sure *or* Not applicable *or* Missing	**97**	**0.78**	**0.04**

[a]The item is repeated again in different contexts (Anxiety item # 10, PTSD item # 39, negative symptom item # 116, ADHD item # 181)
[b]The item is repeated again in a different context (negative symptom item # 117)

51_GUILT (P_DEP51)	**Guilt**	**The patient feels guilty or ashamed of himself/herself for something the patient has done or thought**	***Have you felt guilty or ashamed of yourself for something you have done or thought?*** 0 Patient has no feeling of guilt 1 Patient feels guilty less than half The time 2 Patient feels guilty more than half The time . Not sure *or* Not applicable *or* Missing	**86**	**0.80**	**0.04**
52_SUICD_ THOT (P_DEP52)	**Thoughts of suicide**	**The patient had thoughts, intention or plans to harm or kill himself/ herself during the past month. The patient may have made one or more suicide attempt during the past month**	***Have you had thoughts, intention or plans to harm or kill yourself during the past month?*** ***Have you made a suicide attempt during the past month?*** 0 Patient had no suicidal thoughts or made a suicide attempt during the past month 1 Patient had thoughts, intention or plans to harm self 2 Patient made one recent suicide attempt during the past month 3 Patient made two or more recent suicide attempts during the past month . Not sure *or* Not applicable *or* Missing	**68**	**0.64**	**0.04**
53_CRY_DEP (P_DEP53)	**Crying when depressed**	**Patient has crying spells when depressed**	***Have you cried when depressed?*** 0 Patient has no crying spells 1 Patient has crying spells due to sadness less than half the time 2 Patient has crying spells due to sadness more than half the time . Not sure *or* Not applicable *or* Missing.	**11**	**0.76**	**0.04**

54_FATIGUE (P_DEP54)	**Fatigue and loss of energy**	**Patient feels tired and exhausted during the day, even when he/she sleeps well and does not work very hard.** **Even though patient may feel tired and exhausted, he/she may have no decrease in the three main goal-directed activities in life: school, work, or social activities with other people (item # 114)**	***Have you felt tired and exhausted during the day, even when you slept well and did not work very hard?*** 0 Patient has no fatigue or loss of energy 1 Patient feels tired and exhausted less than half the time 2 Patient feels tired and exhausted more than half the time . Not sure *or* Not applicable *or* Missing	**97**	**0.72**	**0.04**
55_APPT_ LOSS (P_DEP55)	**Loss of appetite when depressed**	**Patient has marked loss of appetite when depressed**	***Have you lost your appetite when depressed?*** 0 Patient had no loss of appetite 1 Patient had marked loss of appetite for 2 weeks or less 2 Patient had marked loss of appetite for more than 2 weeks . Not sure *or* Not applicable *or* Missing	**93**	**0.79**	**0.04**
56_APPT_ INCREASE (P_DEP56)	**Increased appetite when depressed**	**Patient has marked increase of appetite when depressed**	***Has your appetite increased when depressed?*** 0 Patient had no increase of appetite 1 Patient had marked increase of appetite for 2 weeks or less 2 Patient had marked increase of appetite for more than 2 weeks . Not sure *or* Not applicable *or* Missing	**93**	**0.79**	**0.04**
57_WT_LOSS (P_DEP57)	**Weight loss**	**Patient had marked loss of weight when depressed**	***Did you lose weight when depressed?*** 0 Patient had no weight loss or minimal weight loss 1 Patient lost more than 5% of body weight in a month 2 Patient lost more than 15% of body weight in a year . Not sure *or* Not applicable *or* Missing	**62**	**0.71**	**0.04**
58_WT_GAIN (P_DEP58)	**Weight gain**	**Patient had marked weight gain when depressed.**	***Did you gain weight when depressed?*** 0 Patient had no weight gain or minimal weight gain 1 Patient gained more than 5% of body weight in a month 2 Patient gained more than 15% of body weight in a year . Not sure *or* Not applicable *or* Missing	**15**	**0.76**	**0.05**

59_INIT_ INSOMNIA (P_DEP59)	**Initial insomnia**	**Patient has difficulty falling asleep (1 hour or more) more than half the time when depressed**	***Have you had difficulty falling asleep when depressed?*** 0 Patient has no sleeping problems 1 Patient has difficulty falling asleep (1 hour or more) more than half the time when depressed . Not sure *or* Not applicable *or* Missing	**103**	**0.79**	**0.04**
60_MID_ INSOMNIA (P_DEP60)	**Middle insomnia**	**Patient has difficulty staying asleep (awakens and stays awake 1 hour or more) more than half the time when depressed**	***Have you had difficulty staying asleep when depressed?*** 0 Patient has no sleeping problems 1 Patient has difficulty staying asleep (awakens and stays awake 1 hour or more) more than half the time when depressed . Not sure *or* Not applicable *or* Missing	**79**	**0.65**	**0.04**
61_LATE_ INSOMNIA (P_DEP61)	**Late insomnia**	**Patient has early awakenings (at least 2 hours earlier than intended) more than half the time when depressed**	***Have you been waking much earlier than your usual?*** 0 Patient has no sleeping problems 1 Patient has early waking (at least 2 hours) more than half the time when depressed . Not sure *or* Not applicable *or* Missing	**46**	**0.62**	**0.04**
62_HYPER_ SOMNIA (P_DEP62)	**Hypersomnia**	**Patient has excessive sleep (sleeps longer than 12 hours in a 24-hour period including naps) more than half the time**	***Have you been sleeping a lot more than usual when depressed?*** 0 Patient has no hypersomnia 1 Patient has excessive sleep (sleeps longer than 12 hours in a 24-hour period including naps) more than half the time . Not sure *or* Not applicable *or* Missing	**26**	**0.68**	**0.05**
63_ DECREASED_ LIBIDO (P_DEP63)	**Decreased libido**	**Patient has much lower or no interest in sex or sexual activities**	***Has your interest in sex or your sexual activity been less than usual when depressed?*** 0 Patient has no change in sexual activities or interest in sex 1 Patient has much lower or no interest in sex or sexual activities . Not sure *or* Not applicable *or* Missing	**74**	**0.80**	**0.04**
64_ELATED_ MOOD (P_MAN64)	**Elated (euphoric) mood (expansive mood)**	**Elated mood: the patient feels very happy and on top of the world. Expansive mood: the patient feels very happy and excessively friendly towards others**	***Have you sometimes felt very happy, elated, on top of the world without much reason?*** 0 Patient has no elated mood 1 Patient has elated mood less than half the time 2 Patient has elated mood more than half the time . Not sure *or* Not applicable *or* Missing	**71**	**0.75**	**0.04**

65_IRRIT_ MOOD (P_MAN65)	**Irritable mood**	**The patient feels very easily irritated without reason to the point that he/she may shout at people or start arguments or actually become aggressive**	***Have you sometimes felt that you were easily irritated without reason?*** ***Have you found yourself so irritable that you shout at people or start arguments or actually become aggressive?*** 0 Patient has no irritable mood 1 Patient has irritable mood less than half the time 2 Patient has irritable mood more than half the time . Not sure *or* Not applicable *or* Missing	**70**	**0.76**	**0.04**
66_MIXED_ MOOD (P_MAN66)	**Mixed mood (mood lability) [same day mood changes]**	**Patient has periods of *depression and elation or irritability on the same day***	***Have you had mixed mood swings: Periods of depression and elation or irritability on the same day?*** 0 Patient has no mixed mood swings 1 Patient has mixed mood less than half the time 2 Patient has mixed mood more than half the time . Not sure *or* Not applicable *or* Missing.	**41**	**0.58**	**0.05**
67_RACING_ THOT (P_MAN67)	**Racing thoughts**	**The patient has too many different thoughts racing through his/her mind compared with normal**	***Have you felt that you had too many different thoughts racing through your mind compared with normal?*** 0 Patient has no racing thoughts 1 Patient has racing thoughts less than half the time 2 Patient has racing thoughts more than half the time . Not sure *or* Not applicable *or* Missing	**71**	**0.85**	**0.04**
68_PRESS_ SPEECH (P_MAN68)	**Pressured speech**	**Patient has been talking faster than usual during this time (for Example, people said that they were unable to understand the patient because he/she was speaking too fast or the patient felt a pressure to continue talking)**	***Have you been talking faster than usual during this time (for example, people said that they were unable to understand you because you were speaking too fast or you felt a pressure to continue talking)?*** 0 Patient has normal speech 1 Patient has pressured speech less than half the time 2 Patient has pressured speech more than half the time . Not sure *or* Not applicable *or* Missing	**53**	**0.72**	**0.04**
69_FLIGHT_ IDEAS (P_MAN69)	**Flight of ideas**	**Flight of ideas (a combination of pressured speech and derailment) is observed during the clinical interview**	***Flight of ideas (a combination of pressured speech and derailment):*** 0 Patient has no flight of ideas 1 Patient has flight of ideas . Not sure *or* Not applicable *or* Missing	**15**	**0.62**	**0.06**

70_MORE_ ACTIVE (P_MAN70)	**Increase in activities**	**The patient has been more active and more productive than usual at work or school**	***Have you been more active and had more energy than usual?*** ***Did you do more things than usual at work or school?*** 0 Patient has no increased energy 1 Patient has too much energy less than half the time 2 Patient has too much energy more than half the time . Not sure *or* Not applicable *or* Missing	**68**	**0.83**	**0.04**
71_LESS_ SLEEP (P_MAN71)	**Decreased sleep**	**The patient needed to sleep 4 hours or less (in a 24-hour period including naps) and felt rested**	***Have you needed less sleep than usual and without getting tired?*** 0 Patient has normal sleep 1 Patient sleeps 4 hours or less (in a 24-hour period including naps) and feels rested . Not sure *or* Not applicable *or* Missing	**56**	**0.78**	**0.04**
72_ DISTRACTION (P_MAN72)[a]	**Distraction (attention is distracted by environmental noises)**	**The patient is easily distracted by unimportant activities or external noises happening in the surroundings**	***Do you find yourself easily distracted by unimportant activities or external noises happening around you?*** 0 Patient has no distraction 1 Patient has been easily distracted by external stimuli less than half the time 2 Patient has been easily distracted by external stimuli more than half the time . Not sure *or* Not applicable *or* Missing	**63**	**0.79**	**0.04**

[a]The item is repeated again in a different context (ADHD item # 187)

73_GRAND IOSE (P_MAN73)	**Grandiosity**	**The patient feels more self-confident than usual, or he/she has special powers or special abilities**	***Have you felt more self-confident than usual?*** ***Have you felt that you have special powers or special abilities?*** 0 Patient has no grandiosity 1 Patient has grandiose thoughts, but not of a delusional quality . Not sure *or* Not applicable *or* Missing	**40**	**0.81**	**0.04**

74_OVER SPENDING (P_MAN74)	**Overspending (poor judgment in new activities)**	**The patient has poor judgement with regard to engaging in new activities, usually involving money and sexuality.** **Money: Spending more money than he/she could afford, writing bad checks, or investing money foolishly.** **Sexual indiscretions: e.g., having sex in a public setting**	***Have you done something that you regretted later*** **(e.g.,** ***spending a lot of money that you could not afford, writing bad checks, or investing money foolishly, sexual indiscretions)?*** 0 Patient did not go on a spending spree 1 Patient went on a spending spree during manic phase . Not sure *or* Not applicable *or* Missing	**49**	**0.74**	**0.04**
75_HYPER SEXUAL (P_MAN75)	**Hyper sexuality**	**The patient's interest in sex or sexual activity has notably increased**	***Have you found that your interest in sex or your sexual activity has increased much compared with normal?*** 0 Patient has no change in sexual activities or interest in sex 1 Patient has been feeling hypersexual more than usual during manic phase . Not sure *or* Not applicable *or* Missing	**24**	**0.69**	**0.04**
76_CLANG (P_MAN76)	**Clanging**	**Clanging: Words and phrases are associated together inappropriately by similarity in sound rather than meaning.** **Punning: Association by double meaning.** **Assonance: Association by similar syllables**	0 Normal speech 1 Clanging: association by sound 2 Punning: association by double meaning 3 Assonance: association by similar syllables 4 Mixed . Not sure *or* Not applicable *or* Missing	**12**	**0.49**	**0.04**
77_AUD_HAL (P_HAL77)	**Auditory hallucinations (hallucination quality)**	**The patient hears noises (like music, whispering sounds) or voices talking to him/her when there is no one around**	**Do you hear noises (like music, whispering sounds) or voices talking to you when there is no one around?** **Are the voices like a real voice or just thoughts in your mind?** 0 Patient has no auditory hallucinations 1 Patient has auditory hallucinations 2 Patient has auditory hallucinations with command . Not sure *or* Not applicable *or* Missing	**54**	**0.90**	**0.04**

78_FREQ_ AUDH (P_HAL78)	**Frequency of auditory hallucinations**	**The frequency is how many days per month on average the patient hears noises or voices**	**How often do you hear noises (like music, whispering sounds) or voices talking to you when there is no one around?** 0 Patient has no auditory hallucinations 1 Patient has auditory hallucinations (1–4 days / month) 2 Patient has auditory hallucinations (5–15 days/ month) 3 Patient has auditory hallucinations (>15 days/month) . Not sure *or* Not applicable *or* Missing	**54**	**0.93**	**0.05**
79_ DURATION_ AUDH (P_HAL79)	**Hallucination duration**	**The duration is how many hours per day on average the patient hears noises or voices**	**On days when you hear noises or voices, how often do you hear them?** 0 patient has no auditory hallucinations 1 Patient has auditory hallucinations (less than 1 hour/day) 2 Patient has auditory hallucinations (1–4 hours/day) 3 Patient has auditory hallucinations (more than 4 hours/day) . Not sure *or* Not applicable *or* Missing	**46**	**0.92**	**0.05**
80_AUD_ THOT (P_HAL80)	**Audible thoughts**	**Patient experiences auditory hallucinations, with voices speaking his/her thoughts aloud**	***Do you think that your thoughts are so loud that someone close to you can hear what you are thinking?*** 0 Patient has no audible thoughts 1 Patient has audible thoughts . Not sure *or* Not applicable *or* Missing	**7**	**1.00**	**0.05**
81_VOICES_ ARGUE (P_HAL81)	**Voices arguing**	**Two or more hallucinatory voices argue about what the patient is doing or thinking.** **The subject is usually the patient, who is referred to in a third person**	***Do you hear two or more voices that argue about what you are doing or thinking?*** 0 Voices do not argue with the patient 1 Voices argue about what the patient is doing or thinking . Not sure *or* Not applicable *or* Missing	**40**	**0.77**	**0.04**
82_VOICES_ COMMENT (P_HAL82)	**Voices commenting**	**One or more hallucinatory voices comment on what the patient is doing or thinking as they occur**	***Do you hear a voice or voices commenting on what you are doing or thinking?*** 0 Voices do not comment about the patient 1 Voices comment on what the patient is doing or thinking . Not sure *or* Not applicable *or* Missing	**40**	**0.77**	**0.04**

83_INT_HAL (P_HAL83)	**Internal hallucinations**	**The patient hears the voices or noises as coming from inside his/her own head**	***Do you hear the voices or noises inside your head, or as though coming from outside?*** 0 No AH 1 Mostly external hallucinations 2 Almost equal 3 Mostly internal hallucinations . Not sure *or* Not applicable *or* Missing	**50**	**0.84**	**0.04**
84_2X3HAL (P_HAL84)	**Second/third hallucinations**	**The patient hears voices talking directly to him/her (second person) or talking to each other about him/her (third person)**	***Do you hear voices talking directly to you (second person) or talking to each other about you (third person)?*** 0 Voices do not talk to the patient or about the patient 1 Voices talk to the patient directly most of the time 2 Voices talk to the patient directly and talk to each other about the patient 3 Voices talk to each other about the patient most of the time . Not sure *or* Not applicable *or* Missing	**45**	**0.78**	**0.04**
85_OBS_HAL (P_HAL85)	**Observed hallucinations**	**Patient has been observed talking to self, talking to a mirror, or running a conversation with unseen person**	0 Patient has not been observed talking to self 1 Patient has been observed talking to self, talking to a mirror, or running a conversation with unseen person. . Not sure *or* Not applicable *or* Missing	**12**	**0.55**	**0.04**
86_VIS_HAL (P_HAL86)	**Visual hallucinations**	**The patient sees things other people cannot see (e.g., shadows, objects or people)**	***Do you see things other people cannot see* (e.g., *shadows, objects or people)?*** 0 Patient has no visual hallucinations 1 Patient has visual hallucinations . Not sure *or* Not applicable *or* Missing	**27**	**0.81**	**0.04**
87_OLF_HAL (P_HAL87)	**Olfactory hallucinations**	**The patient notices unusual smells that other people do not notice. For example: Patient smells flowers, while no flowers around**	***Do you sometimes notice unusual smells that other people do not notice?*** 0 Patient has no olfactory hallucinations 1 Patient has olfactory hallucinations . Not sure *or* Not applicable *or* Missing	**8**	**0.78**	**0.05**

88_TACT_ HAL (P_HAL88)	**Tactile hallucinations**	**The patient feels strange sensations on his/her body and no clear explanation for them. For example: crawling sensation under the skin, the feeling of being touched and there is no one else around**	***Do you sometimes feel strange sensations on your body and you have no explanation for them?*** 0 Patient has no tactile hallucinations 1 Patient has tactile hallucinations . Not sure *or* Not applicable *or* Missing	**10**	**0.95**	**0.05**
89_SOM_ PASSIVITY (P_DEL89)	***Somatic passivity***	**_Bizarre delusions associated with somatic sensations. _The patient describes bodily sensations (e.g., crawling sensation under the skin, being tortured by electricity, receiving electric shocks, sensation of burning) attributed to an outside person or force**	***Do you feel or have bodily sensations (e.g., something is crawling under your skin) and you think it is caused by an outside person or force?*** 0 Patient has no somatic passivity. 1 Patient has somatic passivity. . Not sure *or* Not applicable *or* Missing.	**7**	**0.58**	**0.04**
90_THOT_ INSERT (P_DEL90)	**Thought insertion**	**An outside person or force is inserting a stream of thoughts to the patient's mind**	***Do you think that thoughts in your mind are not your own thoughts and that they were inserted into your mind by an outside person or force?*** 0 Patient has no delusions of thought insertion. 1 Patient has delusions of thought insertion. . Not sure *or* Not applicable *or* Missing	**16**	**0.76**	**0.04**
***91_THOT_ WITHDR* (P_DEL91)**	***Thought withdrawal***	**An outside person or force is removing or taking thoughts from the patient's mind**	***Do you think that your thoughts were taken out of your mind by an outside person or force?*** 0 Patient has no delusions of thought withdrawal 1 Patient has delusions of thought withdrawal . Not sure *or* Not applicable *or* Missing	**6**	**0.80**	**0.04**
92_THOT_ BROADCAST (P_DEL92)	**Thought broadcasting**	**The patient experiences that his/her thoughts are diffused and broadcast to the outside world**	***Do you think that your thoughts are broadcast so that people are able to know what you are thinking even if they are in different places?*** 0 Patient has no delusions of thought broadcast 1 Patient has delusions of thought broadcast . Not sure *or* Not applicable *or* Missing	**16**	**0.71**	**0.04**

93_PARAND_ DEL (P_DEL93)	**Paranoid/ persecutory delusions**	**Delusion is a false belief that is held by the patient with conviction (firm belief) and despite evidence to the contrary (fixed belief).** **The patient feels that people are against him/her or talking about or laughing at the patient.** **Patient may feel someone is trying to poison or kill the patient**	***Have you felt that people are against you, or talking about you or laughing at you?*** ***Do you think someone is trying to harm you* (e.g., *trying to poison your food or trying to kill you)?*** 0 Patient has no paranoid/persecutory delusions 1 Patient has paranoid/persecutory delusions some of the time 2 Patient has paranoid/persecutory delusions most of the time . Not sure *or* Not applicable *or* Missing	**50**	**0.86**	**0.04**
94_CONSP_ DEL (P_DEL94)	**Conspiracy delusions**	**The patient thinks there is a plot or a conspiracy against him/her by anyone (e.g. a person, FBI, CIA)**	***Do you think there is a plot or a conspiracy against you by anyone* (e.g., *a person, FBI, CIA)?*** 0 Patient has no delusions of conspiracy 1 Patient has delusions of conspiracy some of the time 2 Patient has delusions of conspiracy most of the time . Not sure *or* Not applicable *or* Missing	**49**	**0.84**	**0.04**
95_REF_DEL (P_DEL95)	**Delusions of reference**	**When the patient watches TV, listens to the radio, or reads the newspaper, he/she thinks that special messages are intended specifically for him/her**	***When you are watching TV, listening to the radio, or reading the newspaper, do you think that special messages are intended specifically for you?*** 0 Patient has no delusions of reference 1 Patient has delusions of reference some of the time 2 Patient has delusions of reference most of the time . Not sure *or* Not applicable *or* Missing	**31**	**0.81**	**0.05**
96_READ_ DEL (P_DEL96)	**Delusions of reading thoughts**	**Patient thinks that he/she can read people's minds, or other people can read his/her thoughts**	***Do you think that you can read people's minds?*** ***Do you think that other people can read your thoughts?*** 0 Patient has no delusions of thought reading. 1 Patient has delusions of thought reading. . Not sure *or* Not applicable *or* Missing.	**17**	**0.83**	**0.04**
97_RELIG_ DEL (P_DEL97)	**Religious delusions**	**The patient has unusual religious thoughts, experiences, or practices that most friends or relatives consider very strange.** **The patient may feel that he/she is divine or god**	***Do you have unusual religious thoughts, experiences, or practices that your friends or relatives consider very strange?*** ***Do you feel that you yourself are divine or that you are god?*** 0 Patient has no religious delusions 1 Patient has religious delusions some of the time 2 Patient has religious delusions most of the time . Not sure *or* Not applicable *or* Missing	**17**	**0.80**	**0.04**

98_GRAND_ DEL (P_DEL98)	**Grandiose delusions**	**The patient feels that he/she has special powers or great abilities that most people do not have. The patient may think that he/she is a prominent person in the society**	***Do you feel that you have special powers or great abilities that most people do not have?*** ***Do you think that you are a prominent person in society?*** 0 Patient has no grandiose delusions 1 Patient has grandiose delusions some of the time 2 Patient has grandiose delusions most of the time . Not sure *or* Not applicable *or* Missing	**16**	**0.77**	**0.05**
99_CONTRL_ DEL (P_DEL99)	**Delusions of control**	**The patient experiences that his/her actions, impulses, and emotions are controlled by an outside person or force**	***Do you think that some outside person or force is controlling your actions, impulses or emotions against your will?*** 0 Patient has no delusions of being controlled 1 Patient has delusions of being controlled . Not sure *or* Not applicable *or* Missing	**9**	**0.68**	**0.05**
100_OTHER_ DEL (P_DEL100)	**Other delusions**	**The patient has other strange thoughts or beliefs that other people do not have**	***Do you have any other strange thoughts or beliefs that other people do not have?*** 0 Patient has no other delusions 1 Patient has other delusions . Not sure *or* Not applicable *or* Missing	**12**	**0.40**	**0.05**
101_BIZAR_ DEL (P_DEL101)	**Bizarreness of delusions**	**Delusions are bizarre if they are completely impossible (e.g., patient believes he/she was born on Mars and brought to earth on a spaceship)**	0 Patient has no bizarre delusions 1 Patient has bizarre delusions . Not sure *or* Not applicable *or* Missing	**14**	**0.43**	**0.05**
102_DERAIL (P_DIS102)	**Derailment (loose associations)**	**Derailment (loose associations): Patient's speech shifts to different topics, related or unrelated, but eventually returns to the main topic or may never return to the main topic**	0 Normal speech 1 Patient has derailment (loose associations): speech shifts to different topics, related or unrelated, but eventually comes back to the main topic 2 Patient has severe derailment (loose associations): speech shifts to different topics, mostly unrelated and never comes back to main topic . Not sure *or* Not applicable *or* Missing	**37**	**0.65**	**0.06**

103_ TANGENT (P_DIS103)	**Tangentiality**	**Patient's reply to a question is related in some distant way, or totally unrelated**	0 Normal speech 1 Patient has some tangentiality: replying to a question is related in some distant way 2 Patient has severe tangentiality: replying to a question is totally unrelated . Not sure *or* Not applicable *or* Missing	**28**	**0.57**	**0.06**
104_ INCOHER_SP (P_DIS104)	**Incoherent speech**	**Patient has incoherent speech: Each sentence by itself makes sense. However, the first sentence is unrelated to the next sentence**	0 Normal speech 1 patient has incoherent speech: Each sentence by itself makes sense. However, the first sentence is unrelated to the next sentence . Not sure *or* not applicable *or* missing	**18**	**0.41**	**0.06**
105_ILLOG_ SP (P_DIS105)	**Illogical speech**	**Patient's speech taken together is not logical**	0 Normal speech 1 Patient has illogical speech: taken together, speech is not logical . Not sure *or* Not applicable *or* Missing	**13**	**0.25**	**0.05**
106_WORD_ SALAD (P_DIS106)	**Other disorganized thoughts (e.g., word salad, clanging)**	**Patient has other disorganized thoughts such as world salad (incoherence of speech at the level of the sentence, that is, the first word has nothing to do with the second word) or clanging (words and phrases are associated together inappropriately by similarity in sound rather than meaning)**	0 Normal speech 1 Other disorganized thoughts. . Not sure *or* Not applicable *or* Missing	**39**	**0.65**	**0.04**

107_ AGITATION (P_BEH107)	Agitation	**Patient may be verbally agitated causing people to be annoyed, verbally aggressive causing people to feel insulted or scared, physically agitated toward self-such as pacing, or destructive to objects**	0 Patient has no verbal agitation 1 Patient is **verbally agitated** causing people to **feel annoyed** (e.g., makes loud noises, shouts angrily, constant whining or constant attention seeking) 2 Patient is **verbally aggressive**, causing people to **feel insulted or scared** (e.g., cursing or using foul language, makes threats to others or self) 3 Patient is **physically agitated towards self** (e.g., pacing up and down or disrobing) 4 Patient is **destructive to objects** (e.g., slams doors, throws clothes or objects, kicks wall or furniture, breaks objects, smashes windows) . Not sure *or* Not applicable *or* Missing	**33**	**0.48**	**0.04**
108_ VIOLENCE (P_BEH108)	**Violence toward others**	**Patient is physically violent and threatening towards people without touching victims or the patient touches victims with or without resulting injury**	0 Patient is not violent towards people 1 Patient is **physically violent and threatening towards people without touching** (e.g., makes threatening gesture, swings at people) **2 Patient is physically violent and touches victims with or without resulting injury** (e.g., grabs at clothes, strikes, kicks, pulls hair, attacks) . Not sure *or* Not applicable *or* Missing	**25**	**0.64**	**0.04**
109_ODD_ APPEAR (P_BEH109)	**Odd appearance and behavior**	**Patient wears odd clothes. Social behavior towards others is inappropriate. Sexual behavior towards others is inappropriate**	0 Patient has appropriate appearance and behaviors 1 Patient has inappropriate appearance and behaviors. . Not sure *or* Not applicable *or* Missing	**19**	**0.67**	**0.06**
110_ INAPPRO_ AFFECT (P_BEH110)	**Inappropriate affect**	**Inappropriate affect: The patient's expression of affect is non-congruent with social or emotional context, e.g., laughing when talking about death of a loved one**	0 Patient has appropriate affect 1 Patient has inappropriate affect . Not sure *or* Not applicable *or* Missing	**14**	**0.77**	**0.06**

111_ALOGIA (P_NEG111)	**Alogia**	**Alogia: poverty of speech, or poverty of content of speech**	0 Patient has normal speech 1 Patient has alogia less than half time 2 Patient has alogia more than half time . Not sure *or* Not applicable *or* Missing	**29**	**0.62**	**0.05**
112_ ANHEDONIA (P_NEG112)[a]	**Anhedonia (loss of pleasure and interest)**	**The patient has been unable to experience pleasure and enjoy things that he/she used to enjoy like exercising, enjoying hobbies, or socializing with friends**	***Have you been unable to experience pleasure and enjoy things that you used to enjoy like exercising, enjoying your hobbies, or socializing with friends?*** 0 Patient has no anhedonia 1 Patient has anhedonia less than half the time 2 Patient has anhedonia more than half the time . Not sure *or* Not applicable *or* Missing	**121**	**0.87**	**0.04**
113_FLAT_ AFFECT (P_NEG113)	**Blunted/flat affect (decrease in affective expression) Other descriptors in literature: Apathy, emotional apathy, cmotional blunting, emotional indifference, blunting of emotional tone**	**Decreased facial expression, e.g., not smiling or laughing at a joke, poor eye contact, indifference to things around, loss of emotional reaction and indifference**	0 Patient has broad affect 1 Patient has blunted affect 2 Patient has flat affect . Not sure *or* Not applicable *or* Missing	**42**	**0.68**	**0.05**

[a]The item is repeated again in a different context (depression item # 46)

114_ AVOLITION (P_NEG114)	**Avolition (decrease in goal-directed activities)** ***Other descriptors in literature: apathy, motor apathy, general apathy, lack of drive, lack of energy, lack of interest***	**Decrease in the three main goal-directed activities in life: school, work, or social activities with other people**	0 Patient has normal activities 1 Patient has avolition less than half time 2 Patient has avolition more than half time . Not sure *or* Not applicable *or* Missing	**35**	**0.74**	**0.04**
115 _ASOCIAL (P_NEG115)[a]	**Diminished social interest (asociality)**	**The patient spends less time or shows less interest in activities with friends, family or hobbies that he/she used to enjoy**	***Did you spend less time or show less interest in activities with friends, family or hobbies that you used to enjoy?*** 0 Patient had no significant symptom 1 Patient spends less time or shows less interest in activities with friends, family or hobbies . Not sure *or* Not applicable *or* Missing	**35**	**0.74**	**0.04**
116_POOR_ CONC (P_NEG116)[b]	**Attention impairment (poor concentration)**	**The patient has decreased concentration, and he/she is unable to complete a task (e.g., at work, reading an article, reading a book, or watching a movie), even though the patient was able to do that before**	***Have you found that your concentration has decreased and you are unable to complete a task* (e.g., *at work, reading an article, reading a book, or watching a movie*), *even though you were able to do that before?*** 0 Patient has no concentration problems 1 Patient has difficulty concentrating less than half the time 2 Patient has difficulty concentrating more than half the time . Not sure *or* Not applicable *or* Missing	**41**	**0.92**	**0.12**

[a]The item is repeated again in a different context (PTSD item # 34)
[b]The item is repeated again in different contexts (Anxiety item # 10, PTSD item # 39, depression item # 48, ADHD item # 181)

117_ PSYCHOM_ SLOW (P_NEG117)[a]	**Psychomotor retardation/ slowing**	**Patient is moving slow or talking slow compared to his/her normal. Patient is observed usually sitting or lying down and talking very little**	***Have you felt as though you were talking or moving more slowly than normal for you?*** 0 Patient has normal activity 1 Patient has psychomotor retardation less than half the time 2 Patient has psychomotor retardation more than half the time . Not sure *or* Not applicable *or* Missing	**97**	**0.72**	**0.04**
118_POOR_ CARE (P_NEG118)	**Poor self-care**	**Poor self-care: Patient does not wear proper clothes for the weather, does not shower regularly, and does not eat properly and is very dirty and disheveled**	0 Patient has proper self-care. 1 Patient has poor self-care less than half time 2 Patient has poor self-care more than half time . Not sure *or* Not applicable *or* Missing	**27**	**0.79**	**0.06**

[a]The item is repeated again in a different context (depression item # 49)

119_ALC_ TOL (P_ALC119)	**Alcohol tolerance**	**The patient needed to use a lot more alcohol than he/she previously used to get the same effect (compared when the patient first started to drink). The patient noticed that the same amount of alcohol he/she takes now has less effect than before (compared when the patient first started to drink)**	***Did you use a lot more alcohol than you previously used to get the same effect (compared when you first started to drink)?*** ***Did you notice that the same amount of alcohol you take now has less effect than before (compared when you first started to drink)?*** 0 Patient had no tolerance to alcohol 1 Patient had tolerance to alcohol . Not sure *or* Not applicable *or* Missing	**39**	**0.99**	**0.06**
120_ALC_ WITHDR (P_ALC120)	**Alcohol withdrawal**	**When the patient stopped or cut down on alcohol use, he/she had alcohol withdrawal symptoms. Interviewer gives examples of alcohol withdrawal symptoms**	***When you stopped or cut down on alcohol use, did you have withdrawal symptoms?*** ***(patient gives examples of alcohol withdrawal symptoms).*** 0 Patient had no withdrawal symptoms from alcohol. 1 Patient had withdrawal symptoms from alcohol. . Not sure *or* Not applicable *or* Missing.	**33**	**0.93**	**0.06**

121_ALC_ AVOIDW (P_ALC121)	**Drinking alcohol to avoid withdrawal**	**The patient drinks alcohol to avoid withdrawal symptoms.** **The patient uses benzodiazepines (e.g., Ativan, Klonopin, Xanax) to avoid alcohol withdrawal symptoms**	***Did you drink alcohol to avoid withdrawal symptoms?*** ***Did you use benzodiazepines (e.g., Ativan, Klonopin, Xanax) to avoid withdrawal symptoms?*** 0 Patient did not have to drink alcohol or use benzodiazepines to avoid withdrawal symptoms 1 Patient drank alcohol or used benzodiazepines to avoid withdrawal symptoms . Not sure *or* Not applicable *or* Missing	**29**	**0.96**	**0.06**
122_ UNABLE_ CONTRL_A (P_ALC122)	**Unable to control alcohol**	**The patient drank more alcohol than he/she planned or intended.** **The patient drank alcohol for a longer period of time than he/she planned or intended**	***Did you drink more alcohol than you planned or intended?*** ***Did you drink alcohol for a longer period of time than you planned or intended?*** 0 Patient had control over alcohol drinking 1 Patient was unable to control alcohol drinking . Not sure *or* Not applicable *or* Missing	**51**	**0.96**	**0.06**
123_ UNABLE_ REDUCE_A (P_ALC123)	**Unable to reduce or stop alcohol**	**The patient tried to reduce or stop alcohol use and did not succeed**	***Did you try to reduce or stop alcohol use and not succeed?*** 0 Patient was able to stop or reduce alcohol drinking 1 Patient was unable to stop or reduce alcohol drinking . Not sure *or* Not applicable *or* Missing	**47**	**0.85**	**0.06**
124_TIME_ ALC (P_ALC124)	**Time spent to drink alcohol**	**On days of alcohol use, the patient spends substantial time obtaining, using or recovering from the effect of alcohol.** **Alcohol drinking consumes much of the patient's time**	***On days of alcohol use, did you spend substantial time obtaining, using or recovering from the effect of alcohol?*** ***Did alcohol drinking consume much of your time?*** 0 Patient did not lose substantial time due to alcohol 1 Patient lost substantial time due to alcohol . Not sure *or* Not applicable *or* Missing	**37**	**0.94**	**0.06**
125_FAIL_ OBLIG (P_ALC125)	**Failure to fulfil major obligations**	**The patient's alcohol use resulted in failure to fulfill major role obligations (work, school, or home)**	***Did alcohol use result in failure to fulfill major role obligations (work, school, or home)?*** 0 Alcohol had no effect on work, school, or social obligations 1 Alcohol had negative effect on work, School, or social obligations . Not sure *or* Not applicable *or* Missing	**36**	**0.92**	**0.06**

126_ REDUCE_ SOCIAL (P_ALC126)	**Giving up social or recreational activities**	**The patient's alcohol use resulted in giving up or reducing important social or recreational activities**	***Did alcohol use result in giving up or reducing important social or recreational activities?*** 0 Alcohol use had no effect on social or recreational activities 1 Alcohol use had negative effect on social or recreational activities . Not sure *or* Not applicable *or* Missing	**36**	**0.92**	**0.06**
127_LESS_ WORK (P_ALC127)	**Less time working due to alcohol use**	**Alcohol use resulted in less time working (missing one or more days of work)**	***Did alcohol use result in less time working?*** 0 Alcohol did not result in less time working 1 Alcohol resulted in missing one or more days of work . Not sure *or* Not applicable *or* Missing	**36**	**0.92**	**0.06**
128_WORK_ PROB (P_ALC128)	**Alcohol-related work problems**	**Alcohol use resulted in work-related problems**	***Did alcohol cause any work-related problems?*** 0 Alcohol caused no work problems 1 Alcohol caused work problems . Not sure *or* Not applicable *or* Missing	**29**	**0.83**	**0.06**
129_FIGHT_ ALC (P_ALC129)	**Fighting when intoxicated**	**The patient got in physical fights when intoxicated**	***Did you get in physical fights when intoxicated?*** 0 Patient did not get in physical fights when intoxicated 1 Patient got in physical fights when intoxicated . Not sure *or* Not applicable *or* Missing	**31**	**0.90**	**0.06**
130_FAMILY_ PROBLM (P_ALC130)	**Alcohol-related family problems**	**Alcohol use resulted in family-related problems**	***Did alcohol cause any family problems?*** 0 Alcohol caused no family problems 1 Alcohol caused family problems . Not sure *or* Not applicable *or* Missing	**51**	**0.82**	**0.06**
131_LEGAL_ PROBLM (P_ALC131)	**Alcohol-related legal problems**	**Alcohol use resulted in legal problems**	***Did alcohol cause any legal problems?*** 0 Alcohol caused no legal problems 1 Alcohol caused legal problems . Not sure *or* Not applicable *or* Missing	**29**	**0.92**	**0.06**
132_MED_ PROBLM (P_ALC132)	**Alcohol-induced medical problems**	**Alcohol use resulted in medical problems (e.g., peptic ulcer disease, liver cirrhosis)**	***Did alcohol cause any medical problems* (e.g., *peptic ulcer disease, liver cirrhosis*)?** 0 Alcohol caused no medical problems 1 Alcohol caused medical problems . Not sure *or* Not applicable *or* Missing	**11**	**0.70**	**0.06**

133_ EMOTION_ PROBLM (P_ALC133)	**Alcohol-induced emotional problems**	**Alcohol use resulted in emotional problems (e.g., depression, hallucinations)**	***Did alcohol cause any emotional problems* (e.g., *depression, hallucinations)?*** 0 Alcohol caused no emotional problems 1 Alcohol caused emotional problems . Not sure *or* Not applicable *or* Missing	**24**	**0.90**	**0.06**
134_CONTIN_ ALC (P_ALC134)	**Alcohol use in spite of problems**	**The patient continued to use alcohol even though alcohol caused problems**	***Did you continue to use alcohol even though you had problems?*** 0 Patient had no alcohol problems 1 Patient continued to use alcohol even though alcohol caused problems . Not sure *or* Not applicable *or* Missing	**57**	**0.87**	**0.06**
135_ALC_ HAZARD (P_ALC135)	**Alcohol use in hazardous situations**	**Patient used alcohol in a situation, in which it was physically hazardous (e.g., driving a car or operating machinery)**	***Did you use alcohol in a situation, in which it was physically hazardous* (e.g., *driving a car or operating machinery)?*** 0 Patient did not use alcohol in hazardous situations 1 Patient used alcohol in hazardous situations . Not sure *or* Not applicable *or* Missing	**42**	**0.77**	**0.06**
136_ALC_ BINGE (P_ALC136)	**Alcohol binge**	**The patient goes on binges when he/she kept drinking alcohol for a couple of days or more without sobering up**	***Did you go on binges when you kept drinking alcohol for a couple of days or more without sobering up?*** 0 Patient had no binge problem 1 Patient had binge problem . Not sure *or* Not applicable *or* Missing	**37**	**0.88**	**0.06**
137_ALC_ BLACKOUT (P_ALC137)	**Alcohol blackout**	**The patient had a blackout after drinking so much alcohol that the next day the patient could not remember what he/she said or did**	***Did you have a blackout after drinking so much alcohol that the next day you could not remember what you said or did?*** 0 Patient had no blackout. 1 Patient had blackout . Not sure *or* Not applicable *or* Missing	**53**	**0.98**	**0.06**

138_DRG_ TOL (P_DRG_138)	**Drug tolerance**	**The patient used a lot more of the drug than he/she previously used to get the same effect (compared when the patient first started to use the drug).** **The patient noticed that the same amount of the drug he/she takes now has less effect than before (compared when the patient first started to use the drug)**	***Did you use a lot more of the drug than you previously used to get the same effect (compared when you first started to use the drug)?*** ***Did you notice that the same amount of the drug you take now has less effect than before (compared when you first started to use the drug)?*** 0 Patient had no tolerance to the drug 1 Patient had tolerance to the drug . Not sure *or* Not applicable *or* Missing	**49**	**0.95**	**0.06**
139_DRG_ WITHDR (P_DRG_139)	**Drug withdrawal**	**When the patient stopped or cut down on the drug use, the patient had withdrawal symptoms of the drug.** **(the interviewer gives examples of the drug withdrawal symptoms)**	***When you stopped or cut down on the drug use, did you have withdrawal symptoms? (patient gives examples of the drug withdrawal symptoms).*** 0 Patient had no withdrawal symptoms from the drug 1 Patient had withdrawal symptoms from the drug . Not sure *or* Not applicable *or* Missing	**46**	**0.97**	**0.06**
140_DRG_ AVOIDW (P_DRG_140)	**Using drug to avoid withdrawal**	**The patient had to use the drug to avoid withdrawal symptoms**	***Did you have to use the drug to avoid withdrawal symptoms?*** 0 Patient did not have to use the drug to avoid withdrawal symptoms 1 Patient had to use the drug to avoid withdrawal symptoms . Not sure *or* Not applicable *or* Missing	**40**	**0.94**	**0.06**
141_ UNABLE_ CONTRL_D (P_DRG_141)	**Unable to control drug use**	**The patient used more of the drug than he/she planned or intended to use.** **The patient used the drug for a longer period of time than he/she had planned or intended**	***Did you use more of the drug than you planned or intended to use?*** ***Did you use the drug for a longer period of time than you had planned or intended?*** 0 Patient had control over the drug use 1 Patient used the drug more than what was planned or intended . Not sure *or* Not applicable *or* Missing	**55**	**0.97**	**0.06**

142_ UNABLE_ REDUCE_D (P_DRG_142)	**Unable to reduce or stop drug use**	**The patient tried to reduce or stop the drug use and he/she did not succeed**	***Did you try to reduce or stop the drug use and not succeed?*** 0 Was able to stop or reduce the drug use 1 Patient was unable to stop or reduce the drug use . Not sure *or* Not applicable *or* Missing	**54**	**0.97**	**0.06**
143_TIME_ DRG (P_DRG_143)	**Time spent to use drug**	**On days of drug use, the patient spent substantial time obtaining, using or recovering from the effect of the drug** **The drug use consumed much of the patient's time**	***On days of drug use, did you spend substantial time obtaining, using or recovering from the effect of the drug?*** ***Did drug use consume much of your time?*** 0 Patient did not lose substantial time due to the drug use 1 Patient lost substantial time due to the drug use . Not sure *or* Not applicable *or* Missing	**56**	**0.88**	**0.06**
144_FAIL_ OBLIG (P_DRG_144)	**Failure to fulfil major obligations**	**The drug use resulted in failure to fulfill major role obligations at work, school or home**	***Did the drug use result in failure to fulfill major role obligations at work, school, or home?*** 0 Drug use had no effect on work, school, or social obligations 1 Drug use had a negative effect on work, school, or social obligations . Not sure *or* Not applicable *or* Missing	**50**	**0.95**	**0.06**
145_ REDUCE_ SOCIAL (P_DRG_145)	**Giving up social or recreational activities**	**The patient's drug use resulted in giving up or reducing important social or recreational activities**	***Did the drug use result in giving up or reducing important social or recreational activities?*** 0 The drug had no effect on social or recreational activities 1 The drug had negative effect on social or recreational activities . Not sure *or* Not applicable *or* Missing	**50**	**0.95**	**0.06**
146_LESS_ WORK (P_DRG_146)	**Less time working due to drug use**	**Drug use resulted in less time working (missing one or more days of work)**	***Did drug use result in less time working?*** 0 Drug use did not result in less time working 1 Drug use resulted in missing one or more days of work . Not sure *or* Not applicable *or* Missing	**50**	**0.95**	**0.06**
147_WORK_ PROBLM (P_DRG_147)	**Drug-related work problems**	**Drug use resulted in work-related problems**	***Did drug use cause any work problems?*** 0 Drug use caused no work problems 1 Drug use caused work problems . Not sure *or* Not applicable *or* Missing	**34**	**0.83**	**0.06**

148_FIGHT_ DRG (P_DRG_148)	**Fighting when using drug**	**The patient got in physical fights when using the drug**	***Did you get in physical fights when using the drug?*** 0 Patient did not get in physical fights when using the drug 1 Patient got in physical fights when using the drug . Not sure *or* Not applicable *or* Missing	**22**	**0.80**	**0.06**
149_FAMILY_ PROBLM (P_DRG_149)	**Drug-related family problems**	**Drug use resulted in family-related problems**	***Did drug use cause any family problems?*** 0 Drug use caused no family problems 1 Drug use caused family problems . Not sure *or* Not applicable *or* Missing	**58**	**0.80**	**0.06**
150_LEGAL_ PROBLM (P_DRG_150)	**Drug-related legal problems**	**Drug use resulted in legal problems**	***Did drug use cause any legal problems?*** 0 Drug use caused no legal problems 1 Drug use caused legal problems . Not sure *or* Not applicable *or* Missing	**22**	**0.80**	**0.06**
151_MOOD_ PROBLM (P_DRG_151)	**Drug-induced mood problems**	**Drug use resulted in mood problems (e.g., depression, mood swings)**	***Did drug use cause any mood problems* (e.g., *depression, mood swings)?*** 0 Drug use caused no mood problems 1 Drug use caused mood problems . Not sure *or* Not applicable *or* Missing	**19**	**0.76**	**0.06**
152_ PSYCHOSIS_ PROBM (P_DRG_152)	**Drug-induced psychosis**	**Drug use resulted in psychotic symptoms (e.g., delusions, hallucinations)**	***Did drug use cause any psychotic symptoms* (e.g., *delusions, hallucinations)?*** 0 Drug use caused no psychotic symptoms 1 Drug use caused psychotic symptoms . Not sure *or* Not applicable *or* Missing	**16**	**0.59**	**0.06**
153_CONTIN_ DRUG (P_DRG_153)	**Drug use in spite of problems**	**The patient continued to use the drug even though he/she had problems**	***Did you continue to use the drug even though you had problems?*** 0 Patient had no problems from the drug use 1 Patient continued to use the drug even though the drug caused problems . Not sure *or* Not applicable *or* Missing	**64**	**0.91**	**0.06**

154_DRG_ HAZARD (P_DRG_154)	**Drug use in hazardous situations**	**The patient used the drug in a situation, in which it was physically hazardous (e.g., driving a car or operating machinery)**	***Did you use the drug in a situation, in which it was physically hazardous*** **(e.g.,** ***driving a car or operating machinery)?*** 0 Patient did not use the drug in hazardous situations 1 Patient used the drug in hazardous situations . Not sure *or* not applicable *or* missing	**57**	**0.90**	**0.06**
155_UNDER_ WT (P_EAT155)	**Being underweight**	**The patient has been very thin and could not maintain a minimal normal weight (low weight is defined as a weight that is less than minimally normal)**	***Have you ever been very thin and could not maintain a minimal normal weight?*** ***Have people ever said you weighed much less than normal?*** 0 = Absent or non-significant 1 = Symptoms present . = Not sure *or* Not applicable *or* Missing	**32**	**0.83**	**0.11**
156_WT_ FEELING (P_EAT156)	**Weight affects feelings**	**The patient's weight and shape are very important and affect how he/she feels about himself/herself to the point that the patient does not worry about the health risks of being so little**	***Do you feel that your weight and shape are very important and affect how you feel about yourself to the point that you do not worry about the health risks of being so little?*** 0 = Absent or non-significant 1 =Aymptoms present . =Not sure *or* Not applicable *or* Missing	**50**	**0.75**	**0.12**
157_FEAR_ WT_GAIN (P_EAT157)	**Fear of weight gain**	**The patient has an intense fear of gaining weight or becoming fat, even though he/she is underweight**	***Do you have an intense fear of gaining weight or becoming fat, even though you are underweight?*** 0 =Absent or non-significant 1 =Aymptoms present . =Not sure *or* Not applicable *or* Missing	**20**	**1.00**	**0.12**
158_FASTING (P_EAT158)	**Losing weight by fasting**	**The patient tries to lose weight by fasting (not eating anything at all for at least 24 hours)**	***Do you try to lose weight by fasting (not eating anything at all for at least 24 hours)?*** 0 = Absent or non-significant 1 = Symptoms present . = Not sure *or* Not applicable *or* Missing	**32**	**0.95**	**0.12**
159_ EXERCISE (P_EAT159)	**Losing weight by exercise**	**The patient tries to lose weight by exercising too much (more than 1 hour a day for at least 1 week)**	***Do you try to lose weight by exercising too much (more than 1 hour a day for at least 1 week)?*** 0 = Absent or non-significant 1 = Symptoms present . = Not sure *or* Not applicable *or* Missing	**22**	**0.86**	**0.12**

160_DIET_ PILLS (P_EAT160)	**Losing weight by diet pills**	**The patient tries to lose weight by using diet pills**	***Do you try to lose weight by using diet pills?*** 0 = Absent or non-significant 1 = Symptoms present . = Not sure *or* Not applicable *or* Missing	**22**	**0.97**	**0.12**
161_VOMIT (P_EAT161)	**Losing weight by vomiting**	**The patient tries to lose weight by inducing vomiting**	***Do you try to lose weight by inducing vomiting?*** 0 = Absent or non-significant 1 = Symptoms present . = Not sure *or* Not applicable *or* Missing	**27**	**0.94**	**0.12**
162_ LAXATIVE (P_EAT162)	**Losing weight by laxatives**	**The patient tries to lose weight by taking laxatives or using enemas**	***Do you try to lose weight by taking laxatives or using enemas?*** 0 = Absent or non-significant 1 = Symptoms present . = Not sure *or* Not applicable *or* Missing	**14**	**1.00**	**0.12**
163_OTHER_ METHOD **(P_EAT163)**	***Losing weight by other methods***	**The patient tries to lose weight by taking diuretics or by other methods**	***Do you try to lose weight by taking diuretics?*** ***Do you try to lose weight by other methods?*** 0 = Absent or non-significant 1 = Symptoms present . = Not sure *or* Not applicable *or* Missing	**8**	**1.00**	**0.12**
164_BINGE (P_EAT164)	**Binge-eating**	**The patient has episodes of binge-eating (eating within 1- or 2-hour period what most people would consider an unusually large amount of food)**	***Do you have episodes of binge-eating (eating within 1- or 2-hour period what most people would consider an unusually large amount of food)?*** 0 = Absent or non-significant 1 = Symptoms present . = Not sure *or* Not applicable *or* Missing	**27**	**0.97**	**0.12**
165_BINGE_ FREQ (P_EAT165)	**Binge-eating frequency**	**Binge-eating frequency**	0 None. 1 1–3 times per month. 2 At least once a week for 3 months . Not sure *or* Not applicable *or* Missing	**27**	**0.85**	**0.09**
166_LOSE_ CONTRL (P_EAT166)	**Losing control with binge-eating**	**During the episodes of binge-eating, the patient feels that he/she had lost control and could not stop eating**	***During the episodes of binge-eating, did you feel that you had lost control and could not stop eating?*** 0 = Absent or non-significant 1 = Aymptoms present . = Not sure *or* Not applicable *or* Missing	**17**	**0.96**	**0.12**

167_EAT_ FAST (P_EAT167)	**Eating fast during binge-eating**	**During the episodes of binge-eating, the patient eats much more rapidly than usual**	***During the episodes of binge-eating, did you eat much more rapidly than usual?*** 0 = Absent or non-significant 1 = Symptoms present . = Not sure *or* Not applicable *or* Missing	**16**	**1.00**	**0.12**
168_EAT_ FULL (P_EAT168)	**Eating until uncomfort ably full during binge-eating**	**During the episodes of binge-eating, the patient eats until he/she felt uncomfortably full**	***During the episodes of binge-eating, did you eat until you felt uncomfortably full?*** 0 = Absent or non-significant 1 = Symptoms present . = Not sure *or* Not applicable *or* Missing	**25**	**0.94**	**0.12**
169_EAT_ NOT_ HUNGRY (P_EAT169)	**Eating when not hungry during binge-eating**	**During the episodes of binge-eating, the patient eats a large amount of food when he/she did not feel physically hungry**	***During the episodes of binge-eating, did you eat a large amount of food when you did not feel physically hungry?*** 0 = Absent or non-significant 1 = Symptoms present = Not sure *or* Not applicable *or* Missing	**22**	**0.97**	**0.12**
170_EAT_ ALONE (P_EAT170)	**Eating alone during binge-eating**	**During the episodes of binge-eating, the patient eats alone because he/she was embarrassed by how much he/she was eating**	***During the episodes of binge-eating, did you eat alone because you were embarrassed by how much you were eating?*** 0 = Absent or non-significant 1 = Symptoms present . = Not sure *or* Not applicable *or* Missing	**16**	**0.96**	**0.12**
171_EAT_ DISGUSTED (P_EAT171)	**Feeling disgusted and guilty during binge-eating**	**During the episodes of binge-eating, the patient felt disgusted with himself/herself, depressed or guilty by overeating**	***During the episodes of binge-eating, did you feel disgusted with yourself, depressed or guilty by your overeating*? 0 = Absent or non-significant 1 = Symptoms present . = Not sure *or* Not applicable *or* Missing	**22**	**0.86**	**0.12**
172_EAT_ DISTRESSED (P_EAT172)	**Distressed by overeating during binge-eating**	**During the episodes of binge-eating, the patient felt quite upset or very distressed by overeating**	***During the episodes of binge-eating, did you feel quite upset or very distressed by your overeating?*** 0 = Absent or non-significant 1 = Symptoms present . = Not sure *or* Not applicable *or* Missing	**24**	**0.77**	**0.11**

173_ FASTING_B (P_EAT173)	**Fasting after binge-eating**	**After binge-eating episodes, the patient tries to lose weight by fasting (not eating anything at all for at least 24 hours)**	***After binge-eating episodes, did you try to lose weight by fasting (not eating anything at all for at least 24 hours)?*** 0 = Absent or non-significant 1 = Symptoms present . = Not sure *or* Not applicable *or* Missing	**19**	**0.93**	**0.12**
174_ EXERCISE_B (P_EAT174)	**Exercise after binge-eating**	**After binge-eating episodes, the patient tries to lose weight by exercising too much (more than 1 hour a day for at least 1 week)**	***After binge-eating episodes, did you try to lose weight by exercising too much (more than 1 hour a day for at least 1 week)?*** 0 = Absent or non-significant 1 = Symptoms present . = Not sure *or* Not applicable *or* Missing	**12**	**0.95**	**0.12**
175_DIET_ PILLS_B (P_EAT175)	**Using diet pills after binge-eating**	**After binge-eating episodes, the patient tries to lose weight by using diet pills**	***After binge-eating episodes, did you try to lose weight by using diet pills?*** 0 = Absent or non-significant 1 = Symptoms present . = Not sure *or* Not applicable *or* Missing	**12**	**0.95**	**0.12**
176_ VOMIT_B (P_EAT176)	**Vomiting after binge-eating**	**After binge-eating episodes, the patient tries to lose weight by inducing vomiting**	***After binge-eating episodes, did you try to lose weight by inducing vomiting?*** 0 = Absent or non-significant 1 = Symptoms present . = Not sure *or* Not applicable *or* Missing	**17**	**1.00**	**0.12**
177_ LAXATIVE_B (P_EAT177)	**Taking laxatives after binge-eating**	**After binge-eating episodes, the patient tries to lose weight by taking laxatives or enemas**	***After binge-eating episodes, did you try to lose weight by taking laxatives or enemas?*** 0 = Absent or non-significant 1 = Symptoms present . = Not sure *or* Not applicable *or* Missing	**14**	**1.00**	**0.12**
178_OTHER METHOD_B **(P_EAT178)**	***Other losing weight methods after binge-eating***	**After binge-eating episodes, the patient tries to lose weight by taking diuretics or by other methods**	***After binge-eating episodes, did you try to lose weight by taking diuretics?*** ***Do you try to lose weight by other methods?*** 0 = Absent or non-significant 1 = Symptoms present . = Not sure *or* Not applicable *or* Missing	**9**	**1.00**	**0.12**

179_BINGE_ BHV_FREQ (P_EAT179)	**Binge-eating compensatory behavior frequency**	**Binge-eating compensatory behavior frequency**	0 None 1 1–3 times per month 2 At least once a week for 3 months. . Not sure *or* Not applicable *or* Missing	**25**	**0.87**	**0.09**
180_OTHER_ EATING **(P_EAT180)**	***Other eating behaviors***	**Any other eating behaviors**	***Do you have any other eating behaviors?*** 0 = Absent or non-significant 1 = Symptoms present . = Not sure *or* Not applicable *or* Missing	**4**	**0.39**	**0.09**
181_POOR_ CONC (P_ADHD181)[a]	**Attention impairment (poor concentration)**	**The patient has difficulty paying attention and concentrating when reading an article, watching a TV show or a movie, or doing work or school assignments**	***Do you have difficulty paying attention and concentrating when reading an article, watching a TV show or a movie, or doing your work or school assignments?*** = Absent or non-significant 1 = Patient has poor attention and concentration . = Not sure *or* Not applicable *or* Missing	**41**	**0.92**	**0.12**
182_SUST_ ATTN_ IMPAIR (P_ADHD182)	**Sustained attention impairment**	**The patient has difficulty concentrating on one thing for a long time (e.g., reading a book, writing a letter)**	***Do you have difficulty concentrating on one thing for a long time*** **(e.g.,** ***reading a book, writing a letter)?*** 0 = Absent or non-significant 1 = Patient has difficulty concentrating for a long period of time . = Not sure *or* Not applicable *or* Missing	**39**	**0.95**	**0.12**
183_AVOID_ TASKS (P_ADHD183)	**Avoiding sustained attention tasks**	**The patient avoids tasks that require a lot of concentration at work, school, or home (e.g., reading a book, writing a letter)**	***Do you avoid tasks that require a lot of concentration at work, school, or home*** **(e.g.,** ***reading a book, writing a letter)?*** 0 = Absent or non-significant 1 = Patient avoids tasks that require sustained mental effort . = Not sure *or* Not applicable *or* Missing	**34**	**0.97**	**0.12**
184_ATTN_ SPOKEN (P_ADHD184)	**Attention when spoken to**	**Patient has difficulty concentrating on what people say to him/her, even when they are speaking to the patient directly**	***Do you have difficulty concentrating on what people say to you, even when they are speaking to you directly?*** 0 = Absent or non-significant 1 = Patient has difficulty concentrating on what people say . = Not sure *or* Not applicable *or* Missing	**32**	**0.97**	**0.12**

[a]The item is repeated again in different contexts (Anxiety item # 10, PTSD item # 39, depression item # 48, negative symptom item # 116)

185_ MANAGE_ TIME (P_ADHD185)	**Organization and meeting deadlines**	**The patient has difficulty with tasks that require organization and keeping track of many things all at once (e.g., planning and organizing work duties or household chores). The patient has difficulty managing his/her time (e.g., usually fails to meet deadlines)**	***Do you have difficulty with tasks that require organization and keeping track of many things all at once* (e.g., *planning and organizing your work or household chores)?*** ***Do you have difficulty managing your time* (e.g., *usually fail to meet deadlines)?*** 0 = Absent or non-significant 1 = Patient has difficulty with tasks that require organization or meeting deadlines . = Not sure *or* Not applicable *or* Missing	**30**	**0.82**	**0.12**
186_ CHANGE_ ACTIVITY (P_ADHD186)	**Changing activities**	**The patient changes from one activity to another without finishing the first**	***Do you change from one activity to another without finishing the first?*** 0 = Absent or non-significant 1 = Patient changes from one activity to another without finishing the first . = Not sure *or* Not applicable *or* Missing	**40**	**0.92**	**0.12**
187_ DISTRACTION (P_ADHD187)[a]	**Distraction (attention is distracted by environmental noises)**	**The patient is easily distracted from tasks by activity or noise in the surroundings**	***Are you easily distracted from tasks by activity or noise around you?*** 0 = Absent or non-significant 1 = Patient is easily distracted from tasks by activity or noise around . = Not sure *or* Not applicable *or* Missing	**43**	**0.97**	**0.12**

[a]The item is repeated again in different contexts (manic item # 72)

188_MISPLACE_THINGS (P_ADHD188)	**Misplacing things**	**The patient loses or misplaces things more often than others (e.g., wallets, keys, cell phones)**	***Do you lose or misplace things more often than others* (e.g., *wallets, keys, cell phones)?*** 0 = Absent or non-significant 1 = Patient loses or misplaces things more often than others . = Not sure *or* Not applicable *or* Missing	**43**	**0.94**	**0.12**
189_FORGET_ACTIVITY (P_ADHD189)	**Forgetting daily activities**	**The patient forgets daily activities more often than others (e.g., appointments, paying bills, returning phone calls)**	***Do you forget daily activities more often than others* (e.g., *appointments, paying bills, returning phone calls)?*** 0 = Absent or non-significant 1 = Patient forgets daily activities more often than others . = Not sure *or* Not applicable *or* Missing	**24**	**0.94**	**0.12**
190_LOSE_TRACK (P_ADHD190)	**Losing track**	**The patient loses track of what he/she is doing (e.g., forgets why he/she went to get something)**	***Do you lose track of what you are doing* (e.g., *forget why you went to get something)?*** 0 = Absent or non-significant 1 = Patient loses track of what he/she is doing . = Not sure *or* Not applicable *or* missing	**40**	**0.92**	**0.12**
191_FIDGETY (P_ADHD191)	**Fidgety**	**The patient has difficulty remaining seated (fidgets with hands and feet, squirms, or wiggles in seat) when he/she is expected to remain seated (e.g., in a meeting or a church service)**	***Do you have difficulty remaining seated (fidget with hands and feet, squirm or wiggle in seat) when expected to remain seated* (e.g., *in a meeting or a church service)?*** 0 = Absent or non-significant 1 = Patient fidgets with hands and feet, or wiggles in seat . = Not sure *or* Not applicable *or* Missing	**41**	**0.81**	**0.12**
192_LEAVE_ SEAT (P_ADHD192)	**Leaving seats**	**The patient leaves his/her seat in meetings or other situations (e.g., during an appointment or a church service) where the expectation is to remain seated**	***Do you leave your seat in meetings or other situations* (e.g., *during an appointment or a church service) where you are expected to remain seated?*** 0 = Absent or non-significant 1 = Patient leaves seat in meetings or other situations where expected to remain seated . = Not sure *or* Not applicable *or* Missing	**30**	**0.88**	**0.12**

193_GETUP_ MOVE (P_ADHD193)	**Restlessness/ moving**	**The patient feels restless and fidgety and must get up and move around**	***Do you feel restless, fidgety and you must get up and move around?*** 0 = Absent or non-significant 1 = Patient feels restless, fidgety and must move around . = Not sure *or* Not applicable *or* Missing	**49**	**0.61**	**0.12**
194_HYPER ACTIVE (P_ADHD194)	**Hyperactivity**	**The patient feels overly active and compelled to do things, like he/she is driven by a motor**	***Do you feel overly active and compelled to do things, like you are driven by a motor?*** 0 = Absent or non-significant 1 = Patient feels overly active and compelled to do things . = Not sure *or* Not applicable *or* Missing	**22**	**0.97**	**0.12**
195_WAIT_ LINE (P_ADHD195)	**Waiting in line**	**The patient has difficulty waiting in line for his/her turn when the situation calls for it**	***Is it difficult for you to wait in line for your turn when the situation calls for it?*** 0 = Absent or non-significant 1 = Patient has difficulty waiting in line . = Not sure *or* Not applicable *or* Missing	**23**	**1.00**	**0.12**
196_TALK_ ALOT (P_ADHD196)	**Talking too much**	**The patient thinks he/she talks too much.** **Others say that the patient talks too much**	***Do you think you talk too much?*** ***Do others say that you talk too much?*** 0 = Absent or non-significant 1 = Patient talks too much . = Not sure *or* Not applicable *or* Missing	**12**	**1.00**	**0.12**
197_LOUD_ NOISY (P_ADHD197)	**Loud and noisy**	**The patient thinks that he/she is a loud and noisy person.** **Other people sometimes ask the patient to quiet down or lower his/her voice**	***Do you think that you are a loud and noisy person?*** ***Do other people sometimes ask you to quiet down or lower your voice?*** 0 = Absent or non-significant 1 = Patient or others feel the patient is loud and noisy . = Not sure *or* Not applicable *or* Missing	**22**	**0.58**	**0.11**

198_ IMPULSIVE (P_ADHD198)	**Impulsivity**	**The patient is impulsive (e.g., acts before he/she thinks adequately about consequences of actions)**	***Are you impulsive* (e.g., *act before you think adequately about consequences of actions*)*?*** 0 = Absent or non-significant 1 = Patient is impulsive . = Not sure *or* Not applicable *or* Missing	**41**	**0.92**	**0.12**
199_ DISTURB_ OTHERS (P_ADHD199)	**Disturbing others**	**The patient disturbs others or intrudes on others (e.g., when people are talking or when people are involved in activities)**	***Do you disturb others or intrude on others* (e.g., *when people are talking or when people are involved in activities?*)** 0 = Absent or non-significant 1 = Patient disturbs others or intrudes on others . = Not sure *or* Not applicable *or* Missing	**23**	**0.97**	**0.12**
200_BLURT_ OUT (P_ADHD200)	**Blurt out answers**	**The patient has the tendency to blurt out an answer before another person has finished asking the question**	***Do you have tendency to blurt out an answer before another person has finished asking the question?*** 0 = Absent or non-significant 1 Patient blurts out the answers . = Not sure *or* Not applicable *or* Missing	**32**	**0.89**	**0.12**

[a]Measurement-Based Care (MBC) code
[b]Personalized Medicine in Psychiatry (PMP) code

The same psychopathology item has the same title/subtitle and definition regardless of the diagnosis. For example, the inability to experience pleasure and enjoyments is repeated twice in the SCIP glossary: in item # 46 (in the context of depression) and in item # 112 (in the context of negative symptoms). Similarly, the poor concentration described in the SCIP glossary is repeated in item # 10 (in the context of anxiety), item # 39 (in the context of trauma), item # 48 (in the context of depression), item # 116 (in the context of negative symptoms), and item # 181 (in the context of attention deficit). Regardless of the diagnosis, the SCIP items are transdiagnostic, meaning that they have the same titles/subtitles and definitions. A truly transdiagnostic instrument is a tool that has comprehensive and consistent definitions of psychopathology items, allows for the use of the same items with different diagnoses, and facilitates the measurement of dimensions across different diagnostic categories [24].

The SCIP 30 screening items and 200 psychopathology items make up a standardized and comprehensive collection ("a boilerplate") of adult psychopathology. Researchers can modify and improve the reliability of existing items and add new psychopathology items not currently described in the SCIP "boilerplate" of adult psychopathology. Each of the 230 psychopathology items has 2 codes (column one): a measurement-based care (MBC) code and a personalized medicine in psychiatry (PMP) code. The measurement-based care (MBC) code can be used to streamline research across the globe. The personalized medicine in psychiatry (PMP) code can be used in personalized medicine in psychiatry and will be explained further in Chap. 11. In sum, the SCIP glossary of psychiatric symptoms and signs, as shown in Table 5.1, provides the most comprehensive and consistent psychiatric vocabulary in the literature to date.

References

1. Moore T: The Essential Psychoses and Their Fundamental Syndromes: Studies in Psychology and Psychiatry from the Catholic University of America. Pace EA, editor. Baltimore, Williams and Wilkins; 1933.
2. Kendler, K. S. (2016). The clinical features of mania and their representation in modern diagnostic criteria. *Psychological Medicine, 1-17.*
3. Kendler, K. S. (2016). Phenomenology of schizophrenia and the representativeness of modern diagnostic criteria. *JAMA Psychiatry., 73*, 1082–1092.
4. Guy, W., & Ban, T. (1982). *The AMDP-system. Manual for the assessment and documentation of psychopathology*. Springer.
5. De Leon, J. (2014). A post-DSM-III wake up call to European psychiatry. *Acta psychiatrica Scandinavica., 129*, 76–77.
6. Wing, J. K., Birley, J. L., Cooper, J. E., Graham, P., & Isaacs, A. D. (1967). Reliability of a procedure for measuring and classifying "present psychiatric state". *The British Journal of Psychiatry, 113*, 499–515.
7. Wing, J. K., Henderson, A. S., & Winckle, M. (1977). The rating of symptoms by a psychiatrist and a non-psychiatrist: A study of patients referred from general practice. *Psychological Medicine, 7*, 713–715.

8. Wing, J. K., Nixon, J. M., Mann, S. A., & Leff, J. P. (1977). Reliability of the PSE (ninth edition) used in a population study. *Psychological Medicine, 7*, 505–516.
9. Cooper, J. E., Copeland, J. R., Brown, G. W., Harris, T., & Gourlay, A. J. (1977). Further studies on interviewer training and inter-rater reliability of the Present State Examination (PSE). *Psychological Medicine, 7*, 517–523.
10. Kendell, R. E., Everett, B., Cooper, J. E., Sartorius, N., & David, M. E. (1968). The reliability of the "present state examination". *Social Psychiatry, 3*, 123–129.
11. Luria, R. E., & Berry, R. (1979). Reliability and descriptive validity of PSE syndromes. *Archives of General Psychiatry, 36*, 1187–1195.
12. Luria, R. E., & McHugh, P. R. (1974). Reliability and clinical utility of the "Wing" present state examination. *Archives of General Psychiatry, 30*, 866–871.
13. Farmer, A. E., Katz, R., McGuffin, P., & Bebbington, P. (1987). A comparison between the present state examination and the composite international diagnostic interview. *Archives of General Psychiatry, 44*, 1064–1068.
14. Bebbington, P., Hurry, J., Tennant, C., Sturt, E., & Wing, J. K. (1981). Epidemiology of mental disorders in Camberwell. *Psychological Medicine, 11*, 561–579.
15. Rodgers, B., & Mann, S. A. (1986). The reliability and validity of PSE assessments by lay interviewers: A national population survey. *Psychological Medicine, 16*, 689–700.
16. WHO. (1998). *Schedules for clinical assessment in neuropsychiatry glossary*. World Health Organization.
17. Keshavan, M. S., Clementz, B. A., Pearlson, G. D., Sweeney, J. A., & Tamminga, C. A. (2013). Reimagining psychoses: An agnostic approach to diagnosis. *Schizophrenia Research., 146*, 10–16.
18. Bermanzohn, P. C., Porto, L., Arlow, P. B., Pollack, S., Stronger, R., & Siris, S. G. (2000). Hierarchical diagnosis in chronic schizophrenia: A clinical study of co-occurring syndromes. *SchizophrBull., 26*, 517–525.
19. Hwang, M. Y., & Bermanzohn, P. C. (2001). *Schizophrenia and comorbid conditions: Diagnosis and treatment*. American Psychiatric Press.
20. American Psychiatric, A. (1994). *Diagnostic and statistical manual of mental disorders* (4th Edi ed.). American Psychiatric Association.
21. Keshavan, M. S. (2015). How are endophenotype data best combined with clinical information? *Schizophrenia Bulletin, 41*, S21.
22. Andreasen, N. C., Flaum, M., & Arndt, S. (1992). The Comprehensive Assessment of Symptoms and History (CASH). An instrument for assessing diagnosis and psychopathology. *Archives of General Psychiatry, 49*, 615–623.
23. Moritz, S., Fritzsche, A., Engel, M., Meiseberg, J., Klingberg, S., & Hesse, K. (2018). A plea for a transdiagnostic conceptualization of negative symptoms and for consistent psychiatric vocabulary. *Schizophrenia Research., 204*, 427.
24. Aboraya, A. (2019). A plea for a transdiagnostic tool and consistent psychiatric vocabulary is answered: The Standard for Clinicians' Interview in Psychiatry (SCIP). *Asian Journal of Psychiatry, 46*, 41–43.

Chapter 6
Measurement-Based Care (MBC): Advances in the Twenty-First Century

Introduction

In science, measurement is defined as "rules for assigning numbers to objects in such a way as to represent quantities of attributes" [1]. Measures are the backbone of research. The creation of reliable and valid measures allows for important research, including hypothesis testing and clinical trials, which further advances science and medicine. Major advances in science are preceded by breakthroughs in measurement methods. In the field of psychology, this was demonstrated by the flood of research following the development of intelligence tests and the intelligence quotient in 1912 [1].

In psychiatry, the term measurement-based care (MBC) was coined by Trivedi in 2006 and was defined as "the routine measurement of symptoms and side effects at each treatment visit and the use of a treatment manual describing when and how to modify medication doses based on these measures" [2]. Other authors have offered similar definitions: Harding defined MBC as "enhanced precision and consistency in disease assessment, tracking, and treatment to achieve optimal outcomes" [3]. Arbuckle referred to the term as "a step-by-step approach for assessing, treating, reviewing outcomes and revising treatment in managing medical diseases" [4]. Fortney described MBC as "the systematic administration of symptom rating scales and use of the results to drive clinical decision-making at the level of the individual patient" [5]. Our working definition of MBC in psychiatry is "the use of validated clinical measurement instruments to objectify the assessment, treatment, and clinical outcomes, including efficacy, safety, tolerability, functioning, and quality of life in patients with psychiatric disorders" [6].

Measurement-based care (MBC) refers to two processes: routine *assessments*, such as measuring the severity of symptoms with rating scales, and the use of assessments in *decision-making*. The development of rating scales and standardized diagnostic interviews during the second half of the twentieth century and their

A. S. Aboraya, *Manual for the Standard for Clinicians' Interview in Psychiatry (SCIP)*, Advances in Mental Health and Addiction,
https://doi.org/10.1007/978-3-030-94930-3_6

subsequent use in psychiatric research and clinical trials catalyzed the development and implementation of measurement-based care. With the publication of the DSM-III in 1980 and its widespread use worldwide, psychiatric research and clinical trials flourished as geneticists, pharmacologists, and neuroscientists partnered with investigative psychiatrists [7]. Around the world, clinical trials have assessed the efficacy and safety of new psychotropic medications [8–16]. With the availability of rating scales and standardized diagnostic interviews, the Texas Medication Algorithm Project (TMAP) and the German Algorithm Project (GAP) tested the implementation of measurement-based care in outpatient and inpatient clinical settings and have shown that MBC can positively impact patient outcomes [17, 18]. MBC has been an integral component of randomized clinical trials for decades [19].

The other popular method of caring for patients is the "standard" or "usual" care that has been routinely provided by clinicians. Usual standard of care (USC) for patients involves the same two components of MBC: *assessment and decision-making*. Clinicians, by training, provide care for their patients by assessing psychopathology and subsequently making decisions, without using "rating scales" or "standardized diagnostic interviews." In 1933, Hardcastle et al. studied the present condition of the first 100 patients (adults and children) who attended the department of psychological medicine at Guy's Hospital in London in 1931. Although clinicians in 1933 did not use the Hamilton Depression Rating Scale (HAM-D) or other scales used in current clinical practice, they evaluated patients and grouped them into four main categories: much improved, improved, unchanged, and worse. They decided to admit or treat patients according to these categorizations [20].

Recent research has shown that MBC is superior compared to USC in improving patient outcomes [5, 21–23]. A recent, well-designed, blind-rater, and randomized trial by Guo et al. has shown that MBC is more effective than USC in achieving response and remission and lowering the time to response and remission [24]. *Given the evidence of the benefits of MBC in improving patient outcomes, an important question arises: why has MBC not yet been established as the standard of care in clinical practice?*

This chapter addresses the advantages of MBC, the barriers to implementing MBC in clinical practice, and important contemporary developments in the twenty-first century that are expected to accelerate the adoption of MBC in clinical practice.

Advantages of Measurement-Based Care

Research over the past 20 years has shown that MBC improves the quality of patient care. Leaders in the mental health field have called for the integration of MBC into routine care [5]. As described in our previous manuscript [6], MBC has been shown to:

1. Improve psychotherapy and pharmacotherapy outcomes [5]
2. Monitor symptom reduction in patients with psychiatric disorders such as anxiety, depression, and bipolar disorder [25–27]

3. Identify patients who are improving and those who are deteriorating [5, 28, 29]
4. Improve patient function, satisfaction with care, and quality of life [27, 30]
5. Enhance the therapeutic relationship and communication between providers and patients [5]
6. Improve collaborative care efforts among providers [21, 30]
7. Improve the accuracy of clinical judgment [3, 31]
8. Close the gap between research and practice and move psychiatry into the mainstream of medicine [3]
9. Enhance the clinician's decision-making process [21, 23]
10. Enhance individualized treatment [32]

In addition, there is emerging evidence that clinicians can implement MBC regardless of their theoretical orientation or training background [21]. It is also feasible to implement MBC on a large scale [2, 33–36].

Barriers to Measurement-Based Care

Even though recent research has shown many benefits of MBC compared to usual care, MBC is still not the standard of care in clinical settings, and a very small proportion of clinicians use outcome assessments [3, 37]. Many psychiatric measures with good psychometric properties have been developed and tested over the past decades (e.g., standardized diagnostic interviews, clinician-administered scales, and self-administered scales) [38]. However, most of these measures are used in research and clinical trials but not in clinical settings. A study by Hatfield reported that 37.1% of clinicians use some form of outcome assessments, and 62.9% do not use any outcome measures [23]. Zimmerman found that more than 80% of psychiatrists indicated that they did not routinely use scales to monitor patient outcomes when treating depression [39]. In a survey of psychiatric practitioners, Nasrallah found that 98% of psychiatrists do not use any of the four clinical rating scales that are routinely used in clinical trials and are required for FDA approval of psychiatric medications. These rating scales are the Positive and Negative Syndrome Scale (PANSS), Young Mania Rating Scale (YMRS), Hamilton Depression Rating Scale (HAM-D), and Montgomery-Asberg Depression Rating Scale (MADRS) [40]. The vast majority of those surveyed attributed their avoidance of rating scales to "lack of time." Many other authors have noted that clinicians do not use standardized scales in clinical practice [41–47].

The following barriers to implementing MBC have been identified:

1. Measures are time-consuming to complete (most commonly cited reason by psychiatrists) [39, 40, 45].
2. Measures are designed for research use and not for clinical use [40, 47].
3. Ratings produced by measures may not always be clinically relevant [48, 49].

4. Administering rating scales may interfere with establishing rapport with patients [50].
5. The perception that measures are not more useful than clinical assessment [39, 50].
6. MBC may be perceived as over-systematizing and depersonalizing [3].
7. Some measures, such as standardized diagnostic interviews, can be cumbersome, unwieldy, and complicated [48].
8. Implementing MBC can be costly and requires resources [23].
9. Limited formal training (included in the top two barriers for residents and faculty [23, 50]).
10. Lack of protocols and training manuals [21].
11. Lack of consensus as to which instrument to use for a given disorder [50].
12. Absence of a requirement to use MBC. Few work settings require MBC, and most do not [23, 50].
13. Lack of incentives to use MBC.
14. Providers face complex patients with multiple overlapping comorbidities, which may make implementing MBC more difficult.
15. Some providers may feel that measures "restrict the flexibility and creativity" of the interviewer.

Properties of Clinically Useful Measures in Clinical Practice

To encourage clinicians to use measures in clinical decision-making, measures should have the following basic properties:

1. Efficiency: measures should be brief and not time-consuming for the clinician to complete [3, 51]. A rating scale completed by the clinician should take no more than a few minutes to administer.
2. Measures should have demonstrated reliability and validity evidence [3]
3. Measures should be user-friendly and reflect what clinicians do in clinical settings [51].
4. Self-report scales completed by patients should be brief (no more than 2–3 min to complete) and relatively simple to complete, so that patients are willing to take the test at subsequent visits [52].
5. Measures should be clinically meaningful and useful (covering the criteria and symptom domains of the disorder) [51].
6. Measures should be clinically relevant to decision-making [49].
7. Measures should be easily extractable and not embedded in progress notes [5].
8. Measures should be sensitive to changes induced by medications or psychotherapy [53].

The Development of the Standard for Clinicians' Interview in Psychiatry (SCIP) as a Practical MBC Tool

After I finished my master and doctoral degrees at Johns Hopkins University in 1991, I started psychiatry residency training with a determination to use psychiatric measures in clinical settings. After 10 years of trying to use almost all of the relevant existing scales and standardized diagnostic interviews for adult psychiatric disorders, I concluded that the existing measures were not practical for use in the real world of psychiatric practice. Consequently, I embarked on developing the Standard for Clinicians' Interview in Psychiatry (SCIP) as a tool to be used by clinicians in real clinical settings for assessment and decision-making. In other words, the SCIP was designed from the outset as a measurement-based care tool.

As described in Chap. 2, the SCIP project resulted in four main outcomes (the SCIP Suite):

1. Comprehensive and reliable 230 psychopathology items (Chap. 2).
2. A complete set of 18 clinician-administered (CA) and 15 self-administered (SA) scales (Chap. 4).
3. A comprehensive and consistent psychiatric glossary (Chap. 5).
4. The first comprehensive measurement-based care (MBC) curriculum for clinicians and psychiatric residents (Chap. 9).

Recent Developments Affecting MBC

Two important technological developments of the twenty-first century will accelerate the adoption of MBC in clinical practice:

1. *Electronic Health Records*: Electronic health records (EHR) are being used across clinical settings, from large university institutions to private practices. The federal government has provided financial incentives to private practitioners to use EHR, and most university institutions use advanced EHR [54]. Once MBC tools are identified, they can be uploaded to the EHR and made readily available for clinicians to use. The use of EHR will facilitate implementing MBC [3].
2. *Health Information Technology*: Advances in health information technology such as software programs, handheld devices, web-based training, and videos can certainly facilitate training clinicians and using MBC tools [5, 54, 55]. Currently, psychiatrists record diagnoses, mental status, and other aspects of clinical status in a loose narrative outline. This style of documentation makes it difficult to measure or compare the outcomes of patients as assessed by different clinicians [51]. This current practice will become outdated in the near future as MBC becomes implemented. With the right software and integrated EHR, clinicians should be able to complete a rating scale, calculate the scale score, com-

pare scores on the same scale over time, create graphs, and do analyses with the push of a few buttons.

Owl is one of the leading providers of precision-guided behavioral health solutions with a cloud-based platform that provides clients with a large library of evidence-based measures that are available for use in clinical practice. The Owl platform provides the SCIP scales for their clients to use. By using the Owl platform, clinicians use the SCIP scales to assess psychopathology, and the platform generates scale scores along with severity classifications (e.g., mild, moderate, severe). The platform can also generate visual graphs and scores that show the progress of the patient over time and can be shared with the patient during a visit. This provides the patient and clinician with a measurement feedback system that facilitates decision-making at each visit throughout their treatment. If the patient indicates the potential for self-harm, the platform sends an alert to the clinician and provides resources to the patient. In addition, the platform provides reports that provide views into how the client's patient panel is responding to treatment, and the data can be exported into statistical programs to perform further analyses. Owl maps to existing clinical workflows, which makes it easy for clinicians to use and implement MBC in their practice.

Conclusions

After Robert Spitzer developed the Mental Status Schedule, the first published structured interview in the United States [56], the *New York Post* published an article in 1963 that stated "a young doctor at Columbia University's New York State Psychiatric Institute has developed a tool which may become the psychiatrist's thermometer and microscope and X-ray machine rolled into one" [57]. Five decades later, this statement is still true; measures in psychiatry are the equivalent of a thermometer and a stethoscope to a physician. No measure or scale or diagnostic interview will ever replace a seasoned and experienced clinician who has been evaluating and treating real patients for years. MBC is not intended to replace clinical judgment and cannot be a substitute for an observant and caring clinician [3]. Just as thermometers, stethoscopes, and lab results help other types of physicians to reach accurate diagnoses and provide appropriate care, the use of MBC by psychiatrists will improve the accuracy of diagnoses and improve care outcomes. In essence, MBC aims to get the diagnosis and management right as often and as quickly as possible [3].

Although scientific rules and input from experts were used to create efficient and validated SCIP scales (see Chap. 4), this does not minimize the importance of the psychopathology items that were not included in the final SCIP scales. The core depression scale of the SCIP does not include questions on reduced sexual drive, sleep, and appetite changes. Clinicians need to inquire about these important items because they will impact the clinicians' choice of medications to prescribe for the patient. When teaching and implementing MBC, clinicians should stress the importance of comprehensive psychopathological assessment to avoid limiting psychopathology education to specific diagnostic criteria or certain scales.

Recent studies have shown that the cost of MBC is minimal and that the benefits are huge for patients, providers, and payers [5]. The advantages of MBC outweigh the challenges of its implementation [58]. Moreover, payers and accreditation organizations are demanding the use of MBC in psychiatric practice. It is better for health care providers to develop their own MBC tools rather than have outcome measures imposed on them by payers and regulators [5]. The SCIP scales and glossary are MBC tools for clinicians as described in detail in the manual.

References

1. Nunnally, J. C. (1978). *Psychometric theory*. McGraw-Hill.
2. Trivedi, M. H., Rush, A. J., Wisniewski, S. R., Nierenberg, A. A., Warden, D., Ritz, L., Norquist, G., Howland, R. H., Lebowitz, B., McGrath, P. J., Shores-Wilson, K., Biggs, M. M., Balasubramani, G. K., Fava, M., & Team SDS. (2006). Evaluation of outcomes with citalopram for depression using measurement-based care in STAR*D: Implications for clinical practice. *The American Journal of Psychiatry, 163*, 28–40.
3. Harding, K. J., Rush, A. J., Arbuckle, M., Trivedi, M. H., & Pincus, H. A. (2011). Measurement-based care in psychiatric practice: A policy framework for implementation. *The Journal of Clinical Psychiatry, 72*, 1136–1143.
4. Arbuckle, M. R., Weinberg, M., Kistler, S. C., Cabaniss, D. L., Isaacs, A. J., Sederer, L. I., & Essock, S. M. (2013). A curriculum in measurement-based care: Screening and monitoring of depression in a psychiatric resident clinic. *Academic Psychiatry, 37*, 317–320.
5. Fortney, J. C., Unutzer, J., Wrenn, G., Pyne, J. M., Smith, G. R., Schoenbaum, M., & Harbin, H. T. (2016). A tipping point for measurement-based care. *Psychiatric Services, 68*(2), 179–188. https://doi.org/10.1176/appi.ps.201500439
6. Aboraya, A., Nasrallah, H. A., Elswick, D. E., Ahmed, E., Estephan, N., Aboraya, D., Berzingi, S., Chumbers, J., Berzingi, S., Justice, J., Zafar, J., & Dohar, S. (2018). Measurement-based care in psychiatry-past, present, and future. *Innovations in Clinical Neuroscience, 15*, 13–26.
7. McHugh, P. R. (2005). Striving for coherence: psychiatry's efforts over classification. *Journal of the American Medical Association, 293*, 2526–2528.
8. Fleischhacker, W. W., Gopal, S., Lane, R., Gassmann-Mayer, C., Lim, P., Hough, D., Remmerie, B., & Eerdekens, M. (2012). A randomized trial of paliperidone palmitate and risperidone long-acting injectable in schizophrenia. *The International Journal of Neuropsychopharmacology, 15*, 107–118.
9. Fleischhacker, W. W., McQuade, R. D., Marcus, R. N., Archibald, D., Swanink, R., & Carson, W. H. (2009). A double-blind, randomized comparative study of aripiprazole and olanzapine in patients with schizophrenia. *Biological Psychiatry, 65*, 510–517.
10. Kane, J. M., Eerdekens, M., Lindenmayer, J. P., Keith, S. J., Lesem, M., & Karcher, K. (2003). Long-acting injectable risperidone: Efficacy and safety of the first long-acting atypical antipsychotic. *The American Journal of Psychiatry, 160*, 1125–1132.
11. Kane, J. M., Skuban, A., Ouyang, J., Hobart, M., Pfister, S., McQuade, R. D., Nyilas, M., Carson, W. H., Sanchez, R., & Eriksson, H. (2015). A multicenter, randomized, double-blind, controlled phase 3 trial of fixed-dose brexpiprazole for the treatment of adults with acute schizophrenia. *Schizophrenia Research, 164*, 127–135.
12. Kane, J. M., Zukin, S., Wang, Y., Lu, K., Ruth, A., Nagy, K., Laszlovszky, I., & Durgam, S. (2015). Efficacy and safety of cariprazine in acute exacerbation of schizophrenia: Results

from an international, phase III clinical trial. *Journal of Clinical Psychopharmacology, 35*, 367–373.
13. Nasrallah, H. A., Silva, R., Phillips, D., Cucchiaro, J., Hsu, J., Xu, J., & Loebel, A. (2013). Lurasidone for the treatment of acutely psychotic patients with schizophrenia: A 6-week, randomized, placebo-controlled study. *Journal of Psychiatric Research, 47*, 670–677.
14. Durgam, S., Cutler, A. J., Lu, K., Migliore, R., Ruth, A., Laszlovszky, I., Nemeth, G., & Meltzer, H. Y. (2015). Cariprazine in acute exacerbation of schizophrenia: A fixed-dose, phase 3, randomized, double-blind, placebo- and active-controlled trial. *The Journal of Clinical Psychiatry, 76*, e1574–e1582.
15. Durgam, S., Starace, A., Li, D., Migliore, R., Ruth, A., Nemeth, G., & Laszlovszky, I. (2014). An evaluation of the safety and efficacy of cariprazine in patients with acute exacerbation of schizophrenia: A phase II, randomized clinical trial. *Schizophrenia Research, 152*, 450–457.
16. Meltzer, H. Y., Risinger, R., Nasrallah, H. A., Du, Y., Zummo, J., Corey, L., Bose, A., Stankovic, S., Silverman, B. L., & Ehrich, E. W. (2015). A randomized, double-blind, placebo-controlled trial of aripiprazole lauroxil in acute exacerbation of schizophrenia. *The Journal of Clinical Psychiatry, 76*, 1085–1090.
17. Crismon, M. L., Trivedi, M., Pigott, T. A., Rush, A. J., Hirschfeld, R. M., Kahn, D. A., DeBattista, C., Nelson, J. C., Nierenberg, A. A., Sackeim, H. A., & Thase, M. E. (1999). The Texas medication algorithm project: Report of the Texas consensus conference panel on medication treatment of major depressive disorder. *The Journal of Clinical Psychiatry, 60*, 142–156.
18. Ricken, R., Wiethoff, K., Reinhold, T., Schietsch, K., Stamm, T., Kiermeir, J., Neu, P., Heinz, A., Bauer, M., & Adli, M. (2011). Algorithm-guided treatment of depression reduces treatment costs–results from the randomized controlled German Algorithm Project (GAPII). *Journal of Affective Disorders, 134*, 249–256.
19. Rush, A. J. (2015). Isn't it about time to employ measurement-based care in practice? *The American Journal of Psychiatry, 172*, 934–936.
20. Hardcastle, D. (1934). A follow-up study of one hundred cases made for the department of psychological medicine, Guy's hospital. *Journal of Mental Science, 80*, 536–549.
21. Scott, K., & Lewis, C. C. (2015). Using measurement-based care to enhance any treatment. *Cognitive and Behavioral Practice, 22*, 49–59.
22. Lambert, M. (2001). Psychotherapy outcome and quality improvement: Introduction to the special section on patient-focused research. *Journal of Counseling and Clinical Psychology, 69*, 147–149.
23. Hatfield, D. R., & Ogles, B. M. (2007). Why some clinicians use outcome measures and others do not. *Administration and Policy in Mental Health, 34*, 283–291.
24. Guo, T., Xiang, Y. T., Xiao, L., Hu, C. Q., Chiu, H. F., Ungvari, G. S., Correll, C. U., Lai, K. Y., Feng, L., Geng, Y., Feng, Y., & Wang, G. (2015). Measurement-based care versus standard care for major depression: A randomized controlled trial with blind raters. *The American Journal of Psychiatry, 172*, 1004–1013.
25. Roy-Byrne, P., Craske, M. G., Sullivan, G., Rose, R. D., Edlund, M. J., Lang, A. J., Bystritsky, A., Welch, S. S., Chavira, D. A., Golinelli, D., Campbell-Sills, L., Sherbourne, C. D., & Stein, M. B. (2010). Delivery of evidence-based treatment for multiple anxiety disorders in primary care: A randomized controlled trial. *Journal of the American Medical Association, 303*, 1921–1928.
26. Simon, G. E., Ludman, E. J., Bauer, M. S., Unutzer, J., & Operskalski, B. (2006). Long-term effectiveness and cost of a systematic care program for bipolar disorder. *Archives of General Psychiatry, 63*, 500–508.
27. Bauer, M. S., McBride, L., Williford, W. O., Glick, H., Kinosian, B., Altshuler, L., Beresford, T., Kilbourne, A. M., Sajatovic, M., & Cooperative Studies Program 430 Study Team. (2006). Collaborative care for bipolar disorder: Part II. Impact on clinical outcome, function, and costs. *Psychiatric Services, 57*, 937–945.

28. Hatfield, D., McCullough, L., Frantz, S. H., & Krieger, K. (2010). Do we know when our clients get worse? An investigation of therapists' ability to detect negative client change. *Clinical Psychology & Psychotherapy, 17*, 25–32.
29. Hannan, C., Lambert, M. J., Harmon, C., Nielsen, S. L., Smart, D. W., Shimokawa, K., & Sutton, S. W. (2005). A lab test and algorithms for identifying clients at risk for treatment failure. *Journal of Clinical Psychology, 61*, 155–163.
30. Katon, W. J., Lin, E. H., Von Korff, M., Ciechanowski, P., Ludman, E. J., Young, B., Peterson, D., Rutter, C. M., McGregor, M., & McCulloch, D. (2010). Collaborative care for patients with depression and chronic illnesses. *The New England Journal of Medicine, 363*, 2611–2620.
31. Sapyta, J., Riemer, M., & Bickman, L. (2005). Feedback to clinicians: Theory, research, and practice. *Journal of Clinical Psychology, 61*, 145–153.
32. Trivedi, M. H., & Daly, E. J. (2007). Measurement-based care for refractory depression: A clinical decision support model for clinical research and practice. *Drug and Alcohol Dependence, 88*(Suppl 2), S61–S71.
33. Unutzer, J., Chan, Y. F., Hafer, E., Knaster, J., Shields, A., Powers, D., & Veith, R. C. (2012). Quality improvement with pay-for-performance incentives in integrated behavioral health care. *American Journal of Public Health and the Nation's Health, 102*, e41–e45.
34. Pomerantz, A. S., Kearney, L. K., Wray, L. O., Post, E. P., & McCarthy, J. F. (2014). Mental health services in the medical home in the Department of Veterans Affairs: Factors for successful integration. *Psychological Services, 11*, 243–253.
35. Johnson-Lawrence, V., Zivin, K., Szymanski, B. R., Pfeiffer, P. N., & McCarthy, J. F. (2012). VA primary care-mental health integration: Patient characteristics and receipt of mental health services, 2008–2010. *Psychiatric Services, 63*, 1137–1141.
36. Sachs, G. S. (2004). Strategies for improving treatment of bipolar disorder: Integration of measurement and management. *Acta Psychiatrica Scandinavica, 110*, 7–17.
37. Hatfield, D. O., & B. (2004). The use of outcome measures by psychologists in clinical practice. *Professional Psychology: Research and Practice, 35*, 485–491.
38. Rush, A. J., First, M. B., & Blacker, D. (Eds.). (2000). *Handbook of psychiatric measures*. American Psychiatric Association.
39. Zimmerman, M., & McGlinchey, J. B. (2008). Why don't psychiatrists use scales to measure outcome when treating depressed patients? *The Journal of Clinical Psychiatry, 69*, 1916–1919.
40. Nasrallah, H. (2009). Long overdue: Measurement-based psychiatric practice. *Current Psychiatry, 8*, 14–16.
41. Zimmerman, M. (2014). Measuring outcome in clinical practice. *Psychiatric Times, 31*, 28.
42. Duffy, F. F., Chung, H., Trivedi, M., Rae, D. S., Regier, D. A., & Katzelnick, D. J. (2008). Systematic use of patient-rated depression severity monitoring: Is it helpful and feasible in clinical psychiatry? *Psychiatric Services, 59*, 1148–1154.
43. Gilbody, S. M., House, A. O., & Sheldon, T. A. (2002). Psychiatrists in the UK do not use outcomes measures. National survey. *The British Journal of Psychiatry: The Journal of Mental Science, 180*, 101–103.
44. Bastiaens, L. (2011). Poor practice, managed care, and magic pills: Have we created a mental health monster? *Psychiatric Times, 28*, 1–4.
45. Aboraya, A. (2009). Use of structured interviews by psychiatrists in real clinical settings: Results of an open-question survey. *Psychiatry (Edgmont), 6*, 24–28.
46. Rettew, D. C., Lynch, A. D., Achenbach, T. M., Dumenci, L., & Ivanova, M. Y. (2009). Meta-analyses of agreement between diagnoses made from clinical evaluations and standardized diagnostic interviews. *International Journal of Methods in Psychiatric Research, 18*, 169–184.
47. Busner, J., Kaplan, S. L., Greco, N., & Sheehan, D. V. (2011). The use of research measures in adult clinical practice. *Innovations in Clinical Neuroscience, 8*, 19–23.
48. Aboraya, A., Nasrallah, H., Muvvala, S., El-Missiry, A., Mansour, H., Hill, C., Elswick, D., & Price, E. C. (2016). The standard for clinicians' interview in psychiatry (SCIP): A clinician-administered tool with categorical, dimensional, and numeric output-conceptual development, design, and description of the SCIP. *Innovations in Clinical Neuroscience, 13*, 31–77.

49. Aboraya, A., & Nasrallah, H. A. (2016). Perspectives on the Positive and Negative Syndrome Scale (PANSS): Use, misuse, drawbacks, and a new alternative for schizophrenia research. *Annals of Clinical Psychiatry, 28*, 125–131.
50. Arbuckle, M. R., Weinberg, M., Harding, K. J., Isaacs, A. J., Covell, N. H., Cabaniss, D. L., Essock, S. M., & Sederer, L. I. (2013). The feasibility of standardized patient assessments as a best practice in an academic training program. *Psychiatric Services, 64*, 209–211.
51. Roy-Byrne, P., Dagadakis, C., Ries, R., Decker, K., Jones, R., Bolte, M. A., Scher, M., Brinkley, J., Gallagher, M., Patrick, D. L., et al. (1995). A psychiatrist-rated battery of measures for assessing the clinical status of psychiatric inpatients. *Psychiatric Services, 46*, 347–352.
52. Zimmerman, M., & McGlinchey, J. B. (2008). Depressed patients' acceptability of the use of self-administered scales to measure outcome in clinical practice. *Annals of Clinical Psychiatry, 20*, 125–129.
53. Baer, L. (2015). *Handbook of clinical rating scales and assessment in psychiatry and mental health*. Humana Press.
54. Blumenthal, D. (2009). Stimulating the adoption of health information technology. *The New England Journal of Medicine, 360*, 1477–1479.
55. Long, N. (2008). Closing the gap between research and practice–the importance of practitioner training. *Clinical Child Psychology and Psychiatry, 13*, 187–190.
56. Spitzer, R. L., Fleiss, J. L., Burdock, E. I., & Hardesty, A. S. (1964). The mental status schedule: Rationale, reliability and validity. *Comprehensive Psychiatry, 5*, 384–395.
57. Spitzer, R. L. (1983). Psychiatric diagnosis: Are clinicians still necessary? *Comprehensive Psychiatry, 24*, 399–411.
58. Valenstein, M., Adler, D. A., Berlant, J., Dixon, L. B., Dulit, R. A., Goldman, B., Hackman, A., Oslin, D. W., Siris, S. G., & Sonis, W. A. (2009). Implementing standardized assessments in clinical care: now's the time. *Psychiatric Services, 60*, 1372–1375.

Chapter 7
The Psychiatric Interview Contribution to Measurement-Based Care and Research

The psychiatric interview consists of direct interactions and communication between the patient and the clinician. This interview is the clinician's major source of information for understanding how to care for the patient. Regardless of the interviewer's style or technique, the psychiatric interview is a combination of art and science. The art of the psychiatric interview refers to the interviewer's skills in building rapport with the patient and engaging him/her in the therapeutic process. These skills include the interviewer's ability to show empathy, compassion, and sensitivity to the patient, which enables the patient to trust in the interviewer. The interviewer's demeanor and ability to actively listen to the patient by paying attention to his/her statements and following up on leads are important elements of artful and skillful interviewing. The art of the interview is learned by practice, rather than from reading articles or books. The science of the psychiatric interview refers to the skill of the interviewer to elicit valid and reliable data that can be used for diagnostic, therapeutic, and research purposes. The clinician must balance the need to engage the patient in the therapeutic process with the need to collect diverse data required for clinical, research, and billing purposes.

Shea articulated seven comprehensive goals of the psychiatric interview, which can be organized under the categories of art and science [1]:

Art of the interview:

1. "To establish a sound engagement of the patient in a therapeutic alliance"
2. "To develop an evolving and compassionate understanding of the patient"
3. "To effect some decrease in anxiety in the patient"
4. "To instill hope and ensure that the client will return for the next appointment"

Science of the interview:

1. "To collect a valid database"
2. "To develop an assessment from which a tentative diagnosis can be made"

A. S. Aboraya, *Manual for the Standard for Clinicians' Interview in Psychiatry (SCIP)*, Advances in Mental Health and Addiction,
https://doi.org/10.1007/978-3-030-94930-3_7

3. "To develop an appropriate disposition and treatment plan"

Measurement-based care (MBC) includes two main components: routine initial assessments, such as using diagnostic interviews to make a diagnosis and measuring the severity of illness with rating scales, and the use of measurement to make clinical decisions at the individual level over time. Although it might seem that MBC would be considered part of the science of interviewing, the art of conducting a good interview and establishing trust with the patient is crucial to obtaining valid information. The art and science of the interview are intertwined and are difficult to separate.

The Components of Psychiatric Assessment

The process of psychiatric assessment has three components: the psychiatric interview, the etiological search, and the disorder classification.

A. **The psychiatric interview (dimensional component):** This is the direct psychiatric interview with the patient that produces a broad range of clinical data such as chief complaints, the history of present illness, past psychiatric history, medical history, mental status examination, and other relevant and important data. Individual symptoms, current and past, are evaluated for their presence or absence. These symptoms form the dimensions of psychopathology. To be useful to the clinician, the collected information will need to be organized through the processes of etiological search and disease classification.
B. **Etiological search (etiological component):** As the clinician conducts the interview, he/she explores the potential causes of symptoms. If the patient reports depression and drinks alcohol, the clinician may explore whether the depressed mood is secondary to alcohol use or whether the patient has a dual diagnosis (e.g., alcohol use disorder and major depression). For example, a patient may have had no depressive symptoms prior to alcohol use but may have begun to feel depressed after the alcohol use began. The same patient may stop drinking alcohol and find that his mood returns to normal. This temporal sequence indicates alcohol-induced depression. Another patient may have had months of sobriety (no alcohol or drug abuse), during which he felt depressed, hopeless, and suicidal and met the criteria for major depression, at which point he began to drink alcohol to cope with his depression. This patient may have primary mood disorder and alcohol use disorder (dual diagnoses). Since medical conditions can affect psychiatric presentations, a psychiatrist uses his or her medical knowledge and clinical skills to decide whether any medical conditions might have caused or exacerbated psychiatric symptoms. The clinician may need to order certain labs, urine drug screen, or neuroimaging to confirm or refute an etiological factor.
C. **Disorders classification (categorical component):** The clinician evaluates whether a symptom or cluster of symptoms causes significant distress (Table 7.1)

Table 7.1 A symptom or cluster of symptoms can cause distress to the patient

Codes of distress:
0 No distress
1 Some distress, but manageable
2 Significant distress: the patient is distressed, upset, or bothered by symptom(s) more than half the time

Table 7.2 A symptom or a cluster of symptoms can affect the functioning of the patient

Codes of functional impairment:
0 No effect on social or occupational activities
1 Some impairment in social and occupational activities, but many activities are still intact
2 Significant impairment of most or all social and occupational activities

or functional impairment (Table 7.2). Finally, the clinician utilizes all of the available information to decide whether the patient meets criteria for a psychiatric disorder(s) based on the Diagnostic and Statistical Manual (DSM) or International Classification of Disease (ICD) criteria. Once a diagnosis is established, a treatment plan is formulated for the patient.

Phases of the Psychiatric Interview

A typical psychiatric interview conducted by psychiatrists and other mental health clinicians has three phases.

Phase one (5–10 minutes) The clinician greets the patient, introduces himself/herself, and asks the patient basic demographic questions (age, marital status, education, occupation and living arrangements). The clinician asks about the chief complaint(s) and allows the patient to take the lead by describing the history of the present illness and any recent stressor(s). The clinician observes and listens to the patient, allowing for good rapport to be established, and may write brief notes. The clinician gives attention to the patient in order to maintain good rapport. Questions in this phase tend to be open-ended to allow the patient to talk freely and the interviewer to listen.

Phase two (15–25 minutes) At the beginning of this phase, the clinician should have a good idea about the patient's main problem(s). The clinician takes the lead and asks screening questions covering the main domains of psychopathology. The screening questions cover anxiety, mood, psychosis, alcohol, drugs, somatoform disorders, eating, attention, and hyperactivity. There is no specific order for the screening questions. The clinician may choose an order of questions that allows the interview to flow smoothly and maintains a good rapport with the patient. For example, if the patient's main symptom is depressed mood, it is wise to start with the mood questions and inquire more about anhedonia, elevated mood, and mood swings. Then the clinician can screen for anxiety and psychosis. Another example is as follows: if the patient's main problem is alcohol or drug use, it is wise to start with the alcohol and drug questions and get relevant information as to the extent of the substance use problem. The clinician inquires about a time when the patient was sober for a reasonable amount of time and screens for anxiety, mood, and psychosis symptoms during the time of sobriety. Another example is that if the patient starts the interview with bizarre statements about aliens from Mars invading earth and appears disorganized, the clinician may inquire about delusions and hallucinations. For this patient, the clinician may skip anxiety- and attention-deficit questions because the patient is too disorganized to provide any valid information. In summary, there are no rules or specific orders to be followed in this phase. The clinician utilizes his/her clinical skills, aided by the screening questions, to detect any abnormal psychopathology. It is important to remember that the screening questions represent a review of the main psychopathological domains of adults. It is also important for the clinician not to miss any important areas of psychopathology in this phase. If a patient presents with depressive symptoms and the clinician does not ask about a history of manic episodes, the interview is flawed and may result in misdiagnosis and mistreatment.

Phase three (10–15 minutes) By this phase of the interview, the clinician should have determined diagnostic possibilities. The clinician asks specific closed-ended questions to test whether the patient meets the criteria for a specific disorder, a process called pattern matching or hypothesis testing [2]. During this phase, the clinician determines whether the symptoms cause significant distress or impairment of function. Finally, the clinician determines whether or not the patient has a psychiatric disorder(s) and initiates treatment planning.

It is important to know that the sequence of the three phases described above does not have to be followed in that order. Many psychiatrists like to start by asking patients about the chief complaint(s) and history of present illness at the beginning of the interview, and the demographic information comes later as the interview proceeds. Many psychiatrists do phases two and three together. For example, if the patient describes a depressed mood, the interviewer follows up by asking about depressive symptoms (anhedonia, hopelessness, suicidal thoughts and plans, **etc.*****). Similarly, if the patient reports abuse, the interviewer asks about posttraumatic stress symptoms (bad dreams, nightmares, flashbacks,*** **etc.*****). The technique of conducting phases two and three simultaneously makes the interview proceed smoothly with a natural progression and helps to maintain rapport with the patient. Finally, the interviewer has a lot of freedom as long as he/she conducts an artful and skillful interview that results in valid information, accurate diagnoses, and ultimately proper treatment.***

Inputs and Outputs of the Psychiatric Interview

Inputs result from direct questioning of the patient and can be summarized as:

1. Demographic data and social history
2. History of present illness and past psychiatric history
3. History of suicide and self-injurious behavior
4. Alcohol and drug history
5. Allergies and medications
6. Medical and family history

Outputs are the result of clinician interpretation of the data collected and can be summarized as:

1. Mental status examination
2. Evaluation of past episodes
3. Provisional diagnosis and differential diagnosis
4. Treatment plan

Mental Status Examination

Mental status examination (MSE) is the evaluation of the patient's current state of the cognitive and emotional function and is evaluated throughout the entire interview [2] (Table 7.3).

Table 7.3 Definitions and examples of the main items of the MSE

MSE item	Definition and examples
Appearance	Kempt, unkempt, alert, drowsy, intoxicated, others
Behavior	Cooperative, defensive, guarded, angry, suspicious, calm, tense, pacing, agitated, others
Motor activities	Posture: erect, rigid, relaxed, stooped over, others Gait: normal, shuffling gait, others Abnormal movements: tremors, tics, mannerism, twitches, stereotyped behavior, catatonia, rigidity, others
Speech	Rate: normal, slowed, pressured, monotonous Volume: normal, high, low Content: clear, slurred, coherent, incoherent, rambling, echolalia (repetition of a word or sentence just spoken by another person), stuttering, mute, clanging, distractible, others
Mood	The current state of feeling manifested by thoughts or actions. A patient may express feeling depressed. Another patient may appear very sad without expressing sadness in words A mood can be happy, sad, irritable, labile (changing during the day or from day to day), stable, expansive, others
Affect	Affect is the patient's external facial expression of the mood Affect can be appropriate or inappropriate. Affect range can be full, constricted, blunted, or flat

(continued)

Table 7.3 (continued)

MSE item	Definition and examples
Thought process	Goal-oriented Circumstantiality: excessive details that may be relevant or irrelevant Looseness of association: speech shifts to different topics, related or unrelated Tangentiality: replying to a question is related in some distant way or totally unrelated Thought blocking: sudden cessation of thoughts Perseveration: repetition of a meaningless word or sentence Others
Thought content	Delusions: thoughts characterized by being false, firm (held with conviction) and fixed (held regardless of counter evidence). Types of delusions: paranoid, grandiose, somatic, bizarre, and others Obsession: an intrusive thought or image that does not make sense and keeps coming back to the mind Compulsion: repeating things over and over that can be actions (e.g., checking doors) or mental (e.g., repeating numbers) Suicidal thought: with the intent to die Self-harm thought: without the intent to die Homicidal thoughts toward others
Perception	Hallucinations: subjective perception without stimuli and can be auditory, visual, olfactory, gustatory, or tactile
Cognitive function	Orientation: time, place, person, situation Attention: e.g., counting backward by ones from 57 Calculation: e.g., subtracting 7 from 100 or 3 from 20 General information: e.g., names of the presidents Abstraction: interpretation of proverbs: e.g., how are apple and orange alike? Memory: Immediate memory: registration of information (e.g., repeating three names) Short-term memory: e.g., five-minute recall Long-term memory: recalling events of the past several days, months, or years
Insight	Self-understanding of the illness and need for treatment
Judgment	Patient's ability to make rational decisions

The mental status examination (MSE) contributes to MBC. For example, a 25-year-old male patient may present with depressive symptoms and informs the interviewer that he has been feeling sad most of the time for the past month. The MSE describes the current depressed mood. This information will be reflected in the current episode of depression and rated 2 (depression most of the time).

Evaluation of Past Episodes

Depending upon the clinical presentation of the patient, the clinician may decide to explore past episodes of emotional problems. For the same 25-year-old male patient described above, the clinician may go beyond the current episode of depression and explore other episodes of depression in the past. The clinician should inquire about past episodes of mania. The same patient may tell the interviewer that last year he was feeling extremely happy, euphoric, and on top of the world and that the feeling lasted 10 days, during which he was highly energetic and not sleeping. The interviewer evaluates that manic episode a year ago and may rate a past episode of euphoric mood as 2 (euphoric mood most of the time). Chapter 3 includes the principles of evaluating symptoms and signs and different episodes.

Approaches to Psychiatric Diagnoses

To make a psychiatric diagnosis, the clinician may follow one of the three approaches described in the literature: the "top-down" approach, "bottom-up" approach, and "Bottom First Then Top" (BFTT) approach [3]. **In the top-down approach**, the clinician has a good knowledge of the diagnostic criteria of main psychiatric disorders according to the DSM. The clinician also knows the necessary criteria to make a specific diagnosis. If the patient denies feeling sad and denies anhedonia, the clinician knows in advance that the patient will not meet the criteria for a major depressive episode according to the DSM-5 criteria. In a research setting, the top-down approach is exemplified by the Structured Clinical Interview for DSM-IV Axis I Disorders (SCID-I), where questions are grouped by diagnosis and criteria. If the required criteria for a specific diagnosis are not met, the interviewer skips the remaining questions assessing the other criteria for that diagnosis. For example, if the patient denies depressed mood and anhedonia, the SCID-I instructs the interviewer to skip the remaining questions for the diagnosis of major depression [4]. The top-down approach leads to efficient interviews by focusing on diagnoses, facilitates clinical communication among providers, and improves reliability. On the other hand, diagnostic interviews based upon the top-down approach tend to be biased toward preconceived diagnostic criteria, lack validity, may result in the loss of important information, and need to be updated every time the diagnostic system changes.

In the bottom-up approach, the clinician focuses on a complete and comprehensive assessment of symptoms regardless of the diagnosis. After the assessment of symptoms, the clinician considers a diagnosis based upon the positive symptoms and other relevant data. In a research setting, the bottom-up approach is exemplified by the Schedules for Clinical Assessment in Neuropsychiatry (SCAN); the interview is based upon a comprehensive assessment of symptoms, while being agnostic to diagnosis [5]. After symptom assessment, algorithms are used to make psychiatric diagnoses. The bottom-up approach has the advantage of avoiding biases toward preconceived diagnoses and can survive diagnostic criteria changes. However, the bottom-up approach leads to lengthy interviews and may lack the precision needed to fulfill diagnostic criteria [6].

Seasoned and competent psychiatrists generally use the **"Bottom First Then Top" (BFTT)** approach in diagnostic assessment. An ideal psychiatric diagnostic interview starts with a bottom-up approach: the psychiatrist establishes rapport with the patient and inquires about chief complaint(s) and history of the present illness. The patient is initially allowed to take the lead to express feelings, thoughts, current stressors, and other problems. The psychiatrist continues the bottom-up approach by obtaining a detailed life history, screening for symptoms, examining mental status, exploring potential causes of symptoms, and utilizing records and informants as needed. As the psychiatrist narrows down the potential differential diagnoses, the top-down approach takes over the interview process. The psychiatrist checks the symptoms and decides whether or not the patient meets the diagnostic criteria of a disorder. The psychiatric interview component and the etiological component are mainly bottom-up approaches. The disorder classification component is mainly a top-down approach. ***The motto of the BFTT approach is to listen to and understand the patient first and then focus on making a diagnosis.*** Another term proposed to describe this approach is "**Patient First Then Clinician" (PFTC),** highlighting the importance of listening to and understanding the patient first before making a diagnosis.

The Clinician's Role in Interviewing Patients

Clinicians with experience in the mental health field who regularly complete diagnostic interviews play a pivotal role in gathering valid information from patients. Even though the SCIP manual includes the definitions of 230 psychopathology items and accompanying questions for each item, a clinical interview is not "scripted," and clinicians cannot ask verbatim questions and expect patients to respond in a certain way according to some predefined ratings. As described earlier, the art and science of interviewing are intertwined.

In addition to information from the patient's medical records, there are six direct sources of information that contribute to an assessment of psychopathology:

1. The questions asked by the clinician
2. The clinician's observations of the patient
3. The clinician's provision of examples and clarifications
4. The patient volunteering information, not in response to questions
5. The patient's responses to specific questions
6. The patient's provision of examples and clarifications

Over the course of an artful interview, any of these six sources of information can appear in any order. For instance, a patient may begin the interview by telling the clinician that he has been feeling sad and depressed most of the time after his wife left him 3 months ago and that he is contemplating ending his life by overdosing on his blood pressure medications. The clinician can then ask the patient to give more details, ask further questions, observe the patient, and use his/her skills to gather all the information needed to make a full assessment. Finally, the clinician can make an initial diagnosis and initiate a treatment plan.

The psychopathology item validation (PIV) is a process in which the clinician uses one or more of the six sources of information to reach a reasonably valid rating of the psychopathology item. During the PIV process, the clinician may modify or change the wording of any of the SCIP questions in order to ensure the patient's understanding. The clinician may ask the patient to give examples or provide the patient with examples. The clinician may be satisfied with the patient's own description and rate a psychopathology item without even asking any questions. The clinician may choose to ask questions to clarify the patient's descriptions. For example, in clip #5 (Chapter 10, Video #1), when the patient responded to a question regarding mood fluctuations within a day, the patient also described racing thoughts, although this was not the topic of the original question.

Patient: Yeah. Yesterday, for a period of about 4 hours, I went from depression, to hypomania, to depression, to what I call scatter brained. I get so many thoughts going through my mind that I can't focus on anything. I can't slow anything down enough to grasp one specific thought long enough to get ahold of myself.

In clip #3 (Chapter 10, Video #1), when the patient responded to the depressed mood question by stating that she felt extremely depressed, the patient also described feeling guilty, helpless, and unable to do anything more. The clinician asked if the patient felt depressed most of the time and the patient said yes. The clinician elaborated and asked more about feeling guilty and psychomotor retardation later in the interview.

C: Let's focus on the past month. Have you been feeling sad and depressed?
P1: Yes, extremely. Very guilty. I feel helpless and feel like I can't do anything more. I feel like it's Groundhog Day every day. Same day over and over.
C: So you have been feeling depressed most of the time.
P1: Yes.

Only experienced clinicians can decide to choose one or more of the six sources of information to make a rating. Lay interviewers, without experience in the mental health field, can be trained to use a fully structured interview such as the Diagnostic Interview Schedule (DIS) with a high level of reliability. However, lay interviewers cannot use the PIV process. An experienced clinician, along with utilizing the PIV process, usually produces a reasonably valid assessment of psychopathology. The SCIP 30 screening items and 200 psychopathology items compose a standardized and comprehensive collection ("a boilerplate") of adult psychopathology, which facilitates the clinician's ability to use the PIV process and evaluate the presence or absence of psychopathology during the clinical interview. At the end of the interview, the clinician should be able to describe the patient's mental status and measure the main psychopathology domains.

Conclusions

The journey of psychiatric interviewing starts with greeting the patient and ends with a provisional diagnosis and initiation of a treatment plan. The information technology revolution of the twenty-first century has had a direct impact on psychiatric interviewing. More information is requested and expected by insurers, accreditation agencies, patients, and the public. To ease the burden on clinicians, self-administered scales, completed by patients, have been developed for use in a variety of settings (see Chap. 4). The emergence of MBC, the need to use reliable measures to make individualized decisions, and the need for collaboration among different providers are important developments that require collecting more information from the patient. The clinician is then tasked with the challenge of balancing the need to engage the patient in the therapeutic process (the art of interviewing) and the need to collect more data (the science of interviewing) in order to fulfill clinical, research, and billing purposes.

References

1. Shea, S. C. (1998). *Psychiatric interviewing: The art of understanding*. W.B. Saunders.
2. Carlat, D. J. (1999). *The psychiatric interview*. Lippincott Williams & Wilkins.
3. Aboraya, A., Nasrallah, H., Muvvala, S., El-Missiry, A., Mansour, H., Hill, C., Elswick, D., & Price, E. C. (2016). The standard for clinicians' interview in psychiatry (SCIP): A clinician-administered tool with categorical, dimensional, and numeric output-conceptual development, design, and description of the SCIP. *Innovations in Clinical Neuroscience, 13*, 31–77.
4. Spitzer, R. L., Williams, J. B., Gibbon, M., & First, M. B. (1992). The Structured Clinical Interview for DSM-III-R (SCID). I: History, rationale, and description. *Archives of General Psychiatry, 49*, 624–629.
5. Wing, J., Babor, T., Brugha, T., Burke, J., Cooper, J. E., Giel, R., Jablenski, A., Regier, D., & Sartorius, N. (1990). SCAN. Schedules for clinical assessment in neuropsychiatry. *Archives of General Psychiatry, 47*, 589–593.
6. Ustun, T. B., & Tien, A. Y. (1995). Recent developments for diagnostic measures in psychiatry. *Epidemiologic Reviews, 17*, 210–220.

Chapter 8
Epidemiological Concepts and Measures in Psychiatry

This chapter reviews important basic epidemiological concepts (reliability, validity, and types of measures used in psychiatry).

Epidemiological Concepts

Reliability and Validity

Reliability: Reliability is the consistency and stability of a measurement [1]. Three important types of reliability are described in the literature:

Internal consistency refers to the extent to which individual items are consistent with each other and reflect a single underlying construct [2]. Researchers investigate the correlations between individual items when examining the internal consistency reliability of a rating scale. **Cronbach's alpha** is a statistical measure of internal consistency reliability [3–5]. Cronbach's alpha considers the mean inter-item correlation between the items and its value increases as the average inter-item correlation, and the number of items increase [4]. The reliability of a scale is considered good if Cronbach's alpha is greater than 0.7, moderate if alpha ranges between 0.5 and 0.7, and poor if alpha is less than 0.5 [5].

Inter-rater reliability is the degree to which a measure yields stable scores when administered by different interviewers who are rating the same patient [2]. Inter-rater reliability was used in the SCIP project when patients were interviewed by two or more interviewers at the same time in the same room. The lead interviewer conducted the interview and the other interviewers observed and rated the items during the interview. When the interview concluded, observing interviewers were allowed to ask clarifying questions if needed. All interviewers rated the patient's responses independently and were not allowed to discuss their ratings.

A. S. Aboraya, *Manual for the Standard for Clinicians' Interview in Psychiatry (SCIP)*, Advances in Mental Health and Addiction,
https://doi.org/10.1007/978-3-030-94930-3_8

Inter-rater reliability was measured for the SCIP items using the Kappa statistic [6]. Another method of establishing inter-rater reliability occurs when two or more interviewers watch a videotaped interview of a patient and rate the items independently.

Test-retest reliability is the degree to which a measure yields stable scores when completed at different points in time with patients who are assumed to have maintained their clinical status on the domains being assessed [2]. In the test-retest design, the patient is interviewed once by an interviewer and interviewed again (after a reasonably short period) by the same person, or by a different interviewer. The test-retest design was used in the SCID project [7, 8]. **Both inter-rater and test-retest reliabilities can be measured by the Kappa statistic (K)**, which calculates the proportion of agreement when corrected for chance agreement [9–11]. In general, Kappa values greater than 0.7 indicate good agreement, Kappa values between 0.5 and 0.7 indicate fair agreement, and Kappa values less than 0.5 indicate poor agreement [8].

Validity refers to examining the approximate truth or falsity of scientific propositions [12]. A similar definition of validity is the extent to which obtained measures approximate values of the "true" state of nature [13]. In other words, validity is a representation of "truth" or "ultimate criterion" or "gold standard" as determined by "experts" in the field at one point in time. If experts in the field agree that object A is the ultimate true gold standard, other objects (B, C, D …) will strive to be like A, the true gold standard. By applying this concept in psychiatry, we can identify three types of validity: criterion, content, and construct validity.

Criterion validity is the degree of correlation between a new measure and an established ultimate criterion ("gold standard") measure [2]. Due to the absence of "biological makers" or "definite diagnostic tests" for most mental disorders, expert consensus is often used as the ultimate criterion or the gold standard. Experts may agree that a diagnosis made by experienced psychiatrists who interviewed the patient and family, reviewed the records, and performed necessary labs and neuroimaging is sufficient to establish a valid psychiatric diagnosis. If we develop a screening test to diagnose mental disorders, the validity of the screening test is measured against the psychiatrist's diagnosis, the "gold standard" diagnosis. We can create a 2 × 2 table as follows:

	Psychiatrist diagnosis (gold standard) +	Psychiatrist diagnosis (gold standard) –
Screening test diagnosis +	A	B
Screening test diagnosis -	C	D

Sensitivity is the ability of the test to correctly identify those who have a disease (A/A + C) [14].

Specificity is the ability of the test to correctly identify those who do not have the disease (D/B + D).

Positive predictive value is the proportion of patients who test positive for a disease who actually have the disease (A/A + B).

Negative predictive value is the proportion of patients who test negative for a disease who do not actually have the disease (D/C + D).

Content validity is the extent to which the instrument assesses all relevant or important content or domains [2]. If experts in the field agree that delusions, hallucinations, and disorganized thoughts are the relevant domains of schizophrenia symptoms, then the content validity of a scale designed to assess schizophrenia is measured by the inclusion of symptoms of delusions (such as delusions of paranoia, grandiosity, and reference), hallucinations (auditory, visual, olfactory, etc.), and disorganized thoughts (tangentiality, loose associations, etc.). The diagnostic criteria for psychiatric disorders established by the DSM further facilitate the ability to measure the content validity of a scale or a diagnostic interview [1].

Construct validity was first proposed by Cronbach and Meehl in 1955 and has since become widely accepted by scientists [15, 16]. Construct validity is a complicated process of validating theoretical constructs as proposed by scientists and clinicians. Construct validity is especially important in psychology and psychiatry because we deal with behaviors, traits, and feelings, which are entities that cannot be measured directly. The process of establishing construct validity consists of five steps: careful theory specification, hypothesis derivation and testing, developing a sound research design, examining the degree to which observations confirm hypotheses, and ongoing revisions of both theory and measures [16]. The process of establishing construct validity is complex and involves multiple studies, different methods and designs, and different samples and settings. Developing construct validity may also involve content and criterion validity to further evaluate the hypothetical construct in question. Consequently, there is no single measure of construct validity [17]. A simple definition of construct validity is the extent to which the measure of interest is related to other theoretically related concepts [18]. Ultimately, construct validity boils down to the circumstantial evidence for the usefulness of the construct or the hypothesis under study [18].

In 1970, Robins and Guze articulated the elements of construct validity in psychiatry by proposing five phases to achieve a valid classification of mental disorders: clinical description, laboratory study, exclusion of other disorders, follow-up study, and family study. They applied the criteria to schizophrenia and concluded that "good prognosis schizophrenia" is not "mild schizophrenia," but a different illness [19]. Other authors have added potential validators such as treatment response and diagnostic consistency over time [20–22].

The goals of validity in fields such as chemistry or physics differ from the goals of validity in medicine and psychiatry. In medicine, the clinician's ultimate goal is not a quest of knowledge per se, but the ability to use the available knowledge and skills to prevent and diminish patients' symptoms and impairment [20]. The search for an "ultimate criterion" or "gold standard" or "truth" may be elusive in many instances. For instance, after over a century of research, the true validity of a "schizophrenia spectrum" diagnosis, including whether it consists of one disease or several diseases, is still unknown. Despite this uncertainty, clinicians have been able to provide patients with many therapeutics (medications, therapy, family support, and others) to alleviate the symptoms experienced by patients and minimize the burden on their families. Clinicians continue research to improve the validity of the schizophrenia diagnosis and improve therapeutics for the illness. As Nunnally has said, "Validity usually is a matter of degree rather than an all-or-none property, and validation is an unending process" [18]. I proposed clinically oriented definitions of a validity criterion and gold standard with regard to psychiatric diagnoses. **Validity criterion** is any knowledge, method (such as rating scale or structured interview), or procedure (such as blood test, lumbar puncture, or MRI) that can improve the accuracy of measurement for a disease, syndrome, or disorder; help to rule out other diseases, syndromes, or disorders in the differential diagnosis; or validate a provisional diagnosis of the disease, syndrome, or disorder [23]. **The gold standard in diagnosis** is the standard that utilizes all validity criteria available at the time. In medicine and psychiatry, clinicians should use all available validity criteria to obtain the most accurate diagnosis [24]. Validity is a relative phenomenon, and any knowledge provided by the validity criteria helps researchers and clinicians to validate the construct of the disease, syndrome, or disorder. The psychiatrist who uses his or her clinical skills along with a rating scale can provide a more accurate diagnosis (with greater content validity) relative to a psychiatrist who uses clinical skills alone. Similarly, for example, the neurologist who uses clinical examination, lumbar puncture, and MRI can provide a more accurate diagnosis of multiple sclerosis when compared to a neurologist who uses clinical examination alone.

Validation of diagnostic interviews can be conducted by comparing the agreement between a diagnosis produced by the new instrument and a diagnosis produced by an existing instrument, using Kappa statistic. Another method of validation is to calculate the sensitivity and specificity of the new instrument's diagnosis against the diagnosis of the established instrument or method (i.e., criterion validity). Both methods of validation were used to validate the Mini-International Neuropsychiatric Interview (MINI) and the Standard for Clinicians' Interview in Psychiatry (SCIP) [25, 26].

In the SCIP project, the validity of psychiatric diagnoses produced by the SCIP interview was measured against the psychiatric diagnoses produced by the experienced clinician (EC) and diagnoses produced by the Schedules for Clinical Assessment in Neuropsychiatry (SCAN) [27]. The experienced clinician (EC) diagnoses were done by the unit attending, a Board Certified psychiatrist with 6 years of experience after residency training. The attending examined and treated the patients from admission to discharge at one unit of the William R. Sharpe, Jr. Hospital. The attending ordered psychological testing, labs, and imaging procedures as clinically indicated. The attending interviewed the patients several times a week and may have spoken or met with family members during their hospital stay. The attending discharged the patients when they became stable and dictated discharge summaries. The experienced clinician (EC) diagnoses as dictated in the discharge summaries were used as gold standard diagnoses in the SCIP study. The total number of patients diagnosed by the EC was 80. The author of the manual is a SCAN trainer, and he interviewed 31 patients using the SCAN interview. A total of 31 patients interviewed and diagnosed by the SCAN were combined with the 80 patients who were assessed and diagnosed by the experienced clinician, and both methods of diagnosis were considered to be gold standard diagnoses (111 patients altogether). The same 111 patients were interviewed by other SCIP investigators using the SCIP interview. The SCIP interviewers, the SCAN interviewer, and the attending were blind to each other's diagnoses. The combined EC and SCAN diagnoses allowed a large enough sample size to calculate stable Kappa, sensitivities, and specificities for the 13 main psychiatric diagnoses. The agreement between the SCIP diagnoses and the gold standard diagnoses was calculated using the Kappa statistic. Table 8.1 shows the base rate for each disorder, the number of positive diagnoses (a minimum of ten diagnoses altogether by either rater), the values of stable Kappa, and the standard error (SE) of each Kappa for 13 main psychiatric diagnoses. Kappa was poor (less than 0.5) for three diagnoses: panic, bipolar I, and mixed and schizoaffective disorders. Kappa was fair to good (greater than 0.5) for ten diagnoses: generalized anxiety, posttraumatic stress, major depression, bipolar I, schizophrenia, and alcohol, cannabis, cocaine, opioid, and sedative use disorders. In general, Kappa was fair to good for 77% of the main psychiatric diagnoses. Table 8.1 presents the

Table 8.1 Base rate, number of positive diagnoses, Kappa, Kappa standard error (SE), sensitivity and specificity of SCIP diagnoses against the gold standard diagnoses (diagnoses generated by the SCAN interview and the expert clinician) in patients at the William R. Sharpe, Jr. Hospital

	Diagnosis	Base rate (%)	Number of positive diagnoses	Kappa[a]	SE	Sensitivity (%)	Specificity (%)
1	Generalized anxiety disorder	4.5	11	0.6	0.09	100	94.3
2	Panic disorder with and without agoraphobia	7.2	15	0.45	0.09	62.5	93.2
3	Posttraumatic stress disorder	8.1	11	0.68	0.09	66.7	98
4	Major depression	11	21	0.54	0.09	75	90.9
5	Bipolar I disorder with/without psychosis	9	18	0.51	0.09	70	92.1
6	Bipolar I disorder, mixed, with/without psychosis	5.4	10	0.3	0.09	33.3	96.2
7	Schizoaffective (depressed and bipolar type)	16	20	0.46	0.09	38.9	97.8
8	Schizophrenia	18	30	0.68	0.09	90	89
9	Alcohol use disorder	27	38	0.69	0.09	80	90.1
10	Cannabis use disorder	14	20	0.61	0.09	62.5	95.8
11	Cocaine use disorder	4.5	13	0.52	0.08	100	92.5
12	Opioid use disorder	7.2	13	0.74	0.09	100	95.1
13	Sedative use disorder	6.3	10	0.54	0.09	57.1	97.1

[a]Kappa values were calculated based upon 111 interviews

sensitivities and specificities of the SCIP diagnoses against the gold standard diagnoses. Sensitivities and specificities of SCIP diagnoses against the gold standard diagnoses were poor (less than 50%) in 8%, fair (between 50% and 70%) in 19.0%, and good (greater than 70%) in 73.00%.

In psychiatry, it is common to develop a short screening test (questionnaire) to diagnose a specific mental disorder and to validate the new screening test (screener) against an established criterion/gold standard diagnosis to establish criterion validity [28–31]. The Mini-Mental State Examination (MMSE) is a widely accepted brief screening test for cognitive function and takes 5–10 minutes to complete [30]. Patients who score 23 or less can be referred to psychiatrists who perform extensive clinical assessment, order neuropsychological assessment, and imaging to confirm a diagnosis of dementia. Borson (2003) developed a briefer cognitive screening test (Mini-Cog) composed of two simple tasks (three-item word memory and clock drawing) which takes 2–4 minutes to administer and showed that the Min-Cog has similar sensitivity (76% vs 79%) and specificity (89% vs 88%) compared with the MMSE [28]. Similarly, the Patient Health Questionnaires (PHQ-2 and PHQ-9) were developed to screen for depression in primary care settings [29].

Many adult psychiatric diagnoses have one or more "core," "gate," "necessary," or "stem" criteria that must be met to diagnose the mental disorders [32, 33]. For example, a major depressive episode has two core criteria: depressed mood and anhedonia. At least one of these criteria must be present to diagnose a major depressive episode. For a schizophrenia diagnosis, one or more of the three core criteria (delusions, hallucinations, and disorganized thoughts) is required to diagnose the disorder. For the main adult psychiatric diagnoses (generalized anxiety, panic, post-traumatic stress, major depressive, bipolar, schizoaffective, schizophrenia spectrum, alcohol use, and drug use disorders), there are 16 items that represent the core criteria of the main psychiatric diagnoses. The 16 core criteria are ideal to screen for the major adult psychiatric disorders. **The sensitivities and specificities of the SCIP 16 core screening items (CSI) when compared against the main psychiatric diagnoses are presented in** Table 8.2. Sensitivities and specificities of the SCIP 16 core screening items were good (greater than 70%) in 66% of the items, fair (between 50% and 70%) in 19% of the items, and poor (less than 50%) in 15% of the items. In sum, 85% (27 out of 32) of the sensitivities and specificities of the SCIP 16 core screening items were fair to good. The validity of the SCIP scales was described in our article on measurement-based care [34]. The validity of the SCIP diagnoses were described in detail in this manual and in another manuscript [26]. The validity of the SCIP core screening items are described in this manual. In sum, the SCIP instrument was validated at three levels: scales, diagnoses, and core screening items. Therefore, the SCIP can be considered one of the most validated instruments in the literature to date.

Table 8.2 Sensitivity and specificity of core screening items of the SCIP against psychiatric diagnoses in patients at the William R. Sharpe, Jr. Hospital and Chestnut Ridge Center in the United States

	SCIP item (Symptoms and signs)	Diagnosis	Sensitivity[a] (%)	Specificity[a] (%)
1	Generalized anxiety	Generalized anxiety disorder	81.5	89.6
2	Panic attack	Panic disorder with/without agoraphobia	91.7	92.4
3	Experience traumatic events	Posttraumatic stress disorder	87.7	86.6
4	Re-experience traumatic events	Posttraumatic stress disorder	83.1	95.3
5	Depressed mood	Major depressive disorder, single and recurrent (without psychotic features)	83.6	57.6
6	Anhedonia	Major depressive disorder, single and recurrent (without psychotic features)	63	77.7
7	Elated mood	Bipolar I disorder, with/without psychosis	47.6	86.6
8	Irritable mood	Bipolar I disorder, with/without psychosis	54.8	82.7
9	Mixed mood (same day mood changes)	Bipolar I disorder, mixed, with/without psychosis	76.1	86.8
10	Paranoid delusions	Schizophrenia	61.3	73.8
11	Other delusions	Schizophrenia	41.9	89.9
12	Auditory hallucination	Schizophrenia	50	79.9
13	Visual hallucination	Schizophrenia	16.1	92.3
14	Disorganized thoughts	Schizophrenia	15.3	97
15	Alcohol problems	Alcohol abuse/dependence	63.3	94.3
16	Opioid problem	Opioid abuse/dependence	47.6	98.6

[a]Sensitivity and specificity were calculated based upon 697 interviews

Measures in Psychiatry

Rating Scales and Diagnostic Interviews

Patients with mental disorders present to mental health professionals with a variety of symptoms, seeking help to alleviate their suffering and prevent negative outcomes such as suicide, violence, and future disability. **Rating scales** are designed to measure domains of psychopathology, probe its severity, and evaluate the patient's response to treatment. As described in Chapter One, the first rating scales were developed by Thomas Moore in 1933 and continue to be used today, with hundreds of scales existing to measure many aspects of human psychology.

The science of classification of mental disorders has lagged behind the science of rating scales and expanded during the second half of the twentieth century due to the efforts of the World Health Organization (WHO) and the American Psychiatric Association (APA). The World Health Organization (WHO) published the

International Classification of Diseases (ICD), with the latest version (ICD-10) in 1993 [35]. In the United States, the American Psychiatric Association published the *Diagnostic and Statistical Manual of Mental Disorders* (DSM), with the latest version (*DSM-5*) in 2013 [36]. The publication of the *DSM-III* in 1980 and its widespread acceptance and use globally initiated the development of diagnostic interviews to diagnose mental disorders according to criteria proposed by the DSM and ICD. **Diagnostic interviews** vary from brief screening instruments to more detailed standardized diagnostic interviews (SDIs).

Types of rating scales: There are two types of rating scales: a clinician-administered (CA) scales and self-administered (SA) or self-report (SR) scales. Benefits and drawbacks to each type are noted below:

Pros of Clinician-Administered (CA) Scales

1. Clinician-administered (CA) scales are administered by clinicians who have knowledge and expertise with regard to mental disorders.
2. Clinicians may ask clarifying questions, give examples to the patient if needed, and probe further if the patient's response is inconsistent with available information [37].
3. Clinicians' ratings of symptoms may be more likely to be "valid" compared with self-report of symptoms by patients.

Cons of Clinician-Administered (CA) Scales

1. Clinicians often have their own set of biases based upon their background, theoretical orientation, and training.
2. Clinicians may overestimate the patient's improvement [38].
3. Clinicians must be trained to use and administer the scales.

Pros of Self-Administered (SA) Scales

1. Self-administered scales are inexpensive and efficient to administer, saving professional time needed for administration [39].
2. Patients are more likely to freely answer sensitive and private questions with SA scales.
3. Patients are more likely to freely report progress or lack of progress with SA scales. Patient self-report is universally acknowledged as a valid index of treatment outcome [40].

Cons of Self-Administered (SA) Scales

1. Patients completing SA scales may manipulate the answers for their own reasons. Patients may exaggerate symptoms to receive benefits or to avoid criminal responsibilities in forensic cases. Patients may minimize symptoms to please their providers.
2. Responses on SA scales will vary based upon the patients' reading abilities and level of education.
3. The correlation between self-administered scales and clinician-administered scales is high for anxiety and obsessive-compulsive and depressive disorders

[37, 38, 41]. However, psychotic patients may not be able to complete self-administered scales or assess their own condition [40].

Self-administered (SA) scales are completed by patients before they arrive to the clinic or while they are waiting to be seen in the office. Typically, SA scales are used in outpatient settings and CA scales are used in inpatient settings.

Table 8.3 presents the main 15 adult psychiatric diagnoses and a list of the non-SCIP scales that can be used clinically for each of the disorders. We avoided the

Table 8.3 Recommended rating scales in clinical settings for the main 15 adult psychiatric diagnoses

Psychiatric disorder	Name of the scale and reference	Type of scale (CA/SA)[a]
1. Generalized anxiety	Hamilton anxiety rating scale (HAM-A) 14-item scale [44]	CA
Generalized anxiety	Clinical anxiety Scale (CAS) (6 items from HAM-A) [45]	CA
Generalized anxiety	Clinically useful anxiety outcome Scale (CUXOS) [46]	SA
Generalized anxiety	Generalized anxiety disorder (GAD-7) [47]	SA
2. Panic	Panic disorder severity Scale (PDSS) [48]	CA
3. Phobias	Liebowitz social anxiety Scale [37, 49]	CA/SA
4. Obsessive-compulsive disorder	Yale-Brown obsessive compulsive scale (YBOCS) [50, 51]	CA/SA
5. Posttraumatic stress	Short PTSD rating Scale (SPRINT) [43]	CA
6. Major depressive	Quick inventory of depressive Symptomatology (clinician-rated) (QIDS-C16) [52]	CA
Major depressive	Quick inventory of depressive Symptomatology (self-report) (QIDS-SR16) [52]	SA
Major depressive	Patient health questionnaire (PHQ-9) [53]	SA
Major depressive	Clinically useful depression outcome Scale (CUDOS) [54]	SA
7. Bipolar	Young mania rating Scale (YMRS) [55]	CA
8. Schizophrenia	Psychotic symptom rating Scale (PSYRATS) [56]	CA
Schizophrenia	The brief negative symptom scale (BNSS) [57]	CA
9. Schizoaffective	Depression, mania, and psychotic scales	
10. Alcohol use	Alcohol use disorders identification Test (AUDIT) [58]	CA/SA
11. Drug use	Leeds dependence questionnaire (LDQ) [59]	SA
12. Attention deficit/hyperactivity	Adult ADHD self-report Scale (ASRS) [60, 61]	SA
13. Eating	Eating disorders diagnostic Scale (EDDS) [62]	SA
14. Personality	Standardized assessment of personality—Abbreviated scale (SAPAS) [63]	CA
15. Neurocognitive	The Mini-mental state Examination (MMSE) [30]	CA

[a] *CA* clinician-administered, *SA* self-administered

lengthy and time-consuming scales, as they are not practically feasible to use in clinical settings. As an example, the Clinician-Administered PTSD Scale (CAPS) [42] is considered a gold standard measure to assess and diagnose PTSD, but it takes an hour to administer and not practical to use in clinical settings [17]. The Short PTSD Rating Interview (SPRINT) takes approximately 10 minutes to complete and was included in Table 8.3 [43].

Types of Diagnostic Interviews

Diagnostic interviews vary from brief screening tools (screeners) to more detailed standardized diagnostic interviews (SDIs). Standardized diagnostic interviews (SDIs) are designed to interview the patient, assess symptoms, and diagnose mental disorders according to the diagnostic criteria of the DSM or ICD. Two types of SDIs are described: fully structured and semi-structured.

Fully structured diagnostic instruments are usually administered by lay interviewers after completing the required training. Questions and rules for processing each response are precisely specified [64]. Examples of the fully structured diagnostic tools are the WHO Composite International Diagnostic Interview (CIDI) and the Mini-International Neuropsychiatric Interview (MINI) [25, 65].

Semi-structured diagnostic instruments permit more flexible questions and probes and are typically administered by trained clinicians [64]. Semi-structured interviews allow for considerable variation in the interviewing style and allow clinicians to probe and make a clinical judgment whether the patient's symptoms meet the diagnostic criteria or not [8]. Examples of the semi-structured diagnostic instruments are the Schedules for Clinical Assessment in Neuropsychiatry (SCAN), the Structured Clinical Interview for DSM-IV Axis I Disorders (SCID-I), and the Standard for Clinicians' Interview in Psychiatry (SCIP) [6, 7, 27].

Demonstration of the WHO Composite International Diagnostic Interview

CIDI: Lay interviewers receive 1 or 2 weeks of training and follow detailed instructions on how to conduct the interview and code patients' responses.

Depression example: The first question is about periods of being sad or depressed.

- E1. (READ SLOWLY.) In the past 12 months, have you had a period of 2 weeks or longer when you felt sad or depressed or empty?
- 1. YES
- 5. NO GO TO E2
- 8. DK GO TO E2

- 9. REF GO TO E2
- E1a. Think of the 2 weeks during the past 12 months when this feeling was most persistent. During that 2-week period, did you feel sad or depressed or empty every day, nearly every day, most days, about half the days, or less than half the days? (PROBE DK: What's your best estimate? REPEAT RESPONSE CATEGORIES).
- 1. EVERY DAY, NEARLY EVERY DAY, MOST DAYS
- 4. ABOUT HALF THE DAYS GO TO E2
- 5. LESS THAN HALF THE DAYS GO TO E2
- 8. DK GO TO E2
- 9. REF GO TO E2.
- E2. (READ SLOWLY.) In the past 12 months, have you had a period of 2 weeks or longer when you lost interest in most things like work, hobbies, and other things you usually enjoy?
- 1. YES
- 5. NO GO TO E2.1
- 8. DK GO TO E2.1
- 9. REF GO TO E2.1.

Although this manual is devoted to the SCIP instrument and SCIP scales, clinicians who seek training in MBC need to know other types of scales and measures published in the literature for three main reasons:

A. There are hundreds of scales with good psychometric properties, and clinicians should choose the scales that they feel most comfortable with and that meet their needs in providing care. In Table 8.3, we list the non-SCIP scales that take a relatively short time to administer and can be used in clinical settings.

B. Even though the SCIP 18 CA scales and 15 SA scales cover most adult psychiatric disorders (generalized anxiety, panic, phobia, obsessive-compulsive, post-traumatic stress, depressive, bipolar, schizophrenia, schizoaffective, alcohol use, drug use, attention-deficit hyperactivity, and eating disorders), the SCIP scales do not cover neurocognitive disorders and personality disorders. Readers can choose published scales for neurocognitive and personality disorders such as the scales recommended in Table 8.3.

C. In addition to the measures of psychopathology (rating scales) and diagnostic instruments, the following are examples of other measures used in psychiatry:

   1. **Measures of disabilities:** The Sheehan Disability Scale (SDS) assesses disability across three domains: work, social life, and family life. The SDS is both self-administered and clinician-administered [66–68].
   2. **Measures of function:** The Duke Health Profile is a 17-item self-report measure of function that covers 5 domains: physical health, mental health, social health, perceived health, and disability [69].
   3. **Measures of quality of life:** The WHOQOL-BREF scale is a measure of quality of life across four domains: physical health, psychological health, social relationships, and environment [70].

4. **Measures of patient satisfaction with care:** The Client Satisfaction Questionnaire-8 (CSQ-8) is a self-administered scale with eight questions that measure satisfaction with care across four domains: quality of service, kind of service, outcome, and general satisfaction [71].
5. **Measures of Suicide:** Columbia Suicide Scale [72].
6. **Measures of self-harm:** The Inventory of Statements About Self-Injury (ISAS) is a measure of self-injury without the intent to die [73, 74].
7. **Measures of stress**: The Perceived Stress Scale (PSS) is a 14-item self-report questionnaire that measures the subjective interpretation of life events [75].
8. **Measures of adverse effects of treatment:** Such as the Barnes Akathisia Rating Scale (BARS) and Abnormal Involuntary Movement Scale (AIMS) [76, 77].

Readers are advised to read the *Handbook of Psychiatric Measures* (2000) by the American Psychiatric Association Task Force, chaired by A.J. Rush Jr., which includes more than 240 measures covering adult and child psychiatry disorders [78]. Another good reference for clinically useful scales is the *Handbook of Clinical Rating Scales and Assessment in Psychiatry and Mental Health* by Baer and Blais [17].

References

1. Eaton, W. W. (2012). *Public mental health*. Oxford University Press.
2. Alonso, A., Geys, H., Molenberghs, G., & Vangeneugden, T. (2002). Investigating the criterion validity of psychiatric symptom scales using surrogate marker validation methodology. *Journal of Biopharmaceutical Statistics, 12*, 161–178.
3. Cronbach, L. J. (1951). Coefficient alpha and the internal structure of tests. *Psychometrika, 16*, 297–334.
4. Carmines, E. G., & Zeller, R. A. (1979). *Reliability and validity assessment*. SAGE.
5. Schene, A. H., Koeter, M., van Wijngaarden, K. H. C., Leese, M., Ruggeri, M., White, I. R., & Vazquez-Barquero, J. L. (2000). Methodology of a multi-site reliability study. EPSILON study 3. European psychiatric services: Inputs linked to outcome domains and needs. *The British Journal of Psychiatry Supplement, 39*, s15–s20.
6. Aboraya, A., El-Missiry, A., Barlowe, J., John, C., Ebrahimian, A., Muvvala, S., Brandish, J., Mansour, H., Zheng, W., Chumber, P., Berry, J., Elswick, D., Hill, C., Swager, L., Abo Elez, W., Ashour, H., Haikal, A., Eissa, A., Rabie, M., ... Price, E. (2014). The reliability of the standard for clinicians' interview in psychiatry (SCIP): A clinician-administered tool with categorical, dimensional and numeric output. *Schizophrenia Research., 156*, 174–183.
7. Spitzer, R. L., Williams, J. B., Gibbon, M., & First, M. B. (1992). The structured clinical interview for DSM-III-R (SCID). I: History, rationale, and description. *Archives of General Psychiatry, 49*, 624–629.
8. Williams, J. B., Gibbon, M., First, M. B., Spitzer, R. L., Davies, M., Borus, J., Howes, M. J., Kane, J., Pope, H. G., Jr., Rounsaville, B., et al. (1992). The structured clinical interview for DSM-III-R (SCID). II. Multisite test-retest reliability. *Archives of General Psychiatry, 49*, 630–636.

9. Cohen, J. (1960). A coefficient of agreement for nominal scales. *Educational and Psychological Measurement., 20*, 37–46.
10. Fleiss, J. (1981). *Statistical methods for rates and proportions* (2nd ed.). Wiley.
11. Kraemer, H. P., Periyakoil, V. S., & Noda, A. (2002). Tutorial in biostatistics: Kappa coefficient in medical research. *Statistics in Medicine., 21*, 2109–2129.
12. Cook, T. D., & Campbell, D. T. (1979). *Quasi-experimentation: Design and analysis issues for field settings*. Rand McNally.
13. Hammersley, M. (1987). Some notes on the terms 'validity' and 'reliability'. *British Educational Research Journal., 13*, 73–81.
14. Gordis, L. (1996). *Epidemiology*. Saunders.
15. Cronbach, L. J., & Meehl, P. E. (1955). Construct validity in psychological tests. *Psychological Bulletin, 52*, 281–302.
16. Smith, G. T. (2005). On construct validity: Issues of method and measurement. *Psychological Assessment., 17*, 396–408.
17. Baer, L. (2015). *Handbook of clinical rating scales and assessment in psychiatry and mental health.* Humana Press.
18. Nunnally, J. C. (1978). *Psychometric theory*. McGraw-Hill.
19. Robins, E., & Guze, S. B. (1970). Establishment of diagnostic validity in psychiatric illness: Its application to schizophrenia. *The American Journal of Psychiatry, 126*, 983–987.
20. Kendell, R. E. (1989). Clinical validity. *Psychological Medicine, 19*, 45–55.
21. Kendler, K. S. (1980). The nosologic validity of paranoia (simple delusional disorder). *Archives of General Psychiatry, 37*, 699–706.
22. Kendler, K. S. (1990). Toward a scientific psychiatric nosology. *Strengths and Limitations. Arch Gen Psychiatry., 47*, 969–973.
23. Aboraya, A., & Compton, I. W. (2004). Biological markers and external validators in psychiatry: Progress report on the validity of psychiatric diagnosis. *eCOMMUNITY: International Journal of Mental Health and Addiction., 3*, 1–6.
24. Aboraya, A., France, C., Young, J., Curci, K., & Lepage, J. (2005). The validity of psychiatric diagnosis revisited: The clinician's guide to improve the validity of psychiatric diagnosis. *Psychiatry (Edgmont), 2*, 48–55.
25. Sheehan, D. V., Lecrubier, Y., Sheehan, K. H., Amorim, P., Janavs, J., Weiller, E., Hergueta, T., Baker, R., & Dunbar, G. C. (1998). The Mini-International Neuropsychiatric Interview (M.I.N.I.): The development and validation of a structured diagnostic psychiatric interview for DSM-IV and ICD-10. *The Journal of Clinical Psychiatry, 59*(Suppl 20), 22–33;quiz 34–57.
26. Aboraya, A. (2015). The validity results of the standard for clinicians' interview in psychiatry (SCIP). *Schizophrenia Bulletin., 41*, S103–S104.
27. Wing, J., Babor, T., Brugha, T., Burke, J., Cooper, J. E., Giel, R., Jablenski, A., Regier, D., & Sartorius, N. S. C. A. N. (1990). Schedules for clinical assessment in neuropsychiatry. *Archives of General Psychiatry, 47*, 589–593.
28. Borson, S., Scanlan, J. M., Chen, P., & Ganguli, M. (2003). The mini-cog as a screen for dementia: Validation in a population-based sample. *Journal of the American Geriatrics Society, 51*, 1451–1454.
29. Arroll, B., Goodyear-Smith, F., Crengle, S., Gunn, J., Kerse, N., Fishman, T., Falloon, K., & Hatcher, S. (2010). Validation of PHQ-2 and PHQ-9 to screen for major depression in the primary care population. *Annals of Family Medicine, 8*, 348–353.
30. Folstein, M. F., et al. (1975). "Mini-mental state" a practical method for grading the cognitive state of patients for the clinician. *Journal of Psychiatric Research, 12*, 189–198.
31. Kroenke, K., Spitzer, R. L., & Williams, J. B. (2003). The patient health questionnaire-2: Validity of a two-item depression screener. *Medical Care., 41*, 1284–1292.
32. Hea, W. (1999). Screening for mental disorders: Performance of the composite international diagnostic – Screener (CID–S). *International Journal of Methods in Psychiatric Research., 8*, 59–70.

33. Zimmerman, M., Gorlin, E., Dalrymple, K., & Chelminiski, I. (2017). A clinically useful screen for attention-deficit/hyperactivity disorder in adult psychiatric outpatients. *Annals of Clinical Psychiatry, 29*, 160–166.
34. Aboraya, A., Nasrallah, H. A., Elswick, D. E., Ahmed, E., Estephan, N., Aboraya, D., Berzingi, S., Chumbers, J., Berzingi, S., Justice, J., Zafar, J., & Dohar, S. (2018). Measurement-based care in psychiatry-past, present, and future. *Innovations in Clinical Neuroscience, 15*, 13–26.
35. WHO. (1993). *The ICD-10 classification of mental and behavioral disorders: Diagnostic criteria for research* (10th ed.). World Health Organization.
36. American Psychiatric Association (Ed.). (2013). *Diagnostic and statistical manual of mental disorders* (5th ed.). American Psychiatric Association.
37. Fresco, D. M., Coles, M. E., Heimberg, R. G., Liebowitz, M. R., Hami, S., Stein, M. B., & Goetz, D. (2001). The Liebowitz Social Anxiety Scale: A comparison of the psychometric properties of self-report and clinician-administered formats. *Psychological Medicine, 31*, 1025–1035.
38. Zimmerman, M., Walsh, E., Friedman, M., Boerescu, D. A., & Attiullah, N. (2018). Are self-report scales as effective as clinician rating scales in measuring treatment response in routine clinical practice? *Journal of Affective Disorders, 225*, 449–452.
39. Zimmerman, M., Chelminski, I., Young, D., Dalrymple, K., Walsh, E., & Rosenstein, L. (2014). A clinically useful self-report measure of the DSM-5 anxious distress specifier for major depressive disorder. *The Journal of Clinical Psychiatry, 75*, 601–607.
40. Bilsker, D., & Goldner, E. M. (2002). Routine outcome measurement by mental health-care providers: Is it worth doing? *Lancet, 360*, 1689–1690.
41. Federici, A., Summerfeldt, L. J., Harrington, J. L., McCabe, R. E., Purdon, C. L., Rowa, K., & Antony, M. M. (2010). Consistency between self-report and clinician-administered versions of the Yale-Brown Obsessive-Compulsive Scale. *Journal of Anxiety Disorders, 24*, 729–733.
42. Blake, D. D., Weathers, F. W., Nagy, L. M., Kaloupek, D. G., Gusman, F. D., Charney, D. S., & Keane, T. M. (1995). The development of a clinician-administered PTSD scale. *Journal of Traumatic Stress., 8*, 75–90.
43. Connor, K. M., & Davidson, J. R. (2001). SPRINT: A brief global assessment of post-traumatic stress disorder. *International Clinical Psychopharmacology., 16*, 279–284.
44. Hamilton, M. (1959). The assessment of anxiety states by rating. *The British Journal of Medical Psychology., 32*, 50–55.
45. Snaith, R. P., Baugh, S. J., Clayden, A. D., Husain, A., & Sipple, M. A. (1982). The clinical anxiety scale: An instrument derived from the Hamilton anxiety scale. *The British Journal of Psychiatry, 141*, 518–523.
46. Zimmerman, M., Chelminski, I., Young, D., & Dalrymple, K. (2010). A clinically useful anxiety outcome scale. *The Journal of Clinical Psychiatry, 71*, 534–542.
47. Spitzer, R. L., Kroenke, K., Williams, J. B., & Lowe, B. (2006). A brief measure for assessing generalized anxiety disorder: The GAD-7. *Archives of Internal Medicine, 166*, 1092–1097.
48. Shear, M. K., Brown, T. A., Barlow, D. H., Money, R., Sholomskas, D. E., Woods, S. W., Gorman, J. M., & Papp, L. A. (1997). Multicenter collaborative panic disorder severity scale. *The American Journal of Psychiatry., 154*, 1571–1575.
49. Liebowitz, M. R. (1987). Social phobia. *Modern Problems of Pharmacopsychiatry, 22*, 141–173.
50. Goodman, W. K., Price, L. H., Rasmussen, S. A., Mazure, C., Delgado, P., Heninger, G. R., & Charney, D. S. (1989). The Yale-Brown obsessive compulsive scale. II. Validity. *Archives of General Psychiatry, 46*, 1012–1016.
51. Goodman, W. K., Price, L. H., Rasmussen, S. A., Mazure, C., Fleischmann, R. L., Hill, C. L., Heninger, G. R., & Charney, D. S. (1989). The Yale-Brown obsessive compulsive scale. I. Development, use, and reliability. *Archives of General Psychiatry, 46*, 1006–1011.
52. Rush, A. J., Trivedi, M. H., Ibrahim, H. M., Carmody, T. J., Arnow, B., Klein, D. N., Markowitz, J. C., Ninan, P. T., Kornstein, S., Manber, R., Thase, M. E., Kocsis, J. H., & Keller, M. B. (2003). The 16-Item Quick Inventory of Depressive Symptomatology (QIDS), clinician rating (QIDS-C), and self-report (QIDS-SR): A psychometric evaluation in patients with chronic major depression. *Biological Psychiatry, 54*, 573–583.

53. Kroenke, K., Spitzer, R. L., & Williams, J. B. (2001). The PHQ-9: Validity of a brief depression severity measure. *Journal of General Internal Medicine., 16*, 606–613.
54. Zimmerman, M., Chelminski, I., McGlinchey, J. B., & Posternak, M. A. (2008). A clinically useful depression outcome scale. *Comprehensive Psychiatry, 49*, 131–140.
55. Young, R. C., Biggs, J. T., Ziegler, V. E., & Meyer, D. A. (1978). A rating scale for mania: Reliability, validity and sensitivity. *The British Journal of Psychiatry, 133*, 429–435.
56. Haddock, G., McCarron, J., Tarrier, N., & Faragher, E. B. (1999). Scales to measure dimensions of hallucinations and delusions: The psychotic symptom rating scales (PSYRATS). *Psychological Medicine, 29*, 879–889.
57. Kirkpatrick, B., Strauss, G. P., Nguyen, L., Fischer, B. A., Daniel, D. G., Cienfuegos, A., & Marder, S. R. (2011). The brief negative symptom scale: Psychometric properties. *Schizophrenia Bulletin, 37*, 300–305.
58. Bohn, M. J., Babor, T. F., & Kranzler, H. R. (1995). The Alcohol Use Disorders Identification Test (AUDIT): Validation of a screening instrument for use in medical settings. *Journal of Studies on Alcohol., 56*, 423–432.
59. Raistrick, D., Bradshaw, J., Tober, G., Weiner, J., Allison, J., & Healey, C. (1994). Development of the Leeds Dependence Questionnaire (LDQ): A questionnaire to measure alcohol and opiate dependence in the context of a treatment evaluation package. *Addiction, 89*, 563–572.
60. Adler, L., Kessler, R. C., & Spencer, T. (2003). *Adult ADHD self-report scale-v1.1 (ASRS-v1.1) symptoms checklist*. World Health Organization.
61. Kessler, R. C., Adler, L., Ames, M., Demler, O., Faraone, S., Hiripi, E., Howes, M. J., Jin, R., Secnik, K., Spencer, T., Ustun, T. B., & Walters, E. E. (2005). The World Health Organization Adult ADHD Self-Report Scale (ASRS): A short screening scale for use in the general population. *Psychological Medicine, 35*, 245–256.
62. Stice, E., Telch, C. F., & Rizvi, S. L. (2000). Development and validation of the eating disorder diagnostic scale: A brief self-report measure of anorexia, bulimia, and binge-eating disorder. *Psychological Assessment., 12*, 123–131.
63. Moran, P., Leese, M., Lee, T., Walters, P., Thornicroft, G., & Mann, A. (2003). Standardised Assessment of Personality – Abbreviated Scale (SAPAS): Preliminary validation of a brief screen for personality disorder. *The British Journal of Psychiatry, 183*, 228–232.
64. Rettew, D. C., Lynch, A. D., Achenbach, T. M., Dumenci, L., & Ivanova, M. Y. (2009). Meta-analyses of agreement between diagnoses made from clinical evaluations and standardized diagnostic interviews. *International Journal of Methods in Psychiatric Research, 18*, 169–184.
65. WHO: Compsite International Diagnostic Interview (CIDI). Geneva World Health Organization; 1990.
66. Arbuckle, R., Frye, M. A., Brecher, M., Paulsson, B., Rajagopalan, K., Palmer, S., & Degl', I. A. (2009). The psychometric validation of the Sheehan disability scale (SDS) in patients with bipolar disorder. *Psychiatry Research, 165*, 163–174.
67. Sheehan, D. (1983). *The anxiety disease*. Scribner's.
68. Sheehan, D. V., Harnett-Sheehan, K., & Raj, B. A. (1996). The measurement of disability. *International Clinical Psychopharmacology., 11*(Suppl 3), 89–95.
69. Parkerson, G. R., Jr., Broadhead, W. E., & Tse, C. K. (1990). The Duke Health Profile. A 17-item measure of health and dysfunction. *Medical Care., 28*, 1056–1072.
70. WHO. (1998). Development of the World Health Organization WHOQOL-BREF quality of life assessment. The WHOQOL Group. *Psychological Medicine, 28*, 551–558.
71. Larsen, D. L., Attkisson, C. C., Hargreaves, W. A., & Nguyen, T. D. (1979). Assessment of client/patient satisfaction: Development of a general scale. *Evaluation and Program Planning, 2*, 197–207.
72. Posner, K., Brown, G. K., Stanley, B., Brent, D. A., Yershova, K. V., Oquendo, M. A., Currier, G. W., Melvin, G. A., Greenhill, L., Shen, S., & Mann, J. J. (2011). The Columbia-suicide severity rating scale: Initial validity and internal consistency findings from three multisite studies with adolescents and adults. *The American Journal of Psychiatry., 168*, 1266–1277.

73. Glenn, C. R., & Klonsky, E. D. (2011). One-year test-retest reliability of the Inventory of Statements about Self-Injury (ISAS). *Assessment, 18*, 375–378.
74. Bildik, T., Somer, O., Kabukcu Basay, B., Basay, O., & Ozbaran, B. (2013). The validity and reliability of the Turkish version of the inventory of statements about self-injury. *Türk Psikiyatri Dergisi, 24*, 49–57.
75. Cohen, S., Kamarck, T., & Mermelstein, R. (1983). A global measure of perceived stress. *Journal of Health and Social Behavior, 24*, 385–396.
76. Barnes, T. R. (1989). A rating scale for drug-induced akathisia. *The British Journal of Psychiatry, 154*, 672–676.
77. Guy, W., Ban, T. A., & Wilson, W. H. (1986). The prevalence of abnormal involuntary movements among chronic schizophrenics. *International Clinical Psychopharmacology., 1*, 134–144.
78. Rush, A. J., Jr. (2000). *Handbook of psychiatric measures*. American Psychiatric Association.

Chapter 9
Measurement-Based Care (MBC) Training Curriculum for Mental Health Professionals and Psychiatry Residency Programs

This chapter describes the first comprehensive training curriculum designed for clinicians and psychiatry residents to use scales in clinical settings. As described earlier, the SCIP is the only instrument that includes 18 clinician-administered scales and 15 self-administered scales covering most adult symptom domains: anxiety, obsessions, compulsions, posttraumatic stress, depression, mania, delusions, hallucinations, disorganized thoughts, aggression, negative symptoms, alcohol use, drug use, attention deficit, hyperactivity, anorexia, binge eating, and bulimia. This unique advantage of the SCIP instrument allowed for the development of the first comprehensive curriculum for training clinicians to use scales in clinical settings as described in the chapter. Guidelines for the timing and frequency of scale use in major psychiatric disorders are described at the end of the chapter.

Introduction

Measurement-based care (MBC) is the systematic administration of symptom rating scales and the use of results to drive clinical decision-making at the level of the individual patient [1]. Recent research shows the superiority of MBC compared to usual standard care (USC) in improving patient outcomes [1–4]. A recent, blind-rater and randomized trial by Guo et al. (2015) showed that MBC is more effective than USC both in achieving response and remission and in reducing the time to response and remission [5]. As discussed in Chap. 6, there are barriers to implementing MBC in clinical practice, which made it difficult for practicing psychiatrists and clinicians to implement MBC for decades [4, 6–9]. Consequently, the Standard for Clinicians' Interview in Psychiatry (SCIP) was developed as a measurement-based care tool and was designed to overcome these barriers and make it more feasible to implement MBC in practice [10–15]. The SCIP scales,

A. S. Aboraya, *Manual for the Standard for Clinicians' Interview in Psychiatry (SCIP)*, Advances in Mental Health and Addiction,
https://doi.org/10.1007/978-3-030-94930-3_9

whether clinician-administered (CA) or self-administered (SA), meet the criteria for MBC because they are efficient, reliable, and valid and reflect the decision-making process by which clinicians assess psychiatric disorders [14]. This MBC training curriculum is designed for psychiatrists and mental health professionals such as psychologists, therapists, clinical social workers, counselors, nurses, nurse practitioners, physician assistants, mental health researchers, and others. To ensure that future generations of psychiatrists have adequate training in MBC, a training curriculum for psychiatry residency programs was also developed by the author and is described in this chapter. **To our knowledge, this is the first comprehensive training curriculum designed for clinicians to implement MBC in practice.**

Trainer and Trainee Qualifications

Trainer qualifications Practicing clinicians have tremendous experience in assessing and treating patients with mental disorders. However, most clinicians have not had formal training in MBC. Clinicians and researchers who have knowledge and degrees in research methodology and who have been involved in mental health research (such as clinical trials) are "trainers" by definition. Clinicians who learn and practice the MBC curriculum described below are qualified to be MBC trainers upon the completion of the MBC training requirements.

Trainee qualifications Mental health professionals include psychiatrists, psychiatry residents, clinical psychologists, therapists, clinical social workers, counselors, nurses, nurse practitioners, physician assistants, mental health researchers, and others. At least 2 years of clinical experience, including interviewing skills, and good knowledge of DSM and ICD criteria are recommended as basic qualifications. Experience may involve a variety of settings: inpatient, outpatient, day hospital, or another setting that cares for patients with mental disorders.

MBC training requirements Three requirements need to be fulfilled to complete MBC training:

A. Basic knowledge in three areas: psychopathology assessment, psychiatric interviewing basics, and epidemiological concepts and measures in psychiatry. Readers of the manual can find this information in Chaps. 3, 7, and 8.
B. Watching and practicing ratings of the 12 videotaped films included in the manual.
C. Passing a competency test for MBC training as outlined in Appendix IV.

Components of the Training Curriculum

There are four components of the training curriculum:

1. Principles of rating symptoms and signs.
2. Psychiatric interviewing basics.
3. Epidemiological concepts and types of measures in psychiatry.
4. Training practice in scale use.

Readers of this manual should have finished the first three components of the curriculum: principles of rating symptoms and signs (Chap. 3), psychiatric interviewing basics (Chap. 7), and epidemiological concepts and types of measures in psychiatry (Chap. 8). The training practice in scale use is achieved by watching the 12 videotaped interviews available to the readers of the manual. The 12 full interview films are Video 10.1 (Expert Ratings), Video 10.2 (Panic and Depression), Video 10.3 (ADHD and Depression), Video 10.4 (Alcohol Use Disorder), Video 10.5 (Posttraumatic Stress Disorder), Video 10.6 (Eating Disorders), Video 10.7 (Psychosis and Mania), Video 10.8 (Anxiety and Panic), Video 10.9 (Narcotic Use Disorder and Depression), Videos 10.10, 10.11, and 10.12. Clinicians who are seeking MBC training (trainees) should watch Video 10.1 (Expert Rating) first. Then, trainees can watch the eight videos (Videos 10.2, 10.3, 10.4, 10.5, 10.6, 10.7, 10.8, and 10.9) in any sequence. Each video has three parts: introduction, patient interview, and the expert ratings. Trainees are advised to watch the introduction and the patient interview first and make their own ratings of the interview. Trainees can then watch the expert ratings and compare their own ratings, exploring and explaining any differences. Trainees are expected to rate the last three videos (Videos 10.10, 10.11, and 10.12) on their own and to discuss their ratings with other clinicians.

The SCIP scales and SCIP principles of psychopathology assessment are the focus of this training curriculum. Even if a clinician will be using non-SCIP scales in his/her research project or clinical settings, the first three components of the curriculum (principles of rating symptoms and signs, psychiatric interviewing basics, and epidemiological concepts and measures in psychiatry) are very useful to any clinician, especially those who have minimal or no background in research or epidemiological concepts. If a clinician or a researcher is recruited to do a specific project using a specific tool, such as the Positive and Negative Syndrome Scale (PANSS), the clinician will need to meet the specific training requirements of the PANSS [16]. In Chap. 8, Table 8.3, a list of the non-SCIP scales that can be used clinically for each of the main 15 adult psychiatric diagnoses was presented. For clinicians who are in practice, they can achieve MBC training by reading and practicing the four components of the curriculum as described in the manual. The next step for clinicians is to implement MBC and practice using the scales with their own patients. It is also important to mention that clinicians seeking MBC training are expected to read more relevant articles and books on psychopathology assessment, scales, diagnostic interviews, and types of measures used in psychiatry.

To obtain a formal MBC trainer certificate and 12 continuing medical education (CME) hours, trainees need to complete the following 5 steps:

1. Trainees read the SCIP manual with a focus on Chaps. 3, 7, and 8.
2. Trainees watch Videos 10.1, 10.2, 10.3, 10.4, 10.5, 10.6, 10.7, 10.8, 10.9, and 10.10 and practice ratings by comparing their ratings to the expert ratings.
3. Trainees watch Videos 10.11 and 10.12 and rate positive psychopathology items as it was done in the first ten videos.
4. Trainees complete the MBC competency test outlined in Appendix IV.
5. Trainees send the ratings of Videos 10.11 and 10.12 and the completed MBC competency test to the address in Appendix IV.

Experts will grade trainees' performance and send the MBC certificate and the 12 CME credits to the trainees who pass the evaluation.

MBC Training Curriculum for Psychiatry Residency Programs

As mentioned earlier, one of the important barriers to MBC implementation is the lack of MBC training curriculums available for clinicians. Lack of training was listed among the top two barriers to using MBC for psychiatry residents and faculty [6, 17]. Psychiatry residency training programs do not have specific requirements to evaluate training residents in the use of MBC during residency [18]. M. Arbuckle (2013) was the first educator to develop an MBC curriculum and train third-year residents to screen and monitor patients with depression using the Patient Health Questionnaire (PHQ-9) scale [19]. Given the fact that psychiatry residents are the future pioneers in the mental health field, incorporating MBC in psychiatry residency programs offers a unique opportunity to enhance knowledge and promote the adoption of MBC [4]. However, the implementation of an MBC curriculum in psychiatry residency must consider the special circumstances of residency programs, including the time constraints of residents' schedules, the rotation of residents in other specialties, the didactics required to meet program accreditation requirements, and other factors. Therefore, the MBC curriculum for clinicians described above was adapted for implementation in psychiatry residency programs. The author of the manual led the implementation of MBC in residency programs at West Virginia University (WVU) and Delaware Psychiatric Center (DPC) in 2019 and is ongoing. This is a summary of MBC training curriculum adapted for psychiatry residency.

Principles of Using the MBC Scales in Psychiatry Residency Training

The following principles are recommended to ensure that the implementation of MBC curriculum does not affect the normal operation of clinical care:

1. First and most importantly, clinicians (including attendings and psychiatry residents) are the architects of patient care. Clinicians conduct comprehensive assessments of patients including etiological, medical, social, environmental, and other factors that may contribute to mental disorders. They subsequently use this information to formulate diagnosis(es) and initiate treatment plans. The use of scales and measures is not intended to replace clinical judgment [4]. Rather, measures are one tool, among many, that clinicians may use to improve their quality of care.
2. Residents will use the scales with all appropriate patients with the goal of improving patient care. Consequently, no Institutional Review Board (IRB) approval or consent is necessary.
3. Residents can choose to use the scales with patients who they think will benefit from them most. Some patients who tend to exaggerate or minimize symptoms or who are especially uncooperative may not benefit from using the scales. Patients with limited cognitive abilities, such as patients with Alzheimer's disease or intellectual developmental disorders (IDDs), may not be appropriate for using the scales.
4. Residents will make every effort to use the scales when time and opportunity permit. In certain busy rotations and emergency situations, residents may not have time to use the scales, which is totally acceptable.
5. Recommendations for the timing and frequency of scale use with various diagnoses are outlined below. However, residents should decide on the timing and frequency of scale use during individual encounters based upon the patient's unique conditions, response to treatment, overall progress, and setting (inpatient, day hospital, or outpatient). In other words, scale use is individualized.
6. Only self-administered scales will be used in outpatient settings due to time limitations. The patient may complete the self-administered scale while he/she is in the waiting area. The resident can also give the scale to the patient in the office to complete while the resident is discussing the case with the attending. In both situations, the resident will not spend extra time administering the scales. The patient's completed self-administered scales will be available for the resident to use in clinical decisions pertaining to the patient. The SCIP scales have been uploaded into Epic electronic health records (EHR) at WVU, and the scales are completed electronically.
7. Clinician-administered scales are ideal for use in inpatient settings. Ideally, a scale is administered upon admission and is repeated weekly and upon discharge. For example, a patient admitted due to severe depression and a suicide attempt will require the SCIP depression scale or the PHQ-9 upon admission. These measures would be repeated weekly and prior to discharge to monitor the patient's progress.

8. Residents should use their skills of rapport-building, empathy, and flexibility in order to avoid a rigid interview. The resident may choose to interview the patient without using a computer. Following the encounter, the clinician may enter the scale data into the electronic health records (EHR).
9. Residents should not schedule patients only to administer scales. Scale administration should follow the usual patient schedule and should not increase the frequency of patients' visits.

MBC Teaching Materials

The four components of the training curriculum described above were reorganized in the following format for residency programs: 2 instruction manuals, 4 self-reading lectures, and the same 12 videotaped interviews (the same 12 video films mentioned above). The two instruction manuals are the SCIP instruction manual, which describes the SCIP method of psychiatric assessment, and the MBC instruction manual for residency programs, which describes the residents' responsibilities and expectations in MBC implementation [11].

The four self-reading lectures were prepared by the first author and cover the first three components of the curriculum (principles of rating symptoms and signs, psychiatric interviewing basics, and epidemiological concepts and types of measures in psychiatry). The titles of the four self-reading lectures are as follows:

1. The psychiatric interview contributions to MBC
2. Measures in psychiatry
3. Descriptive psychopathology
4. MBC tools

The four self-reading lectures cover topics including measures in psychiatry, psychiatric interview contributions to MBC, descriptive psychopathology, screening of psychopathology, types of psychopathology, principles of assessment of symptoms and signs, evaluation of distress and function, stages of psychiatric diagnosis, advantages of MBC, barriers to MBC, criteria of MBC tools, clinician-administered scales, self-administered scales, and examples of MBC tools.

All MBC teaching materials (2 instruction manuals, 4 self-reading lectures, and 12 videotaped interviews) should be saved on the shared drive of the institution so that all residents and attendings can have access to the MBC teaching materials.

Annual Learning and Implementation of MBCs

First-Year Residents.
MBC self-reading: The SCIP Instruction Manual (1 hour of reading) and Video 10.1 (45 minutes video).

MBC didactics: None.

MBC scale practice: None.

Second-Year Residents.
MBC self-reading: Self-reading lecture #1 (psychiatric interview contributions to MBC) and self-reading lecture #2 (measures in psychiatry). Both self-reading lectures take 2 hours of reading in 1 year.

MBC didactics: Two didactic lectures per year (review of MBC principles).

MBC scale practice: Second-year resident can try practice scales with two patients per 1-month rotation on inpatient units (e.g., adult and dual diagnosis units).

Third-Year Residents.
MBC self-reading: Self-reading lecture #3 (descriptive psychopathology) and self-reading lecture #4 (MBC tools). Both self-reading lectures take 2 hours of reading in 1 year.

MBC didactics: Two didactic lectures per year (review of MBC principles and residents' experience in using scales).

MBC scale practice: Residents choose two appropriate patients to complete the self-administered scales per week in the outpatient clinic.

Fourth-year residents Senior residents usually do electives and see patients in different settings (inpatients, day hospitals, and outpatients). Fourth-year residents should use the scales more often with appropriate patients and when time permits.

The main goal of MBC implementation in residency is to teach residents the principles of MBC and give them a chance to practice scales when they have the time and the appropriate patients. The hope is that when they finish residency and launch their career, MBC use will be part of their approach to comprehensive patient assessment and care.

Recommendations for the Timing and Frequency of Using Scales

In general, a scale can be administered as a baseline assessment even if the patient is stable and has no symptoms or minimal symptoms. Later on, if the same patient develops new symptoms, experiences a relapse of symptoms, or has a change in the mental status, the clinician repeats the scale or use a different scale. If the clinician decides to start the patient on a new medication (e.g., for a major depressive episode), the clinician needs to administer a depression scale to measure the depressive episode. The clinician can repeat the depression scale on the next visit or 6–8 weeks later to assess progress.

Detailed recommendations for the timing and frequency of scale use with different psychiatric disorders are presented in Table 9.1. It is important to remember that the timing and frequency will vary across patients, even among those with the same diagnosis. Therefore, the use of scales is individualized.

Table 9.1 Guidelines for the timing and frequency of using the MBC scales

Diagnosis	Scale(s)	When to administer the scale(s)
Generalized anxiety	SCIP anxiety scale	**Outpatient setting (self-administered scales)** 1. Baseline or first assessment opportunity 2. Every 6 months 3. Each time the patient starts a new antianxiety medication 4. Repeat 6–8 weeks from starting a new antianxiety medication. Typically, that will be the next outpatient scheduled visit 5. When there is a change in mental status or the clinician thinks there is a need to repeat the anxiety scale
Major depression	SCIP depression scale	**Outpatient setting (self-administered scales)** 1. Baseline or first assessment opportunity 2. Every 6 months 3. Each time the patient starts a new antidepressant 4. Repeat 6–8 weeks from starting a new antidepressant medication. Typically, that will be the next outpatient scheduled visit 5. When there is a change in mental status or the clinician thinks there is a need to repeat the depression scale **Inpatient or day hospital setting** 1. Upon admission to inpatient or day hospital 2. Upon discharge from inpatient or day hospital
Bipolar disorder	SCIP mania scale	**Outpatient setting (self-administered scales)** 1. Baseline or first assessment opportunity 2. Every 6 months 3. Each time the patient starts a mood stabilizer 4. Repeat 6–8 weeks from starting a new mood stabilizer. Typically, that will be the next outpatient scheduled visit 5. When there is a change in mental status or the clinician thinks there is a need to repeat the mania scale **Inpatient or day hospital setting** 1. Upon admission to inpatient or day hospital 2. Upon discharge from inpatient or day hospital

(continued)

Table 9.1 (continued)

Diagnosis	Scale(s)	When to administer the scale(s)
Obsessive compulsive disorder (OCD)	SCIP OCD scale	**Outpatient setting (self-administered scales)** 1. Baseline or first assessment opportunity 2. Every 6 months 3. Each time the patient starts a new medication for OCD 4. Repeat 6–8 weeks from starting a new medication for OCD. Typically, that will be the next outpatient scheduled visit 5. When there is a change in mental status or the clinician thinks there is a need to repeat the OCD scale
Posttraumatic stress disorder (PTSD)	SCIP PTSD scale	**Outpatient setting (self-administered scales)** 1. Baseline or first assessment opportunity 2. Every 6 months 3. Each time the patient starts a new medication for PTSD 4. Repeat 6–8 weeks from starting a new medication for PTSD. Typically, that will be the next outpatient scheduled visit 5. When there is a change in mental status or the clinician thinks there is a need to repeat the PTSD scale
Schizophrenia	**Three core schizophrenia scales:** 1. SCIP delusion scale 2. SCIP hallucination scale 3. SCIP disorganization scale **Other scales used in schizophrenia:** 1. SCIP negative scale 2. SCIP aggression scale	**Outpatient setting (self-administered scales)** **Administer the three core schizophrenia scales** 1. Baseline or at-first assessment opportunity 2. Every 6 months 3. Each time the patient starts a new antipsychotic medication 4. Repeat 6–8 weeks from starting a new antipsychotic medication. Typically, that will be the next outpatient scheduled visit 5. When there is a change in mental status or the clinician thinks there is a need to repeat the schizophrenia scales **Inpatient or day hospital setting** 1. Administer the three core schizophrenia scales upon admission to inpatient or day hospital 2. Administer the three core schizophrenia scales upon discharge from inpatient or day hospital **Administering the SCIP negative scale and the SCIP aggression scale** 1. Baseline or first assessment opportunity (inpatient, day hospital, or outpatient setting) 2. Every 6 months or if clinically indicated (inpatient, day hospital, or outpatient setting)

(continued)

Table 9.1 (continued)

Diagnosis	Scale(s)	When to administer the scale(s)
Schizoaffective disorder, depressed type	SCIP depression scale	1. Follow schizophrenia guidelines 2. Use depression scale as clinically indicated
Schizoaffective disorder, bipolar type	SCIP mania scale	1. Follow schizophrenia guidelines 2. Use mania scale as clinically indicated
Alcohol use disorder	SCIP alcohol scale	1. Once as a baseline (inpatient, day hospital, or outpatient setting) 2. Repeat alcohol scale if clinically indicated (inpatient, day hospital, or outpatient setting)
Drug use disorder	SCIP drug scale	1. Once as a baseline (inpatient, day hospital, or outpatient setting) 2. Repeat drug scale if clinically indicated (inpatient, day hospital, or outpatient setting)
Attention deficit hyperactivity disorder (ADHD)	SCIP ADHD scale	**Outpatient setting (self-administered scales)** 1. Once as a baseline 2. Repeat every 6 months 3. One time when the patient starts a new medication for ADHD 4. Repeat 6–8 weeks from starting a new medication for ADHD. Typically, that will be the next outpatient scheduled visit 5. One time when there is a change in mental status or the clinician thinks there is a need to repeat the ADHD scale
Eating disorders	SCIP anorexia, binge eating, and bulimia scales	**Outpatient setting (self-administered scales)** 1. Once as a baseline 2. Repeat every 6 months 3. One time when there is a change in mental status or the clinician thinks there is a need to repeat the eating disorders scales
Other scales	For example, PHQ-9	Scales will be used as clinically indicated

Details of implementing MBC in psychiatry residency programs at West Virginia University (WVU) and Delaware Psychiatric Center (DPC) were published in *Annals of Clinical Psychiatry* [20]. Psychiatry residency program directors who are interested in implementing the MBC curriculum can contact the manual author to obtain the MBC teaching materials.

References

1. Fortney, J. C., Unutzer, J., Wrenn, G., Pyne, J. M., Smith, G. R., Schoenbaum, M., & Harbin, H. T. (2016). A tipping point for measurement-based care. *Psychiatric Services, 2016*, appips201500439.
2. Scott, K., & Lewis, C. C. (2015). Using measurement-based care to enhance any treatment. *Cognitive and Behavioral Practice, 22*, 49–59.
3. Trivedi, M. H., & Daly, E. J. (2007). Measurement-based care for refractory depression: A clinical decision support model for clinical research and practice. *Drug and Alcohol Dependence, 88*(Suppl 2), S61–S71.
4. Harding, K. J., Rush, A. J., Arbuckle, M., Trivedi, M. H., & Pincus, H. A. (2011). Measurement-based care in psychiatric practice: A policy framework for implementation. *The Journal of Clinical Psychiatry, 72*, 1136–1143.
5. Guo, T., Xiang, Y. T., Xiao, L., Hu, C. Q., Chiu, H. F., Ungvari, G. S., Correll, C. U., Lai, K. Y., Feng, L., Geng, Y., Feng, Y., & Wang, G. (2015). Measurement-based care versus standard care for major depression: A randomized controlled trial with blind raters. *The American Journal of Psychiatry., 172*, 1004–1013.
6. Hatfield, D. R., & Ogles, B. M. (2007). Why some clinicians use outcome measures and others do not. *Administration and Policy in Mental Health, 34*, 283–291.
7. Hatfield, D. O., & B. (2004). The use of outcome measures by psychologists in clinical practice. *Professional Psychology: Research and Practice., 35*, 485–491.
8. Zimmerman, M., & McGlinchey, J. B. (2008). Why don't psychiatrists use scales to measure outcome when treating depressed patients? *The Journal of Clinical Psychiatry, 69*, 1916–1919.
9. Nasrallah, H. A. (2009). Long overdue: Measurement-based psychiatric practice. *Current Psychiatry., 8*, 14–16.
10. Aboraya, A. (2015). The validity results of the standard for clinicians' interview in psychiatry (SCIP). *Schizophrenia Bulletin., 41*, S103–S104.
11. Aboraya, A. (2016). Instruction manual for the standard for Clinicians' interview in psychiatry (SCIP). *Innovations in Clinical Neuroscience., 13*, 41–77.
12. Aboraya, A., El-Missiry, A., Barlowe, J., John, C., Ebrahimian, A., Muvvala, S., Brandish, J., Mansour, H., Zheng, W., Chumber, P., Berry, J., Elswick, D., Hill, C., Swager, L., Abo Elez, W., Ashour, H., Haikal, A., Eissa, A., Rabie, M., … Price, E. (2014). The reliability of the standard for clinicians' interview in psychiatry (SCIP): A clinician-administered tool with categorical, dimensional and numeric output. *Schizophrenia Research., 156*, 174–183.
13. Aboraya, A., Nasrallah, H., Muvvala, S., El-Missiry, A., Mansour, H., Hill, C., Elswick, D., & Price, E. C. (2016). The Standard for Clinicians' Interview in Psychiatry (SCIP): A clinician-administered tool with categorical, dimensional, and numeric output-conceptual development, design, and description of the SCIP. *Innovations in Clinical Neuroscience, 13*, 31–77.
14. Aboraya, A., Nasrallah, H. A., Elswick, D. E., Ahmed, E., Estephan, N., Aboraya, D., Berzingi, S., Chumbers, J., Berzingi, S., Justice, J., Zafar, J., & Dohar, S. (2018). Measurement-based care in psychiatry-past, present, and future. *Innovations in Clinical Neuroscience, 15*, 13–26.
15. Aboraya, A., & Nasrallah, H. A. (2016). Perspectives on the positive and negative syndrome scale (PANSS): Use, misuse, drawbacks, and a new alternative for schizophrenia research. *Annals of Clinical Psychiatry, 28*, 125–131.
16. Kay, S. R., Opler, L. A., & Fiszbein, A. (1987). *The positive and negative syndrome scale (PANSS) rating manual*. San Rafael.
17. Arbuckle, M. R., Weinberg, M., Harding, K. J., Isaacs, A. J., Covell, N. H., Cabaniss, D. L., Essock, S. M., & Sederer, L. I. (2013). The feasibility of standardized patient assessments as a best practice in an academic training program. *Psychiatric Services, 64*, 209–211.
18. Baker M. Measurement-based care and psychiatric education: Are we doing enough? Psychiatric News. 2015;50:ISSN 0033-2704.

19. Arbuckle, M. R., Weinberg, M., Kistler, S. C., Cabaniss, D. L., Isaacs, A. J., Sederer, L. I., & Essock, S. M. (2013). A curriculum in measurement-based care: Screening and monitoring of depression in a psychiatric resident clinic. *Academic Psychiatry, 37*, 317–320.
20. Aboraya, et al. (2021). Measurement-based care training curriculum in psychiatry residency programs: I: Description of the curriculum and demonstration of implementation. *Annals of Clinical Psychiatry., 33*(3), 168–179.

Chapter 10
Case Demonstrations for Using the SCIP as a Measurement-Based Care Tool in Clinical Practice: Transforming Normal Psychiatric Interviews into Data

This chapter includes the transcripts of 15 videotaped interviews conducted with real patients by the author and colleagues at West Virginia University. All patients had the capacity to provide consent for the interviews to be videotaped and used for teaching purposes. The written consent form indicated that patients could refuse to answer any question, could stop the interview anytime, and could withdraw and transcend their consent in the future if they choose to do so. Patients were never coached as to how to answer any questions and interviewers were instructed to conduct the interviews as they would in a real setting. We are grateful to the patients who were willing to participate in the films.

The first 12 full interview films are video #1 (Expert Ratings), video #2 (Panic and Depression), video #3 (ADHD and Depression), video #4 (Alcohol Use Disorder), video #5 (Post-Traumatic Stress Disorder), video #6 (Eating Disorders), video #7 (Psychosis and Mania), video #8 (Anxiety and Panic), video #9 (Narcotic Use Disorder and Depression), video # 10, video # 11, and video #12. Video #13, video #14, and video #15 are more practice videos.

Readers should watch video #1 (Expert Rating) first. Video #1 describes the principles of rating symptoms and signs of psychopathology and includes 7 videoclips with 14 SCIP questions and their ratings. We recommend that readers begin with video #1 to master the principles of rating psychopathology. Then, readers can watch the eight videos (videos #2 to 9) in any sequence. Each video has three parts: introduction, patient interview, and the expert ratings. Readers are advised to watch the introduction and the patient interview first and make their own ratings of the interview. Readers can then watch the rest of the videotape, compare their own ratings to the expert ratings, and explore and explain any differences. Readers can watch and rate the last six videos (videos #10, 11, 12, 13, 14, 15) on their own.

Supplementary Information The online version contains supplementary material available at [https://doi.org/10.1007/978-3-030-94930-3_10]. The videos can be accessed by scanning the related images with the SN More Media App.

A. S. Aboraya, *Manual for the Standard for Clinicians' Interview in Psychiatry (SCIP)*, Advances in Mental Health and Addiction,
https://doi.org/10.1007/978-3-030-94930-3_10

Video #1: Experts' Ratings

Video #1 has seven interview clips and ratings' explanations in-between.

Clip #1: Beginning the Interview and Establishing Rapport with the Patient

Clip #1 Transcript

Clinician (C) **Patient (P)**

C: My name is Dr. Zafar. I'm one of the chief residents in psychiatry. I appreciate you coming in and being able to help us out. Tell me, where are you from?
P: Blacksville, WV.
C: Born and raised in the Blacksville area?
P: Born in Morgantown, yeah.
C: Grew up with both mom and dad, or with grandparents?
P: Uh, mostly my mom.
C: Mostly your mom, okay. Any brothers and sisters?
P: Two older brothers and one younger sister.
C: Okay. Are you close with them?
P: No.
C: Okay. How far did you go in school?
P: I graduated in the 12th grade, now I work.
C: What kind of work have you done so far?
P: I did a bit of concrete work, but I've been in the coal mine for about 8 years now.
C: So heavy construction type of work.
P: Yeah.
C: Okay, alright. So tell me a little bit about what brought you to the hospital.
P: Mainly depression. I've been depressed for quite a while now, mainly struggling with it for the past year. Just got a lot on my mind, and it led up to suicidal thoughts.
C: I'm glad you came in for the help.

Clip #1 comments**:** *Good introduction by Dr. Zafar to establish rapport with the patient.*

Clip #2: Three Patients

Clip #2 Transcript

Clinician (C)

Patient 1 (P1)

C: You mentioned you also have anxiety for several hours during the day. Describe to me your anxiety. Do you worry too much about things? Explain to me about anxiety.

P1: Somebody has asked me more than several times if there's something in my life that's causing it. It's nothing like that. It's just that I'm generally anxious and nervous. Kind of frightened, if you're in a constant state of that and there is no reason for it.

C: And there's no reason for it. Okay. And you think it is more than most people? Most people have some anxiety here and there, but you think yours is worse than most?

P1: Yes, this is absolutely something that I have been medicated for. This is not a typical everyday type of deal. Something is definitely wrong, just now I know that hopefully I'm not going to die from it.

Patient 2 (P2)

C: Think about the past month, did you have difficulty paying attention and concentrating on what you are doing?

P2: Yes.

C: And a little bit, or a big problem?

P2: Enough for me to notice it.

C: Okay. And do you have difficulty concentrating for a long time on something like reading a book or watching a movie?

P2: Definitely, more so with reading a book. Watching a movie keeps my attention a little bit better.

C: Okay. But you think it is a problem compared to most people?

P2: Yes.

Patient 3 (P3):

C: Do you get startled often?

P3: Yes. Sometimes. That varies a little bit. Not significantly, but enough that I notice it, okay?

Clip #2 Ratings

Patient 1 (P1)

GAD1. Generalized anxiety	*Score*
Have you had excessive worry and anxiety for long periods of time** (e.g., **for hours each day lasting several months), <u>not</u> just during panic attacks?** ***Is it difficult to control the anxiety? 0 Patient has no generalized anxiety or nonsignificant. 1 Patient has generalized anxiety. . Not sure *or* not applicable *or* missing.	*1*

Patient 2 *(P2)*

ATT1. Attention impairment/poor concentration	*Score*
Do you have difficulty paying attention and concentrating when reading an article, watching a TV show or a movie, or doing your work or school assignments? 0 Absent or nonsignificant. 1 Patient has poor attention and concentration. . Not sure *or* not applicable *or* missing.	*0*
ATT2. Sustained attention impairment	
Do you have difficulty concentrating on one thing for a long time (e.g., ***reading a book, writing a letter)?*** 0 Absent or nonsignificant. 1 Patient has difficulty concentrating for a long period of time. . Not sure *or* not applicable *or* missing.	*1*

Patient 3 (P3):

PTSD15. Startle response	*Score*
Did you feel jumpy and easily startled? ***Were you easily scared or did you make a sudden movement or jump when you heard noises or if you were caught by surprise?*** 0 Patient had no significant symptom. 1 Patient feels jumpy and has a startle response. . Not sure *or* not applicable *or* missing.	*0*

Clip #3: Three Patients

Clip #3 Transcript

Clinician (C)

Patient 1 (P1)

C: Let's focus on the past month. Have you been feeling sad and depressed?
P1: Yes, extremely. Very guilty. I feel helpless and feel like I can't do anything more. I feel like it's Groundhog Day every day. Same day over and over.

C: So you have been feeling depressed most of the time.
P1: Yes.
C: And in the past month, were you able to enjoy your life as usual or were you not enjoying your life?
P1: No, I don't enjoy much.

Patient 2 (P2)

C: Questions about activities. When you have time, what do you like to do for fun to enjoy yourself? What do you like to do?
P2: I really enjoy reading. I like to study theology, that's about it really.

C: How about sports?
P2: I used to run, kind of got out of shape in college, but I do enjoy it every now and then on a warm day.
C: Do you like to watch TV/movies?
P2: Yes, occasionally my wife and I will have a movie night, but with two kids now it's a bit harder.
C: The time in the past when you were feeling very depressed, were you able to enjoy your fun activities?
P2: No, I really wasn't. I got bad enough to where that had consumed my life and I couldn't understand why. Even if I had a general sense of sadness, it still takes over your mind. Therefore you can't enjoy something as simple as your favorite cup of coffee because you're just sad about the fact that you can't have it, because it might lead to panic.
C: So when you're feeling really sad and depressed you don't enjoy anything?
P2: I wouldn't say anything. It just definitely affects everything and there are a few things I might enjoy.
C: So you enjoy some things.
P2: Yes.

Patient 3 (P3)

C: When you feel depressed, do you find you are able to enjoy things?
P3: I don't enjoy normal things that I normally would.
C: Do you enjoy anything?
P3: Not really. I feel pretty bad. I don't know why. I know I should be thankful; I try to be thankful, but it still just doesn't click inside me. I don't know why I feel the way I do.

Clip #3 Ratings

<u>Patient 1</u>

D1. Depressed mood	***Score***
Have you been feeling sad, depressed or in low spirits? 0 Patient has no depressed mood. 1 Patient has depressed mood less than half the time. 2 Patient has depressed mood more than half the time. . Not sure *or* not applicable *or* missing.	*2*
D2. Anhedonia (loss of pleasure and interest)	
Have you been unable to experience pleasure and enjoy things that you used to enjoy like exercising, enjoying your hobbies, or socializing with friends? 0 Patient has no anhedonia. 1 Patient has anhedonia less than half the time. 2 Patient has anhedonia more than half the time. . Not sure *or* not applicable *or* missing.	*1*

Patient 2

D2. Anhedonia (loss of pleasure and interest)	*Score*
Have you been unable to experience pleasure and enjoy things that you used to enjoy like exercising, enjoying your hobbies, or socializing with friends? 0 Patient has no anhedonia. 1 Patient has anhedonia less than half the time. 2 Patient has anhedonia more than half the time. . Not sure *or* not applicable *or* missing.	*1*

Patient 3

D2. Anhedonia (loss of pleasure and interest)	*Score*
Have you been unable to experience pleasure and enjoy things that you used to enjoy like exercising, enjoying your hobbies, or socializing with friends? 0 Patient has no anhedonia. 1 Patient has anhedonia less than half the time. 2 Patient has anhedonia more than half the time. . Not sure *or* not applicable *or* missing.	*2*

Clip #4: One Patient

Clip #4 Transcript

Clinician (C) Patient (P)

C: Think about a time when you had a big manic episode. Were you feeling very happy and on top of the world, or very angry and irritable.

P: Both. Sometimes I'd be very happy and expansive, and sometimes I've been more angry and paranoid against people, but also still always the really lot of energy.

C: Which one was more common? Feeling very happy or very irritable?

P: Most of them there was some combination. Some happiness, but whenever anybody got in my way, I would very easily become irritable.

C: Did you also find that your mood would change in the same day, like 1 hour you're feeling happy and the next you feel angry or then you feel sad? Did your mood change in the same day?

P: Yeah, I've had days like that before where it just was all over the place. Like in the morning, I'd be very happy and just cheerful, and then by evening I'd feel down or...you know, and it was like a roller coaster.

C: So the time where you feel very happy, how long would it last? Two days? Five days? A week?

P: Well...sometimes it could last as long as 3–4 days. But after that it would change to more irritation. Then I'd be irritable for several days.

Clip #4 Ratings

M1. Expansive (elated) mood	***Score***
Have you sometimes felt very happy, elated, on top of the world without much reason? 0 Patient has no elated mood. 1 Patient has elated mood less than half the time. 2 Patient has elated mood more than half the time. . Not sure *or* not applicable *or* missing.	*1*
M2. Irritable mood	
Have you sometimes felt that you were easily irritated without reason? ***Have you found yourself so irritable that you shout at people or start arguments or actually become aggressive?*** 0 Patient has no irritable mood. 1 Patient has irritable mood less than half the time. 2 Patient has irritable mood more than half the time. . Not sure *or* not applicable *or* missing.	*1*
M3. Mixed mood (mood lability)	
Have you had mixed mood swings: periods of depression and elation or irritability on the same day? 0 Patient has no mixed mood swings. 1 Patient has mixed mood less than half the time. 2 Patient has mixed mood more than half the time. . Not sure *or* not applicable *or* missing.	*1*

Clip #5: One Patient

Clip #5 Transcript

Clinician (C) **Patient (P)**

P: The mood changes just go all over the place. Right now, I'm all right. We get back over to the building again, I can't tell you where I'm gonna be. I may be okay, I may be pissed off, I may be depressed.

C: So it fluctuates within a day for you.

P: It fluctuates within an hour, okay. Depending on what's going on. My meds are all screwed up. The more screwed up they are, the more screwed up my head gets.

C: So you're trying to get that in check.

P: Yeah. Yesterday, a period of about 4 hours, I went from depression to hypomania, to depression, to what I call scatter brained. I get so many thoughts going through my mind that I can't focus on anything. I can't slow anything down enough to grasp one specific thought long enough to get ahold of myself.

Clip #5 Ratings

M3. Mixed mood (mood lability)	***Score***
Have you had mixed mood swings: periods of depression and elation or irritability on the same day? 0 Patient has no mixed mood swings. 1 Patient has mixed mood less than half the time. 2 Patient has mixed mood more than half the time. . Not sure *or* not applicable *or* missing.	*1*
M4. Racing thoughts (observed as flight of ideas)	
Have you felt that you had too many different thoughts racing through your mind compared with normal? 0 Patient has no racing thoughts. 1 Patient has racing thoughts less than half the time. 2 Patient has racing thoughts more than half the time. . Not sure *or* not applicable *or* missing.	*1*

Clip #6: One Patient

Clip #6 Transcript

Clinician (C) Patient (P)

C: In the past month, did you have any time where you could hear voices talking at you that nobody else could hear?

P: Pretty much every day.

C: Okay. And the voices sometimes ask you to do something, do this or that?

P: Yeah.

C: Can you give me an example of what the voices ask you to do?

P: Sometimes disgusting things.

C: And you don't do those things?

P: No, if I did, it would be bad.

C: All right, okay. So you can hear them every day?

P: Several times a day.

C: Several times a day, okay. And in 1 day, on average, how much time do you hear the voices? For 1 hour or 2 hours?

P: Maybe an hour, hour and a half.

C: Okay, very good.

Clip #6 Ratings

HAL1. Auditory hallucinations	*Score*
Do you hear noises (like music, whispering sounds) or voices talking to you when there is no one around? Are the voices like a real voice or just thoughts in your mind? 0 Patient has no auditory hallucinations. 1 Patient has auditory hallucinations. 2 Patient has auditory hallucinations with command. . Not sure *or* not applicable *or* missing.	*2*
HAL2. Frequency of auditory hallucinations	
How often do you hear noises (like music, whispering sounds) or voices talking to you when there is no one around? 0 Patient has no auditory hallucinations. 1 Patient has auditory hallucinations (1–4 days/month). 2 Patient has auditory hallucinations (5–14 days/month). 3 Patient has auditory hallucinations (≥15 days/month). . Not sure *or* not applicable *or* missing.	*3*

HAL3. Hallucination duration	
On days when you hear noises or voices, how often do you hear them? 0 Patient has no auditory hallucinations. 1 Patient has auditory hallucinations (less than 1 hour/day). 2 Patient has auditory hallucinations (1–4 hours/day). 3 Patient has auditory hallucinations (more than 4 hours/day). . Not sure *or* not applicable *or* missing.	*2*

Clip #7: One Patient

Clip #7 Transcript

Clinician (C) Patient (P)

C: For the past month, did you have any thoughts like somebody is after you or trying to harm you?

P: Well, I had paranoid thoughts about this woman that lives in my building. I thought she was trying to do things to be mean to me.

C: Okay. How do you know her? Who is she?

P: She has an apartment in the same building that I live in.

C: Ah, okay. Does she work there?

P: She's the backup manager.

C: Okay, I see. Did you have any thoughts that she was trying to harm you, like poison your food or anything like that?

P: No, I thought she was using her backup key as a manager to come into my apartment and damage my belongings.

C: That's what you thought.

P: Yeah.
C: But she never did that?
P: Oh yes she did!
C: Oh, she did?
P: Yeah, she actually did, but I can't get anyone in my building to believe me. They all think I'm just cuckoo.
C: Okay, and she came into your apartment and broke up your stuff?
P: Well she like cut my clothing, stole money.
C: Okay, okay.

Clip #7 Ratings

DEL5. Paranoid/persecutory delusions	***Score***
Have you felt that people are against you, talking about you, or laughing at you? Do you think someone is trying to harm you (e.g., trying to poison your food or trying to kill you)? 0 Patient has no paranoid/persecutory delusions. 1 Patient has paranoid/persecutory delusions some of the time. 2 Patient has paranoid/persecutory delusions most of the time. . Not sure *or* not applicable *or* missing.	***0***

Video #2: Panic and Depression

Transcription of Interview #2 (C = Clinician; P = Patient)

C: And do you, have you ever had any panic attacks?
P: Yes.
C: Describe to me your panic attacks.
P: Umm the last panic attack, the big panic attack I had whenever we were in Florida during the hurricane in the beginning of September. I had a big panic attack worrying about trying to get home when all that our flight was canceled. I felt like I couldn't breathe; my chest was heavy, sweating. I just felt like everything was closing in. I was just having a terrible time. Seeing and just couldn't picture everything around me just felt like it was falling apart.
C: And how long did that panic attack last?
P: It lasted a good while. For me it felt like forever, but my husband and kids said it was just probably about a good hour. I went to lie down; I took some medicine and went to lie down, and they said I was probably in there for maybe an hour or two. Then I felt better.
C: Okay.
P: But to me, it felt like it was all day.

C: Right, I understand of course. And how did you come back from Florida? Did you drive?

P: We had to drive unfortunately because our flight was canceled, and luckily, we did find a rental, but we had to drive so that drive was very stressful and very hard.

C: Right, right, very good. I'm glad you came home before the hurricane hits.

P: Yes.

C: And in general, how often do you get a panic attack? Like once a week?

P: I normally get them once a week

C: Okay, alright.

P: Yes.

C: Let me ask you some questions about the depression. And you mentioned that let's focus about the past month, you know have you been feeling sad and depressed for the past month?

P: Yes, extremely. Sad umm very guilty, like guilt feelings. I just feel like helpless and just feel like um I just feel like I can't do anything more. I feel like its Groundhog Day every day. Like it's the same day over and over.

C: So, you have been feeling depressed most of the time?

P: Yes.

C: Okay, again for the past month were you able to enjoy your life as usual or you were not enjoying your life?

P: No, I don't enjoy it, no.

C: And, again for the past month do you feel hopeless about your future?

P: I…no I didn't see much of a future. Um, I don't see. When I look towards the future, I see gray and just dark; it doesn't seem fun.

C: Do you sometimes feel like there is hope in life and hope in the future?

P: I pray but I don't see anything, I'm hoping maybe.

C: Right that's good at least there is some hope.

P: Yeah.

C: And for the past month also, were you able to focus and concentrate on what you are doing as usual or you had difficulty concentrating?

P: No, I have difficulty the concentration yeah. It is focusing, trying to remember, I'm scattered brain. Yeah, it's all there.

C: And you mentioned the word feeling guilty, do you feel guilty?

P: I feel guilty, yes, a lot.

C: A lot?

P: Yes.

C: Or a little bit?

P: I do all the time for if it's the little things. If I didn't, if I forgot to leave something for the kids that I told them I was going to do, I will feel guilty for a week. Anything small up to something big that's.

C: And for the past month, did you feel that you were slow like ah you were moving slow, talking slow, like feeling that everything is slow, or your energy was like normal?

P: It was definitely slow. I feel like I'm always slow. I'm always taking ten steps slower than everyone else. Everyone just saying hurry up mom, hurry up let's go. I just feel like I have no energy. No desire.

C: How about your ability to make decisions? Are you able to make decisions or somewhat affected?

P: I am always indecisive always don't. Never really know what to. If I make a decision, then I'm always, I don't know. I don't like to make decisions.

C: Okay, alright. And how about feelings of having thoughts about harming yourself in the past month?

P: I don't think of harming myself, I mean there are thoughts of I can't do this anymore or there are thoughts of I don't think I can go through another day of this the same thing, but I never physically ever get anything to harm myself.

C: And you never had any intention that you wanted to end your life?

P: No.

C: Okay and let me ask you a few more questions. Have you had any time where you would hear voices talking to you when there is nobody around?

P: No.

C: Have you ever had any time when you would see things that nobody else could see?

P: No.

C: Okay, have you had any thoughts that somebody is trying to harm you? Like poison your food or anything like that?

P: No.

C: Okay, when you watch the TV, do you sometimes feel that the TV is referring to you or talking to you in person or anything like that?

P: No.

Video #2 Ratings

PAN1. Panic attacks (without phobias)	*Score*
Have you gotten suddenly anxious and frightened for a short period of time (up to 60 minutes)? ***During that time, did you feel that your heart was racing or pounding, or did you start shaking or sweating, or did you feel you were choking?*** 0 Patient had no panic attacks. 1 Patient had panic attacks. . Not sure *or* not applicable *or* missing.	1

D1. Depressed mood	*Score*
Have you been feeling sad, depressed, or in low spirits? 0 Patient has no depressed mood. 1 Patient has depressed mood less than half the time. 2 Patient has depressed mood more than half the time. . Not sure *or* not applicable *or* missing.	*2*
D2. Anhedonia (loss of pleasure and interest)	

Have you been unable to experience pleasure and enjoy things that you used to enjoy like exercising, enjoying your hobbies, or socializing with friends? 0 Patient has no anhedonia. 1 Patient has anhedonia less than half the time. 2 Patient has anhedonia more than half the time. . Not sure or not applicable or missing.	*1*
D3. Hopelessness	
Have you felt hopeless about your future? 0 Patient is not hopeless. 1 Patient feels hopeless less than half the time. 2 Patient feels hopeless more than half the time. . Not sure or not applicable or missing.	*1*
D4. Attention impairment/poor concentration	
Have you found that your concentration has decreased and you are unable to complete a task* (e.g., *at work, reading an article, reading a book, or watching a movie), even though you were able to do that before? 0 Patient has no concentration problems. 1 Patient has difficulty concentrating less than half the time. 2 Patient has difficulty concentrating more than half the time. . Not sure or not applicable or missing.	*1*

D5. Psychomotor slowing/retardation	
Have you felt as though you were talking or moving more slowly than normal for you when depressed? 0 Patient has normal activity. 1 Patient has psychomotor retardation less than half the time. 2 Patient has psychomotor retardation more than half the time. . Not sure or not applicable or missing.	*2*
D6. Worthlessness (low self-esteem)	
Have you felt that you are a worthless person in the society or a failure? 0 Patient has no feeling of worthlessness. 1 Patient feels worthless less than half the time. 2 Patient feels worthless more than half the time. . Not sure or not applicable or missing.	***Missing***
D7. Excessive guilt	
Have you felt guilty or ashamed of yourself for something you have done or thought? 0 Patient has no feeling of guilt. 1 Patient feels guilty less than half the time. 2 Patient feels guilty more than half the time. . Not sure or not applicable or missing.	*2*
D8. Other depressive symptoms	
0 Absent. ***1 Present (specify).*** ***. Not sure or not applicable or missing.***	*1*
D9. Suicidal ideation during the past month	

Have you had thoughts about harming or killing yourself? ***0 Patient had no suicidal ideation.*** ***1 Patient had suicidal ideation.*** ***. Not sure or not applicable or missing.***	*0*
D10. Suicidal intention during the past month	
Have you had the intention to carry out the suicidal thoughts? 0 Patient had no suicidal intention. 1 Patient had suicidal intention. . Not sure or not applicable or missing.	*0*
D11. Suicidal plans during the past month	
Have you had specific suicidal plans? 0 Patient had no suicidal plans. 1 Patient had suicidal plans. . Not sure or not applicable or missing.	*0*

D12. Suicidal attempt during the past month	
Have you made a suicide attempt during the past month? 0 Patient made no suicide attempt during the past month. 1 Patient made one recent suicide attempt during the past month. 2 Patient made two or more recent suicide attempts during the past month. . Not sure or not applicable or missing.	*0*
D13. Delusions associated mainly with depressed mood:	
0 Absent. 1 Present. . Not sure or not applicable or missing.	*0*
D14. Hallucinations associated mainly with depressed mood:	
0 Absent. 1 Present. . Not sure or not applicable or missing.	*0*
Depression score = 10 (severe)	

Video #3: ADHD and Depression

Transcription of Interview #3 (C = Clinician; P = Patient)

C: Hello, I am Dr. Aboraya and I want to thank you again for coming. As I explained to you, this interview will be videotaped and used for teaching purposes.

P: No problem.

C: Now, can you tell me more about yourself. Where do you live and who lives with you?

P: I live with my dad in Morgantown.

C: Okay, alright. And you've been in the hospital for how many days?

P: I think 4 days.

C: And what are the main problems that brought you into the hospital?

P: Mainly depression and a bit of impulsive behavior.

C: Okay. And when you say impulsive behavior, can you tell me more about that?

P: It's a symptom of ADHD and I tend to do things before I realize that I'm doing them. An idea will pop into my head and it'll happen.

C: How long have you had these problems?

P: Mainly my entire life.

C: Okay. And have you had any treatment for them before?

P: I was on Ritalin for about 4 years from 8 years old to 12 years old. My mom took me off the treatment.

C: But you still have the same problems until now?

P: Yeah but I've grown a bit out of the hyperactivity but I still have issues with it.

C: Let me explain a couple things. Some patients have bipolar disorder, they have mood swings and at one time they feel sad and depressed, and other times they feel on top of the world and have tons of energy and don't sleep. That's not the ADHD that you are talking about?

P: No.

C: Okay. And for ADHD usually the patient also does other things, like he does one thing and then before he finishes he goes and does something else.

P: Oh yeah I'm horrible about that. If I'm painting a room or something, I can't paint one wall. I'll do a little bit here and there.

C: And you have trouble concentrating on what you are doing?

P: Not really because sometimes I get super focused and forget everything else.

C: I will ask you now more specific questions about the attention problems and hyperactivity. Think about the past month. Did you have difficulty paying attention and concentrating on what you are doing?

P: Yes.

C: A little bit, or a big problem?

P: Enough for me to notice it.

C: And how about difficulty concentrating for a long time on something like reading a book or watching a movie?

P: Definitely. I have hard time reading a book for sure. Watching a movie keeps my attention a little bit better.

C: But you think it is a problem compared to most people?

P: Yes.

C: And do you avoid tasks that require mental effort?

P: Sometimes, depends on my mood.

C: So if you had a task you need to do, you try to avoid it because it requires a lot of attention?

P: Mhhm, certain things.

C: Do you have difficulty concentrating on what people are saying to you?

P: Sometimes. Then other times, like my ex-wife used to hate it because I'd be watching TV and listening to what she was saying, but she thought I couldn't repeat exactly what she said.

C: But you don't think it's a big problem?

P: Not really.

C: You have difficulty with tasks requiring organization?
P: Yes, I'm a very unorganized person.
C: Okay, give an example?
P: Whenever I worked for General Dynamics, my desk was a mess. It was an organized mess to me.
C: Do you have difficulty planning or organizing things at work?
P: It really depends on how well it holds my attention.
C: Do you change from one activity to another before finishing the first one?
P: Yes.
C: A lot?
P: If I get bored, I will spend 5 minutes on each DVD at my house, rather than watching a full one.
C: Okay. And are you easily distracted by noises around you?
P: I wouldn't say I'd be totally distracted, but if I heard a noise behind me right now I'd definitely turn around and look.
C: But you don't think it's a big problem?
P: No.
C: Do you lose or misplace things more often than other people?
P: Yes.
C: Give me an example.
P: When I was doing plumbing work, I would lose my tools everywhere and they'd be right here in front of my face.
C: Did it affect your work?
P: Yes.
C: And do you forget your daily activities more than most people?
P: Yes, especially when a new task is added for that day.
C: Do you think it's a minor problem or a big problem?
P: I'd say in the middle somewhere.
C: Okay. Do you sometimes lose track of what you are doing?
P: Yes, horribly.
C: Do you have difficulty remaining seated?
P: It depends on where I'm at. Like I have a bad problem with standing and eating. Most people sit down and eat. Depends on my mood and where I'm at.
C: Okay. But if you were to go listen to a lecture, are you able to stay in the lecture until it's over?
P: I could stay in the lecture but I would definitely be up and down or moving in my seat.
C: Do you fidget?
P: Yes.
C: Do you think being fidgety is more of a problem for you?
P: I wouldn't necessarily say it's a problem, just something to keep me going.
C: So it doesn't affect your function?
P: No.
C: And if you need to go to the church and stay until the service is over, are you able to do that?

P: Yes.
C: And do you feel restless, fidgety, like you have to get up and move?
P: Yes, at times.
C: It's not a big problem?
P: I wouldn't say it's problematic for me but it can be problematic for other people around me.
C: Do you feel overly active?
P: At times. I'm horrible about cleanliness and I need to be super focused on it.
C: But it's not a big problem?
P: It can be at times, especially if I have a guest over then I get into that kind of a mode.
C: Okay. Is it difficult for you to wait in line or for your turn?
P: Not really because I just start fidgeting.
C: But if you have to wait in line to buy a ticket or something…
P: It would depend on what it was for.
C: Do you feel that you talk too much?
P: I've been known to be very loquacious.
C: Do you think you are loud and noisy?
P: Yes.
C: Why?
P: I tend to speak very loudly.
C: Is it causing a problem?
P: Not to me, but other people.
C: Do you feel impulsive?
P: Extremely. That's why I ended up here.
C: Give me an example.
P: Well actually the reason why I ended up in the hospital was because I was in Kroger and I'm half-blind and I got upset with myself and I just randomly threw my cell phone across the aisle and I could have hit somebody.
C: And what happened in that situation?
P: I ended up going home and thinking about what could have happened and thought maybe I should get a handle on things.
C: And that's why you came to the hospital?
P: Yes.
C: Do you disturb others or intrude on others?
P: I've been known to do it. I wouldn't say it's a super big problem but I do interrupt people.
C: Okay, but you can control it if you want.
P: Sometimes.
C: Do you have a tendency to blurt out answers before the person even finished the question?
P: Yes.
C: Is it a big problem?
P: Sometimes, because I don't give anybody an opportunity to talk.
C: Well, you're doing okay with me asking the questions now.

P: I'm trying very hard.

C: Thank you very much. So you are saying that you were in Kroger and you threw your phone and then went home and thought maybe you needed help.

P: Yes.

C: But is there anything else that brought you in?

P: I have a lot of health conditions. I've never actually had the feeling of wanting to blow my brains out, but I have thought that if I stopped taking my medication I would go very quickly.

C: How old are you?

P: 32.

C: And you've had a stroke?

P: I had two strokes last year. That's why I wear glasses and why I'm half-blind.

C: Obviously when you are young and have medical problems, it affects your mood.

P: Yes, it does a good job of bringing me down quickly.

C: Right, I understand. So have you been feeling sad and depressed?

P: Yes.

C: And how long have you been feeling sad and depressed?

P: Since October, middle of October 2015. That was when I had my first pulmonary embolism.

C: Okay. Right. So a couple of years?

P: Yes.

C: If you think about the past month, have you also been feeling depressed?

P: Yes, it's gotten really bad this past month.

C: Did you feel sad and depressed most of the time?

P: Yes.

C: That's why you came in also?

P: Yes.

C: I'm going to ask more questions about feeling sad. Think about the past month. The past month, did you feel like you were enjoying life?

P: I feel like I don't care or enjoy it.

C: Before you were able to enjoy things?

P: Yes.

C: What did you like to do for fun?

P: Video games, I like to shoot, hunt, listening to nature.

C: And you don't enjoy that anymore?

P: I don't feel like going outside or doing anything.

C: For the past month, did you feel hopeless about your future?

P: Yes. A lack of motivation to do anything.

C: Do you feel hopeless most of the time?

P: Yes.

C: How about your ability to focus over the past month?

P: It's been lessened. I notice it, but I don't think anyone else would. So a mild problem.

C: Do you feel like you are talking or walking slow?

P: I walk very slow for some reason. I tend to lag behind.

C: What about your speech?
P: I don't think I've been slow but I've been slower formulating what I say.
C: Did you feel worthless over the past month?
P: Yes and no. I do feel I have skills, it's more of just being down and not wanting to use skills.
C: How about feeling guilty?
P: Yes. All the time.
C: What do you feel guilty about?
P: I'm also a recovering drug addict and I've done things to people because of that.
C: When did you stop using?
P: April 2016.
C: So for the past year, you didn't use drugs?
P: No.
C: What about alcohol?
P: I do drink.
C: Is it a problem for you?
P: Over the past few years, no. At one point it was for me.
C: For the past year, how often did you drink alcohol?
P: Once a week.
C: Has alcohol affected your life over the past year?
P: No.
C: For the past month, any thoughts of suicide?
P: Yes.
C: What did you think?
P: I call it painting the wall red. I wouldn't do that to my family members that would be responsible for cleaning up my mess.
C: But you didn't in the past month try to kill yourself?
P: No.
C: Have you ever tried to kill yourself?
P: No.
C: For the past month, did you really have the intention to do yourself in?
P: I would like to think I wouldn't. But with how impulsive I can be I'm not sure I can give a straight or direct answer.
C: I understand. Have you ever had a time when you would hear voices talking to you that nobody else can hear?
P: No.
C: What about seeing things others can't see?
P: No.
C: Have you have had a time where you thought someone was after you?
P: No.
C: When you watch the TV, do you think it's talking to you?
P: No.
C: I ask a lot of questions about feeling sad. Some people feel the opposite of depression. They feel on top of the world without reason. They may go without sleep and talk fast. That is called a manic episode. Have you ever had anything like that?

P: No.
C: Do you have any questions for me?
P: No, thank you.

Video #3 Ratings

ATT1. Attention impairment/poor concentration	***Score***
Do you have difficulty paying attention and concentrating when reading an article, watching a TV show or a movie, or doing your work or school assignments? 0 Absent or nonsignificant. 1 Patient has poor attention and concentration. . Not sure *or* not applicable *or* missing.	*0*
ATT2. Sustained attention impairment	
Do you have difficulty concentrating on one thing for a long time* (e.g., *reading a book, writing a letter)? 0 Absent or nonsignificant. 1 Patient has difficulty concentrating for a long period of time. . Not sure *or* not applicable *or* missing.	*1*
ATT3. Avoiding sustained attention tasks	
Do you avoid tasks that require a lot of concentration at work, school, or home* (e.g., *reading a book, writing a letter)? 0 Absent or nonsignificant. 1 Patient avoids tasks that require sustained mental effort. . Not sure *or* not applicable *or* missing.	*1*
ATT4. Attention when spoken to	
Do you have difficulty concentrating on what people say to you, even when they are speaking to you directly? 0 Absent or nonsignificant. 1 Patient has difficulty concentrating on what people say. . Not sure *or* not applicable *or* missing.	*0*
ATT5. Organization and meeting deadlines	
Do you have difficulty with tasks that require organization and keeping track of many things all at once* (e.g., *planning and organizing your work or household chores)? Do you have difficulty managing your time* (e.g., *usually fail to meet deadlines)? 0 Absent or nonsignificant. 1 Patient has difficulty with tasks that require organization or meeting deadlines. . Not sure *or* not applicable *or* missing.	*0*
ATT6. Changing activities	
Do you change from one activity to another without finishing the first? 0 Absent or nonsignificant. 1 Patient changes from one activity to another without finishing the first. . Not sure *or* not applicable *or* missing.	*1*

ATT7. Distraction (attention is distracted by environmental noises)	
Are you easily distracted from tasks by activity or noise around you? 0 Absent or nonsignificant. 1 Patient is easily distracted from tasks by activity or noise. . Not sure *or* not applicable *or* missing.	***0***
ATT8. Misplacing things	
Do you lose or misplace things more often than others do (e.g., ***wallets, keys, cell phones)?*** 0 Absent or nonsignificant. 1 Patient loses or misplaces things more often than others do. . Not sure *or* not applicable *or* missing.	***1***
ATT9. Forgetting daily activities	
Do you forget daily activities more often than others do (e.g., ***appointments, paying bills, returning phone calls)?*** 0 Absent or nonsignificant. 1 Patient forgets daily activities more often than others do. . Not sure *or* not applicable *or* missing.	***1***
ATT10. Losing track	
Do you lose track of what you are doing (e.g., ***forget why you went to get something)?*** 0 Absent or nonsignificant. 1 Patient loses track of what he or she is doing. . Not sure *or* not applicable *or* missing.	***1***
Attention problems score = 6 (moderate)	

HYP1. Fidgety	***Score***
Do you have difficulty remaining seated (fidget with hands and feet, squirm or wiggle in seat) when expected to remain seated (e.g., ***in a meeting or a church service)?*** 0 Absent or nonsignificant. 1 Patient has difficulty remaining seated when expected to. . Not sure *or* not applicable *or* missing.	***0***
HYP2. Leaving seats	
Do you leave your seat in meetings or other situations (e.g., ***during an appointment or a church service) where you are expected to remain seated?*** 0 Absent or nonsignificant. 1 Patient leaves seat in meetings or other situations when expected to remain seated. . Not sure *or* not applicable *or* missing.	***0***
HYP3. Restlessness/moving	
Do you feel restless, fidgety, and you must get up and move around? 0 Absent or nonsignificant. 1 Patient feels restless, fidgety, and must move around. . Not sure *or* not applicable *or* missing.	***1***
HYP4. Hyperactivity	
Do you feel overly active and compelled to do things, like you are driven by a motor? 0 Absent or nonsignificant. 1 Patient feels overly active and compelled to do things. . Not sure *or* not applicable *or* missing.	***1***
HYP5. Waiting in line	

Is it difficult for you to wait in line for your turn when the situation calls for it? 0 Absent or nonsignificant. 1 Patient has difficulty waiting in line. . Not sure *or* not applicable *or* missing.	*0*
HYP6. Talking too much	
Do you think you talk too much? ***Do others say that you talk too much?*** 0 Absent or nonsignificant. 1 Patient talks too much. . Not sure *or* not applicable *or* missing.	*0*

HYP7. Loud and noisy	
Do you think that you are a loud and noisy person? ***Do other people sometimes ask you to quiet down or lower your voice?*** 0 Absent or nonsignificant. 1 Patient or others feel the patient is loud and noisy. . Not sure *or* not applicable *or* missing.	*1*
HYP8. Impulsivity	
Are you impulsive (**e.g.,** ***act before you think adequately about consequences of actions)?*** 0 Absent or nonsignificant. 1 Patient is impulsive. . Not sure *or* not applicable *or* missing.	*1*
HYP9. Disturbing others	
Do you disturb others or intrude on others (**e.g.,** ***when people are talking or when people are involved in activities?)*** 0 Absent or nonsignificant. 1 Patient disturbs others or intrudes on others. . Not sure *or* not applicable *or* missing.	*0*
HYP10. Blurt out answers	
Do you have tendency to blurt out the answer before another person has finished asking the question? 0 Absent or nonsignificant. 1 Patient blurts out the answers. . Not sure *or* not applicable *or* missing.	*0*
Hyperactivity score = 4 (moderate)	

D1. Depressed mood	***Score***
Have you been feeling sad, depressed, or in low spirits? 0 Patient has no depressed mood. 1 Patient has depressed mood less than half the time. 2 Patient has depressed mood more than half the time. . Not sure *or* not applicable *or* missing.	*2*
D2. Anhedonia (loss of pleasure and interest)	

Have you been unable to experience pleasure and enjoy things that you used to enjoy like exercising, enjoying your hobbies, or socializing with friends? 0 Patient has no anhedonia. 1 Patient has anhedonia less than half the time. 2 Patient has anhedonia more than half the time. . Not sure *or* not applicable *or* missing.	*1*
D3. Hopelessness	
Have you felt hopeless about your future? 0 Patient is not hopeless. 1 Patient feels hopeless less than half the time. 2 Patient feels hopeless more than half the time. . Not sure *or* not applicable *or* missing.	2
D4. Attention impairment/poor concentration	
Have you found that your concentration has decreased and you are unable to complete a task* (e.g., *at work, reading an article, reading a book, or watching a movie), even though you were able to do that before? 0 Patient has no concentration problems. 1 Patient has difficulty concentrating less than half the time. 2 Patient has difficulty concentrating more than half the time. . Not sure *or* not applicable *or* missing.	*0*
D5. Psychomotor slowing/retardation	
Have you felt as though you were talking or moving more slowly than normal for you when depressed? 0 Patient has normal activity. 1 Patient has psychomotor retardation less than half the time. 2 Patient has psychomotor retardation more than half the time. . Not sure *or* not applicable *or* missing.	*1*
D6. Worthlessness (low self-esteem)	
Have you felt that you are a worthless person in the society or a failure? 0 Patient has no feeling of worthlessness. 1 Patient feels worthless less than half the time. 2 Patient feels worthless more than half the time. . Not sure *or* not applicable *or* missing.	*0*

D7. Excessive guilt	
Have you felt guilty or ashamed of yourself for something you have done or thought? 0 Patient has no feeling of guilt. 1 Patient feels guilty less than half the time. 2 Patient feels guilty more than half the time. . Not sure *or* not applicable *or* missing.	2
D8. Other depressive symptoms	
0 Absent. 1 Present (specify). . Not sure *or* not applicable *or* missing.	*0*
D9. Suicidal ideation during the past month	

Have you had thoughts about harming or killing yourself? 0 Patient had no suicidal ideation. 1 Patient had suicidal ideation. . Not sure *or* not applicable *or* missing.	***1***
D10. Suicidal intention during the past month	
Have you had the intention to carry out the suicidal thoughts? 0 Patient had no suicidal intention. 1 Patient had suicidal intention. . Not sure *or* not applicable *or* missing.	***Not sure***
D11. Suicidal plans during the past month	
Have you had specific suicidal plans? 0 Patient had no suicidal plans. 1 Patient had suicidal plans. . Not sure *or* not applicable *or* missing.	***1***
D12. Suicidal attempt during the past month	
Have you made a suicide attempt during the past month? 0 Patient made no suicide attempt during the past month. 1 Patient made one recent suicide attempt during the past month. 2 Patient made two or more recent suicide attempts during the past month. . Not sure *or* not applicable *or* missing.	***0***
D13. Delusions associated mainly with depressed mood	
0 Absent. 1 Present. . Not sure *or* not applicable *or* missing.	***0***
D14. Hallucinations associated mainly with depressed mood	
0 Absent. 1 Present. . Not sure *or* not applicable *or* missing.	***0***
Depression score = 10 (severe)	

Video #4: Alcohol Use

Transcription of Interview #4 (C = Clinician; P = Patient)

C: You mentioned you would drink a couple of beers at home. Do you drink on a regular basis?

P: On day shift I drink maybe ten beers at night. On the weekends I drink quite a bit more.

C: How much is quite a bit more?

P: 20, 25 alcoholic beverages.

C: Okay. Some people often tell me that if they don't drink, the next day, they get the shakes, tremors, and they get sweaty. What kind of symptoms have you had along that line?

P: I've had the shakes.

C: Ever had a seizure following drinking?

P: No.
C: Ever feel like things are crawling on your skin if you don't drink for a day or two?
P: Yeah, like mostly shakiness.
C: For how long have you been drinking the 7–10 beers?
P: Probably within the last year.
C: So one year consecutively? And has it been increasing?
P: Yeah definitely.
C: What did it start with?
P: Started with a couple weeks ago, then it seemed like more where I was drinking and I started not staying at home and started drinking more with my friends.
C: Do you get blacked out when you drink?
P: I have before.
C: What about in the past 3–4 months?
P: No, I never drink and drive or anything like that.
C: Ever got a DUI or gotten in trouble because of the drinking?
P: No.
C: Do you describe yourself as a happy drunk, angry drunk, or quiet drunk?
P: Happy.
C: Do you like the taste of alcohol?
P: Yes.
C: What does it do for you?
P: Relaxes me after working all day; I usually drink a few and play with my kids and then fall asleep.
C: Do you view your drinking as a problem?
P: No, nobody has ever complained about it. I don't let it interfere with what I'm doing.
C: Do you ever feel like it interferes with your work the next day?
P: I don't feel like it interferes with it, but I know it's one thing that interferes with my relationship.
C: Has your wife complained about it?
P: She's never complained, but I don't want it to become an issue with enough that's already been going on.
C: In terms of, do you feel like with drinking, what's the most time you've gone without drinking? Was it hours, days, weeks? In the past 5 months?
P: I can go all week without it on my midnight and afternoon shifts.
C: So now it sounds like you're doing a little bit of all types of shifts every day.
P: Yeah.
C: When was the last time you went a 2- to 3-day period without drinking?
P: The last time I was on afternoon shift.
C: When was that?
P: Three weeks ago probably.
C: How many days did you go without drinking?
P: Five days.
C: How were those 5 days for you?

P: I looked forward to the weekend. It never interfered, but I knew eventually it would.
C: Ever use anything else with drinking? Medications or street drugs?
P: I take blood pressure medicine and medicine for heartburn, as well as Prozac for depression.
C: Which came first in your mind, the depression or the drinking?
P: The depression.
C: What age did you start drinking first?
P: I started at a young age. Probably partied and stuff at 15 or 16.
C: When did you get to the point where you were drinking every night?
P: Within the last year.
C: So you're 27 now, right?
P: Yes.
C: So it's been about 11 years of on and off drinking, but it's been troublesome in the past year.
P: Yes.
C: Any other drugs like Xanax, Klonopin?
P: No.
C: Any other street drugs?
P: I've experimented with marijuana when I was younger.
C: But nothing recently?
P: No.
C: What about tobacco?
P: No.
C: So to summarize things, your drinking worsened as your depression has worsened.
P: Yes, definitely.
C: And it sounds like you view it to an extent as that it may be a problem and creating trouble in your relationship with your wife.
P: Yes, and the time where I should be trying to work on things with my wife, I'm going to get beer or thinking about drinking.
C: So you do crave alcohol.
P: Yes.

Video #4 Ratings

ALC1. Tolerance	***Score***
Did you use a lot more alcohol than you previously used to get the same effect (compared when you first started to drink)? ***Did you notice that the same amount of alcohol you take now has less effect than before (compared when you first started to drink)?*** 0 Patient had no tolerance to alcohol. 1 Patient had tolerance to alcohol. . Not sure *or* not applicable *or* missing.	Missing

ALC2. Withdrawal	
When you stopped or cut down on alcohol use, did you have withdrawal symptoms? (interviewer gives examples of alcohol withdrawal symptoms) 0 Patient had no withdrawal symptoms from alcohol. 1 Patient had withdrawal symptoms from alcohol. . Not sure *or* not applicable *or* missing.	*1*
ALC3. Failure to fulfill major obligations	
Did alcohol use result in failure to fulfill major role obligations (work, school, or home)? 0 Alcohol had no effect on work, school, or social obligations. 1 Alcohol had negative effect on work, school, or social obligations. . Not sure *or* not applicable *or* missing.	*0*
ALC4. Social, interpersonal problems due to alcohol	
Did alcohol cause any social or interpersonal problems* (e.g., *work problems, school problems, relationship problems, family problems, legal problems, physical fights)? 0 Alcohol caused no social or interpersonal problems. 1 Alcohol caused social or interpersonal problems. . Not sure *or* not applicable *or* missing.	*1*
ALC5. Alcohol use in spite of problems	
Did you continue to use alcohol even though you had problems? 0 Patient had no alcohol problems. 1 Patient continued to use alcohol even though alcohol caused problems. . Not sure *or* not applicable *or* missing.	*1*
ALC6. Alcohol use in hazardous situations	
Did you use alcohol in a situation, in which it was physically hazardous* (e.g., *driving a car or operating machinery)? 0 Patient did not use alcohol in hazardous situations. 1 Patient used alcohol in hazardous situations. . Not sure *or* not applicable *or* missing.	*0*

ALC7. Alcohol blackout	
Did you have a blackout after drinking so much alcohol that the next day you could not remember what you said or did? 0 Patient had no blackout. 1 Patient had blackout. . Not sure *or* not applicable *or* missing.	*1*
ALC8. Other alcohol problems	
Did you have any other problems due to alcohol use? 0 No. 1 Yes (craving). . Not sure *or* not applicable *or* missing.	*1*
Alcoholism score = 5 (moderate)	

Video #5: PTSD

Transcription of Interview #5 (C = Clinician; P = Patient)

C: I just wanted to thank you for participating with us. This interview will help future trainees and give them some standardized approaches for identifying different pathologies. We understand you have some problems with trauma in childhood, and we wanted to talk about that if you're okay with that.

P: That's fine.

C: Thank you for participating.

C: Have you witnessed or experienced a traumatic event that you were involved in or that was threatened to you? This can be physical abuse, sexual abuse, a terrorist attack, natural disaster. Has anything like that happened to you?

P: Probably too many to count. From my earliest one that I recall was 4 years old. I was sexually abused by a babysitter.

C: I assume when that happened you had some pretty intense fear and feelings of helplessness.

P: I did, but I never told anyone about it.

C: So a lot of these events were kept hidden for a while out of fear, or were you threatened by someone?

P: I wasn't threatened, I was offered an escape from my own life. That's why I participated.

C: Is it fair to say it was more than one event in childhood? You had more than one intense experience?

P: Yes.

C: With regard to these events, do you have a lot of recurring memories of things that happened?

P: I do. I have a lot of nightmares.

C: Okay. How often do you get nightmares? Is this a nightly thing?

P: Maybe four out of seven nights.

C: That's a lot of nights.

P: Oh yes. It makes you trepidatious about going to sleep.

C: It's almost better to stay awake than fall asleep and have to deal with nightmares.

P: Absolutely. Yes.

C: So nightmares are pretty often and I assume they've offered you medicines, or hopefully you've tried some medicines?

P: I haven't brought them up. I've been under psychiatric care since 1968, but I never brought some of these things up until this trip.

C: Well hopefully we'll be able to help address that. In terms of other issues related to your traumas, do you have flashbacks of the events, like re-experiencing them like you're back in that time and place?

P: I do. I smell sometimes the weather will bring these things back. Something on television. Not too long ago I saw a catalogue. I tried to commit suicide when I was 4, I tried to drink something that had a skull and crossbones. I hadn't seen this particular cleaning element in years, and I saw it in a catalogue and I actually got physically sick.

C: So all that time and it brought you right back to where you were.

P: Seventy years later.

C: Not only were you traumatized by things that happened to you, but when you tried to hurt yourself that was traumatic as well.

P: Yes because I was scared to death that if I didn't get it cleaned up, my mother would kill me when she got home which was ridiculous because I was only 4.

C: In terms of other symptoms, do you try to avoid thinking about things, avoiding the thoughts or feelings associated with what happened?

P: Yes, I stayed on pills for many many years just so I would be numb.

C: Try to kind of numb down those thoughts.

P: Yes.

C: Do you also try to avoid people, places, or things that trigger those events? You mentioned the cleaning supplies, that's probably something you would anticipate would bring back memories, but do you try to avoid other things that could spark those memories?

P: I isolate myself.

C: Sort of general avoidance of things.

P: Absolutely.

C: That must be pretty hard. It's hard to feel well when you're isolating all the time from others.

P: A little bit. It's starting to get to me now.

C: Are there any times when your memory is kind of fuzzy of what happened? Like you see pieces of what happened but the full picture is not clear?

P: For approximately 10 years, I lost a whole 10 years. Then a few years ago, I had some traumatic things happen, and all of a sudden, it came back and I was writing on anything I could get my hands on for about 48 hours. It was like I needed to regurgitate all that stuff that had been locked up for so long.

C: I can tell it's hard to think about it even now.

P: Yes.

C: You mentioned that isolation is a problem. Did you find, too, that you were spending less time with family and friends and things that you liked to do because of what happened? Like your trauma was keeping you back from doing things you would want to do?

P: I don't do anything with family and I don't have many friends. I just work. My work is my life. And with Alzheimer's patients, it's not as though I have any feedback from what I give out in the daytime, other than their comfort or their amusement or whatever it might be.

C: Do you feel in some ways that what happened to your trauma has left you feeling cut off or isolated or distant from other people?

P: Absolutely. Yes. For years and years.

C: How about in terms of emotionally? Do you feel that there's a numbness to your emotions as a result of what's happened?

P: Yeah.

C: *So is it hard for you to experience feeling loved or happiness? Just sort of numbed out? Sounds like you've sort of numbed out with medicines too.*

P: *I did for some time. I had my last medications like that 3 years ago, but I still don't get involved with people or situations. I just work and stay to myself. The light of my life is the day hospital.*

C: *It's a good program.*

P: *It really is.*

C: *As a result of it, you mentioned that you kind of fear sleeping sometimes because of the nightmares. Do you have any issues with falling asleep or staying asleep as a result of what's happened?*

P: *Absolutely, yes. Because I'll have dreams and wake up and then I can't get back to sleep.*

C: *A lot of it does have to do with the nightmares, and they've been so pervasive for so long.*

P: *Yes. And they all weren't from back then. They're just about five really traumatic events, and it may be the one from 21 years ago. So it's different for different times.*

C: *So you never really know what you're going to dream about but it's not going to be something good.*

P: *It's usually not.*

C: *Okay. Do you have periods where you get really irritable with people or have sudden outbursts of anger? Some of these symptoms happen to most people, some of them are only for a select few.*

P: *Not generally. I don't let myself do that, but once in a while, it might be with someone from the water department or someone totally isolated from me ordinarily. Someone came to give me physical therapy not too long ago and I was not too nice to her. I apologized. I just don't do well around people a lot.*

C: *Do you ever feel that you have to be more alert or watchful of things around you? So like staying on edge, making sure nothing bad will happen.*

P: *Yes. For 21 years, I didn't go in my living room; I was frightened because something had happened in the house. Just recently I started to go into the living room, thanks to the help that I get at the day hospital. I wouldn't go outside or anything. Just to go to work or to the grocery store.*

C: *Do you think that you also have any issues with your concentration? Like it's difficult to focus on the moment because the past is hampering your abilities to do things?*

P: *Indeed it is. For a long time, I couldn't read. My reading and vocabulary have always been quite good, but I couldn't read a paragraph and realize what it was saying. I would have to read it over and over and over. Just recently I have gotten to where I could read again.*

C: *So like your focus was off for no good reason.*

P: *Absolutely.*

C: *That's difficult. Besides the focus being off and being on edge all the time, do you feel that you're more easily startled or more jumpy about things, like loud noises?*

P: I talked about that yesterday with my pastor. Not too long ago, every time he would walk up behind me as I worked in the church by myself, he would walk up behind me and I would scream bloody murder. He'd say "What's the matter?" Then my daughter came to live with me for 3 years when she started to get sick. She would walk past me in the hallway and I would scream. She'd say "Mom you must be crazy!" You're just on edge. You don't know whether to fight or to run.

C: Are there any other symptoms that you've noticed, anything else? I understand low mood is a problem for you as well. Anything else that you've noticed as a result of the traumas that you've experienced that has affected your life?

P: I don't trust people like I would like to. Sometimes I would like to have a friend. They find it difficult to believe here in the hospital that I had no one to bring me clothes, but they can't understand how isolated I am that my only outlet is my patients who have Alzheimer's and can't drive and are only at home. They had a really hard time understanding that. There is no one, but I've done that to myself and I know that.

C: So just to kind of summarize, you've certainly had enough bad experiences in early childhood and throughout adulthood. Clearly they've affected your functioning in many ways. It's been hard for you to make friends, you tend to isolate a lot, nightmares are chronically a problem. You easily startle around people and it's affected your ability to concentrate on things. You spend a lot of time trying to avoid these feelings and numb you down as best you could.

P: Yes. My appetite is something else too. Food is my lover, my confidante, my best friend, and that's disgusting. I've gained so much weight. I've had two major surgeries to lose weight.

C: We're glad that you're here and glad that you're getting help. We really appreciate you helping us out. Hopefully this helps people in the future with training.

Video #5 Ratings

PTSD1. Witness or experience traumatic events	***Score***
Have you ever witnessed or experienced a traumatic event that involved actual or threatened death or serious injury to you or someone else (e.g., physical or sexual abuse, rape, terrorist attack, natural disaster, war…)? ***Did you feel intense fear and helplessness?*** 0 Patient had no traumatic events. 1 Patient has experienced one traumatic event. 2 Patient has experienced several traumatic events. . Not sure *or* not applicable *or* missing.	*2*
PTSD2. Distressing recollection of events	
Did you have recurrent upsetting memories (distressing recollection) of the event? 0 Patient had no significant symptom. 1 Patient has recurrent upsetting memories (distressing recollection) of the event. . Not sure *or* not applicable *or* missing.	*1*
PTSD3. Bad dreams or nightmares	

Did you have recurrent upsetting dreams or nightmares of the event? 0 Patient had no significant symptom. 1 Patient has recurrent upsetting dreams and nightmares of the event. . Not sure *or* not applicable *or* missing.	*1*
PTSD4. Flashbacks	
Did you have a sense or feeling that the event was happening again: the sense of reliving the event (flashbacks), auditory/visual hallucinations related to the event, or body/somatosensory experiences of the event? 0 Patient had no significant symptom. 1 Patient has a sense or feeling that the event is happening again, the sense of reliving the event (flashbacks). . Not sure *or* not applicable *or* missing.	*1*
PTSD5. Avoidance of thoughts or feelings	
Did you try to avoid thoughts and feelings associated with the event? 0 Patient had no significant symptom. 1 Patient tries not to think about the event. . Not sure *or* not applicable *or* missing.	*1*

PTSD6. Avoidance of people, places, and activities	
Did you try to avoid things that reminded you of the event (such as certain people, certain places, or some activities)? 0 Patient had no significant symptom. 1 Patient avoids things that are reminders of the event (such as certain people, certain Places, or some activities). . Not sure *or* not applicable *or* missing.	*1*
PTSD7. Amnesia	
Did you have difficulty remembering some or all important aspects of the event? 0 Patient had no significant symptom. 1 Patient has difficulty remembering some or all important aspects of the event. . Not sure *or* not applicable *or* missing.	*1*
PTSD8. Diminished social interest (asociality)	
Did you spend less time or show less interest in activities with friends/family or hobbies that you used to enjoy due to the event? 0 Patient had no significant symptom. 1 Patient spends less time or shows less interest in activities with friends/family or hobbies due to the event. . Not sure *or* not applicable *or* missing.	*1*
PTSD9. Detachment and isolation	
Did you feel distant, cut off, or isolated from other people due to the event? 0 Patient had no significant symptom. 1 Patient feels distant, cut off, or isolated from other people due to the event. . Not sure *or* not applicable *or* missing.	*1*
PTSD10. Diminished emotional feelings (diminished experience of emotions)	

Did you feel emotionally numb? ***Did you have trouble experiencing feelings (happiness, love feelings) due to the event?*** 0 Patient had no significant symptom. 1 Patient feels emotionally numb. Patient has trouble experiencing feelings (such as happiness or love feelings) due to the event. . Not sure *or* not applicable *or* missing.	***1***
PTSD11. Insomnia	
Did you have difficulty falling or staying asleep due to the event? 0 Patient had no significant symptom. 1 Patient has difficulty falling or staying asleep due to the event. . Not sure *or* not applicable *or* missing.	***1***

PTSD12. Anger	
Did you have periods of irritability or sudden outbursts of anger due to the event? 0 Patient had no significant symptom. 1 Patient has periods of irritability or sudden outbursts of anger due to the event. . Not sure *or* not applicable *or* missing.	***0***
PTSD13. Attention impairment/poor concentration	
Did you have difficulty concentrating due to the event? 0 Patient had no significant symptom. 1 Patient has difficulty concentrating due to the event. . Not sure *or* not applicable *or* missing.	***1***
PTSD14. Hypervigilance	
Did you feel very alert or watchful of things going on around you even when there was no need to be? 0 Patient had no significant symptom. 1 Patient feels very alert or watchful of things going on around even when there is no need to be. . Not sure *or* not applicable *or* missing.	***1***
PTSD15. Startle response	
Did you feel jumpy and easily startled? ***Were you easily scared or did you make a sudden movement or jump when you heard noises or if you were caught by surprise?*** 0 Patient had no significant symptom. 1 Patient feels jumpy and has a startle response. . Not sure *or* not applicable *or* missing.	***1***
PTSD16. Other PTSD symptoms	
0 No. 1 Yes (specify). . Not sure *or* not applicable *or* missing.	***1***
PTSD score = 16 (severe)	

Video #6: Eating Disorders

Transcription of Interview #6 (C = Clinician; P = Patient)

C: We just want to thank you for coming and participating in this video. We are hoping it will help provide instruction for other trainees in the future. Just a few things to start. Have you had problems with binge eating in the past, like episodes where you would eat a lot more than other people would in a 1- or 2-hour period?

P: Yes.

C: Okay. So is this something that would happen pretty often, like on average once a week or multiple times a week?

P: Yes. Multiple times a week.

C: How long have you been struggling with this?

P: Probably 10 years.

C: So this isn't anything new for you, it's been going on for a while?

P: Yes.

C: When you're in one of these episodes where you're eating a lot, do you feel like you kind of lose control and you can't really stop once you start?

P: I feel like I know that I'm not hungry, but I feel like I'm starving and I just want to keep eating and eating. And then I get sick. Not like throw-up sick, but like…ugh.

C: Physically ill? Like "why did I do that" kind of thing?

P: Yes.

C: When you're in one of these episodes, do you find that you're not only eating more but that you're eating faster than you normally would? So you're shoveling it in basically, just going to town?

P: Yes.

C: You've already kind of said this, but you get to the point where you're uncomfortably full, kind of beyond the normal cessation of a meal?

P: Yes.

C: When you have these kinds of episodes, are you eating even when you're not physically hungry? So just, like, the food is there and the opportunity arises and you're eating?

P: Yes.

C: Okay. When you're doing these, or after the fact, do you get to the point where you feel physically or emotionally disgusted with yourself?

P: Yes.

C: Okay. So a lot of guilt that goes along with this?

P: Oh yeah.

C: How did this all start originally?

P: I don't know. I think I did this even, my mom says, like when I was younger, but I was skinny for years. Even after I had kids, I was thin, and I just didn't really think it was a problem at all, and then of course when I gained a lot of weight, it may not be all that, but I took it as a symptom that maybe I shouldn't be doing this.

C: So you, baseline, you were always thin, then you got married and had kids. How old were they when you started eating like this?

P: Probably little. The youngest was probably two or so.

C: So pretty early on. Was it after your husband and you decided that you weren't going to have more kids, was it kind of around that time?

P: I think it was even after that.

C: Okay. Sometimes looking at causality, what kind of brought these things on is important. Looking for in the future ways to avoid backsliding, as they say. So when you are in one of these episodes of binge eating, do you feel pretty upset and distressed? You already said you feel disgusted with yourself, but do you also get in an emotionally distressed state?

P: Yeah.

C: Okay. Is there any kind of compensatory behavior after binge eating, like anything you try to do to undo what you've done eating-wise?

P: Not really, I just feel awful.

C: Okay. Well, some people when they binge eat, afterwards they will excessively try dieting or fasting or sometimes using laxatives. Is that something you've ever done before?

P: No.

C: Okay. Any diet pills that you've taken, not prescribed?

P: No.

C: Okay. What about in terms of after binging, did you ever try making yourself vomit?

P: Oh no. I don't ever want to vomit, ever. That will never be a problem, haha.

C: Okay. What about trying to take laxatives or diuretics?

P: No.

C: Okay. So yours is more, you binge eat, you lose control while you binge eat, you feel terrible afterwards, but you're not necessarily doing anything to undo what you've done?

P: Right.

C: Okay. Any other behavior that you do after the fact? Kind of weird relationships with food you can think of?

P: Not that I can think of.

C: You mentioned when you were younger that you were always thin growing up. How tall are you now?

P: Five foot one.

C: Okay. How much do you weigh these days?

P: I haven't weighed myself recently. I want to say around 210.

C: You were heavier in the past, your highest weight was 240 or so?

P: My highest weight was up to 254.

C: Okay. What's your lowest weight that you've ever been, once you were fully grown?

P: After I had my kids even, I got back down to 127 or something like that.

C: So that was your baseline. Have you ever been very thin and couldn't maintain a minimal low weight? Like you were so small that you couldn't even hit an average weight?

P: No.

C: Okay. Did you ever have people growing up say that you weighed much less than normal?

P: No.

C: Do you feel that your weight and shape were ever very important to the point where they affected how you feel about yourself?

P: Now, yes.

C: Okay. Back then?

P: No.

C: And you were never so small in size that it affected your health and you had problems with your menstrual cycle or things like that?

P: No.

C: Okay. Did you ever have an intense fear of gaining weight when you were a normal weight?

P: No.

C: Did you ever try to have to lose weight when you were younger by fasting?

P: No.

C: Okay. What about with over exercising? Was that ever a problem where you'd gain some weight and try to undo it?

P: No.

C: And no problem with diet pills in the past? And you already said you don't like vomiting, haha.

P: Right.

C: Neither do I. Especially the sound of it, that's the worst. No laxatives or anything?

P: No.

C: Okay. So really normal weight throughout most of life, married and had kids, a couple years later is when binge eating became a problem and got to the point where several times a week you would eat, even if you weren't hungry, until you were too full. It got to the point where you gained weight but we're trying to address it now.

P: Yes.

C: Well thank you for helping us out and hopefully you continue to work with me.

Video #6 Ratings

EATING1. Binge eating	***Score***
Do you have episodes of binge eating (eating within 1- or 2-hour period what most people would consider an unusually large amount of food)? 0 Absent or nonsignificant. 1 Symptoms present. . Not sure *or* not applicable *or* missing.	*1*

EATING2. Binge eating frequency	
0 None. 1 1–3 times per month. 2 At least once a week for 3 months. . Not sure *or* not applicable *or* missing.	*2*
EATING3. Losing control with binge eating	
During the episodes of binge eating, did you feel that you had lost control and could not stop eating? 0 Absent or nonsignificant. Symptoms present. . Not sure *or* not applicable *or* missing.	*1*
EATING4. Eating fast during binge eating	
During the episodes of binge eating, did you eat much more rapidly than usual? 0 Absent or nonsignificant. 1 Symptoms present. . Not sure *or* not applicable *or* missing.	*1*
EATIG5. Eating until uncomfortably full during binge eating	
During the episodes of binge eating, did you eat until you felt uncomfortably full? 0 Absent or nonsignificant. 1 Symptoms present. . Not sure *or* not applicable *or* missing.	*1*

EATING6. Eating when not hungry during binge eating	
During the episodes of binge eating, did you eat a large amount of food when you did not feel physically hungry? 0 Absent or nonsignificant. 1 Symptoms present. . Not sure *or* not applicable *or* missing.	*1*
EATING7. Eating alone during binge eating	
During the episodes of binge eating, did you eat alone because you were embarrassed by how much you were eating? 0 Absent or nonsignificant. 1 Symptoms present. . Not sure *or* not applicable *or* missing.	***Missing***
EATING8. Feeling disgusted and guilty during binge eating	
During the episodes of binge eating, did you feel disgusted with yourself, depressed or guilty by your overeating? 0 Absent or nonsignificant. 1 Symptoms present. . Not sure *or* not applicable *or* missing.	*1*
EATING9. Distressed by overeating during binge eating	
During the episodes of binge eating, did you feel quite upset or very distressed by your overeating? 0 Absent or nonsignificant. 1 Symptoms present. . Not sure *or* not applicable *or* missing.	*1*
Binge eating score = 9	

Video # 7: Psychosis and Mania

Transcription of Interview #7 (C = Clinician; P = Patient)

C: Give me some information about yourself. Where do you live and who lives with you?
P: I live in an apartment alone in a high-rise building downtown.
C: You've been coming here for some years?
P: Many years.
C: What are the reasons that you come here for?
P: Mainly for management of my medications.
C: Let me ask you some questions and focus on the past month. Have you had any time when you heard voices that no one else could hear?
P: Pretty much every day.
C: Okay. Do the voices sometimes ask you to do something?
P: Yeah.
C: Can you give me an example?
P: Sometimes to do disgusting things.
C: And you don't listen to the voices?
P: No, no.
C: So you hear the voices every day?
P: Several times a day.
C: In 1 day, on average, how much time do you hear the voices?
P: Maybe an hour, hour and a half.
C: Do you sometimes hear a voice that comments on what you say or do?
P: Yeah, comments on my behavior or thinking.
C: Can you give me an example?
P: It might say "you're feeling sorry for yourself" or "that dress doesn't look good on you."
C: Do you hear one voice or several voices?
P: Mostly one. Same one, mostly all the time.
C: Is it a man's voice or woman's voice?
P: Male.
C: Do you recognize that person's voice? Is it a person you know?
P: It's a voice in the past, when I've been unwell, I thought it was a demon.
C: Do you sometimes see things that others can't?
P: That only happened when I was extremely sick.
C: I'm going to ask you some other questions about the past month. Did you have any thoughts that someone was after you or trying to harm you?
P: I had paranoid thoughts about this woman who lives in my building. I thought she was trying to do things to be mean to me.
C: Okay. How do you know her? Who is she?
P: She has an apartment in the same building. She's the backup manager.
C: But you think she is trying to harm you?

P: Oh, no. I thought she was using her backup key to come in my apartment and damage my belongings.

C: That's what you thought. But she never did that?

P: Oh yes she did! But I can't get anyone to believe me.

C: Okay. What did she do?

P: She cut my clothing, stole money.

C: For the past month, do you think your thoughts are not your own thoughts and that someone else put them there?

P: Not in the last month, but years ago I had those beliefs.

C: For the past month, did you think someone was taking thoughts out of your mind?

P: Not in the last month, but I have in the past.

C: Did you feel like your thoughts were broadcast over the past month?

P: No, I never thought that.

C: Did you feel that there was a plot or conspiracy against you?

P: Oh no.

C: Did you feel that when you watched the TV that the TV is sending a special message to you?

P: Not in the past month, but back in 1981 I thought the radio stations were playing special songs for me. I thought that for months and months.

C: I understand that you have been sober for…

P: 13.5 years.

C: Good for you. You also mentioned that in the past you had mood swings.

P: Yes.

C: What does "manic episode" mean to you?

P: I was very hyperactive and I had a lot of energy. I couldn't sit still, I hardly slept at all. I spent a lot of money.

C: Think about that time. During that time, were you feeling very very happy? Or did you feel angry and irritable?

P: I've had both. Sometimes the episode would be where I would be very happy and expansive. And sometimes I've had them where I've been angry and paranoid. Most of the time it's some combination of the two. Some happiness, but whenever anybody got in my way, I would easily become irritable.

C: Did you also feel that your mood changed in the same day? Like one hour you feel happy and then you feel sad?

P: Yeah, I've had days like that before. Like in the morning I'll be very happy, and then by evening I feel down. Like a roller coaster.

C: The time when you feel very happy, how long does it last?

P: Sometimes it could last as long as 3 or 4 days. But after that it would change to irritation for several days.

C: During that time of feeling happy or irritable, did you feel that your mind was racing?

P: Yes, exactly. Too many thoughts and they were very fast thoughts.

C: Did you feel this way the whole day?

P: All day, for days. Too many thoughts, too fast to even talk about them.

C: During that time, did you also feel that your speech was different?

P: *Yes, faster than usual.*

C: *Also during that time, did you feel easily distracted by any noise?*

P: *Yes, definitely. In fact I was so distracted that, I normally read a lot, but I couldn't concentrate when I would try to read. I'd read one paragraph, and the cat jumping off the couch would distract me, and then I'd start thinking…I couldn't concentrate on anything.*

C: *Did you also feel like you had too much energy?*

P: *Yes. I couldn't sit still. My boyfriend and I would be watching TV and I couldn't sit still. I couldn't just sit and watch a movie.*

C: *Did you feel that you had a special power or talent?*

P: *I've had thoughts like that but I was very unwilling to tell anyone about that because I knew if I told anyone that they would think I was off my rocker.*

C: *Give me an example of the kind of thoughts you would have.*

P: *There were a few occasions where I'd have hyperactivity and thought I was on a mission from God. Like I had a special mission to accomplish.*

C: *At the same time, did you spend more money than you should?*

P: *Yes, I'm on social security and I get a check that has to last all month, but I'd spend it all in the first 2 weeks and have nothing left.*

C: *Buying things you don't need?*

P: *Yes. I'd go to the mall and buy a bunch of jeans that I don't need.*

C: *How was your sleep during this time?*

P: *I wouldn't sleep very much, 2–3 hours, but I wouldn't be tired at all.*

C: *When you had this manic episode, did you feel paranoid?*

P: *I had a few thoughts about that. A few times I thought a witch was trying to kill me and one of my friends knocked on the door and I wouldn't go because I thought he was part of it!*

C: *During that time, did you hear any voices?*

P: *Whenever I have a mood swing, it makes the voices worse. I don't know what the ratio is for that, but it makes the other problem worse.*

C: *Did you have any other symptoms during the manic phase?*

P: *I was never hungry. I lost weight. I would always lose weight when I was manic if it went on for a while. The manic episodes usually last 3 months and I'd lose about 10 pounds.*

C: *Any other symptoms?*

P: *I know people would get really annoyed with me. I talk constantly, won't shut up, call people up at 3 AM, wake them up, haha.*

C: *Okay. Thank you again for answering these questions.*

Video #7 Ratings

HAL1. Auditory hallucinations	***Score***
Do you hear noises (like music, whispering sounds) or voices talking to you when there is no one around? ***Are the voices like a real voice or just thoughts in your mind?*** 0 Patient has no auditory hallucinations. 1 Patient has auditory hallucinations. 2 Patient has auditory hallucinations with command. . Not sure *or* not applicable *or* missing.	*2*
HAL2. Frequency of auditory hallucinations	
How often do you hear noises (like music, whispering sounds) or voices talking to you when there is no one around? 0 Patient has no auditory hallucinations. 1 Patient has auditory hallucinations (1–4 days/month). 2 Patient has auditory hallucinations (5–14 days/month). 3 Patient has auditory hallucinations (≥15 days/month). . Not sure *or* not applicable *or* missing.	*3*
HAL3. Hallucination duration	
On days when you hear noises or voices, how often do you hear them? 0 Patient has no auditory hallucinations. 1 Patient has auditory hallucinations (less than 1 hour/day). 2 Patient has auditory hallucinations (1–4 hours/day). 3 Patient has auditory hallucinations (more than 4 hours/day). . Not sure *or* not applicable *or* missing.	*2*
HAL4. Audible thoughts	
Do you think that your thoughts are so loud that someone close to you can hear what you are thinking? 0 Patient has no audible thoughts. 1 Patient has audible thoughts. . Not sure *or* not applicable *or* missing.	*Missing*
HAL5. Voices arguing	
Do you hear two or more voices that argue about what you are doing or thinking? 0 Voices do not argue with the patient. 1 Voices argue about what the patient is doing or thinking. . Not sure *or* not applicable *or* missing.	*Missing*
HAL6. Voices commenting	
Do you hear a voice or voices commenting on what you are doing or thinking? 0 Voices do not comment about the patient. 1 Voices comment on what the patient is doing or thinking. . Not sure *or* not applicable *or* missing.	*1*
HAL7. Visual hallucinations	
Do you see things other people cannot see (e.g., shadows, objects or people)? 0 Patient has no visual hallucinations. 1 Patient has visual hallucinations. . Not sure *or* not applicable *or* missing.	*0*
HAL8. Observed hallucinations	

0 Patient has not been observed talking to self. 1 Patient has been observed talking to self, talking to a mirror, or running a conversation with unseen person. . Not sure *or* not applicable *or* missing.	***0***
HAL9. Other hallucinations (olfactory, gustatory, tactile)	
Do you sometimes notice unusual smells that other people do not notice, experience strange tastes in your mouth, or feel strange sensations on your body? 0. Patient has no other hallucinations. 1. Patient has other hallucinations (olfactory, gustatory, or tactile hallucinations). . Not sure *or* not applicable *or* missing.	***Missing***
Hallucinations score during the past month = 8 (moderate)	

DEL1. Somatic passivity (bizarre delusions associated with somatic sensations)	***Score***
Do you feel or have a bodily sensation (e.g., something is crawling under your skin) and think it is caused by an outside person or force? 0 Patient has no somatic passivity. 1 Patient has somatic passivity. . Not sure *or* not applicable *or* missing.	***Missing***
DEL2. Delusions of thought insertion	
Do you think that thoughts in your mind are not your own thoughts and that they were inserted into your mind by an outside person or force? 0 Patient has no delusions of thought insertion. 1 Patient has delusions of thought insertion. . Not sure *or* not applicable *or* missing.	***0***
DEL3. Delusions of thought withdrawal	
Do you think that your thoughts were taken out of your mind by an outside person or force? 0 Patient has no delusions of thought withdrawal. 1 Patient has delusions of thought withdrawal. . Not sure *or* not applicable *or* missing.	***0***
DEL4. Delusions of thought broadcasting	
Do you think that your thoughts are broadcast so that people are able to know what you are thinking, even if they are in different places? 0 Patient has no delusions of thought broadcast. 1 Patient has delusions of thought broadcast. . Not sure *or* not applicable *or* missing.	***0***
DEL5. Paranoid/persecutory delusions	
Have you felt that people are against you, talking about you, or laughing at you? Do you think someone is trying to harm you (e.g., trying to poison your food or trying to kill you)? 0 Patient has no paranoid/persecutory delusions. 1 Patient has paranoid/persecutory delusions some of the time. 2 Patient has paranoid/persecutory delusions most of the time. . Not sure *or* not applicable *or* missing.	***0***
DEL6. Delusions of conspiracy	

Do you think there is a plot or a conspiracy against you by anyone* (e.g., *a person, FBI, CIA)? 0 Patient has no delusions of conspiracy. 1 Patient has delusions of conspiracy some of the time. 2 Patient has delusions of conspiracy most of the time. . Not sure *or* not applicable *or* missing.	*0*

DEL7. Delusions of reference	
When you are watching TV, listening to the radio, or reading the newspaper, do you think that special messages are intended specifically for you? 0 Patient has no delusions of reference. 1 Patient has delusions of reference some of the time. 2 Patient has delusions of reference most of the time. . Not sure *or* not applicable *or* missing.	*0*
DEL8. Other delusions	
Do you have any other strange thoughts or beliefs that other people do not have? 0 Patient has no other delusions. 1 Patient has other delusions. . Not sure *or* not applicable *or* missing.	*0*
DEL9. Bizarreness of delusions (delusions are bizarre if they are completely impossible* (e.g., *patient believes he/she was born on Mars and brought to earth on a spaceship))	
0 Patient has no bizarre delusions. 1 Patient has bizarre delusions. . Not sure *or* not applicable *or* missing.	*0*
Delusions score during the past month = 0	

M1. Expansive (elated) mood	***Score***
Have you sometimes felt very happy, elated, on top of the world without much reason? 0 Patient has no elated mood. 1 Patient has elated mood less than half the time. 2 Patient has elated mood more than half the time. . Not sure *or* not applicable *or* missing.	*1*
M2. Irritable mood	
Have you sometimes felt that you were easily irritated without reason? ***Have you found yourself so irritable that you shout at people or start arguments or actually become aggressive?*** 0 Patient has no irritable mood. 1 Patient has irritable mood less than half the time. 2 Patient has irritable mood more than half the time. . Not sure *or* not applicable *or* missing.	*1*
M3. Mixed mood (mood lability)	
Have you had mixed mood swings: periods of <u>depression and elation or irritability on the same day?</u> 0 Patient has no mixed mood swings. 1 Patient has mixed mood less than half the time. 2 Patient has mixed mood more than half the time. . Not sure *or* not applicable *or* missing.	*1*

M4. Racing thoughts (observed as flight of ideas)	
Have you felt that you had too many different thoughts racing through your mind compared with normal? 0 Patient has no racing thoughts. 1 Patient has racing thoughts less than half the time. 2 Patient has racing thoughts more than half the time. . Not sure *or* not applicable *or* missing.	*2*
M5. Pressured speech	
Have you been talking faster than usual during this time (**e.g.,** ***people said that they were unable to understand you because you were speaking too fast or you felt a pressure to continue talking)?*** 0 Patient has normal speech. 1 Patient has pressured speech less than half the time. 2 Patient has pressured speech more than half the time. . Not sure *or* not applicable *or* missing.	*1*

M6. Distraction (attention is distracted by environmental noises)	
Do you find yourself easily distracted by unimportant activities or things happening around you? 0 Patient has no distraction. 1 Patient has been easily distracted by external stimuli less than half the time. 2 Patient has been easily distracted by external stimuli more than half the time. . Not sure *or* not applicable *or* missing.	*1*
M7. Increase in activities	
Have you been more active and had more energy than usual? ***Did you do more things than usual at work, school, or socially?*** 0 Patient has no increased energy. 1 Patient has too much energy less than half the time. 2 Patient has too much energy more than half the time. . Not sure *or* not applicable *or* missing.	
M8. Grandiosity	
Have you felt more self-confident than usual? ***Have you felt that you have special powers or special abilities?*** 0 Patient has no grandiosity. 1 Patient has grandiose thoughts, but not of a delusional quality. . Not sure *or* not applicable *or* missing.	
M9. Overspending (poor judgment in new activities)	
Have you done something that you regretted later (**e.g.,** ***spending a lot of money that you could not afford, writing bad checks, or investing money foolishly, sexual indiscretions)?*** 0 Patient did not go on a spending spree. 1 Patient went on a spending spree during manic phase. . Not sure *or* not applicable *or* missing.	*1*
M10. Decreased sleep	
Have you needed less sleep than usual and without getting tired? 0 Patient has normal sleep. 1 Patient sleeps 4 hours or less (in a 24-hour period including naps) and feels rested. . Not sure *or* not applicable *or* missing.	*1*

M11. Other symptoms (e.g., hypersexuality, aggressive driving, illegal drug use, or gambling)	
0 Absent. 1 Present (losing weight in a manic episode). . Not sure *or* not applicable *or* missing.	*1*

M12. Delusions associated mainly with manic episode	
0 Absent. 1 Present. . Not sure *or* not applicable *or* missing.	*1*
M13. Hallucinations associated mainly with manic episode	
0 Absent. 1 Present. . Not sure *or* not applicable *or* missing.	*1*
Mania score (a previous manic episode) = 15 (severe)	

Video # 8: Anxiety and Panic

Transcription of Interview #8 (C = Clinician; P = Patient)

C: Tell me where do you live and who lives with you?

P: I live in Headsville, WV. I live with my wife and two sons.

C: What are the main reasons that brought you into the hospital?

P: The main reason I came into the hospital is because my anxiety and the anxiety attacks I had developed to the point where it was almost impossible for me to function in daily life. I knew I had to get help, so we called the Chestnut Ridge Center, and they said the best way to get help would be to come to the ER.

C: I'm glad you came here for help. You mentioned anxiety and panic attacks. Let me describe to you panic attack and tell me whether this happen to you or not. A panic attack is when you feel very anxious and frightened all of a sudden and it happens very fast. If you're very frightened, sometimes you can feel the shakes. Tell me more about what happens to you.

P: I'll have a long-standing sort of panic state that can build into a panic attack like what you just described. When I've come into the hospital for a panic attack before, I became very panicked to the point where I felt numb because I was losing oxygen because I couldn't breathe. It's common for me to live in a continuous state of being frightened. I can't get a cup of coffee because it might kill me. I can't take a shower because I might suffocate. Things like that. There are things like that which trigger a slow incline into a panic attack. They're not usually just onset, right away, but once it does happen it's almost impossible to stop.

C: So you feel anxious most of the time, and then at some point you get a panic attack?

P: Yes, over the past year and a half this has been getting worse. I might be anxious and nervous for hours on end with no real reason. Anything under the sun can be a trigger. And then it can directly lead to a panic attack.

C: Describe for me the last panic attack you had.

P: The last time I had a full one it was several days ago. I was at my house and it got to the point where I could not breathe. We had to call an ambulance and they took me to Western Health System, the closest hospital to us, and I had a panic attack in the ambulance as well.

C: How long did the panic attack last?

P: It felt like it lasted forever, but it probably only lasted, the worst part, about 5–10 minutes, but leading into it, there was a steady rise of breathing issues for about 10 minutes, and then after I started to come down, there was about 10 minutes of more breathing issues. Within that 5–10 minute mark was when it was the worst.

C: On average, how often do you get panic attacks?

P: I would say, at this point, before I came to the facility, they were happening almost several times a day.

C: After the panic attack is finished, do you worry about having another panic attack?

P: Yes, that happens constantly. I have a constant fear of having another panic attack and a constant fear of death and suffocating because of it.

C: Okay. And do you do anything to stop the panic attack? Like take a deep breath?

P: Yes, I try. However, I've found that my triggers are sometimes very ridiculous. Sometimes breathing too deeply sets it off. I've found that a nice walk around the house and trying to focus on something else can help. That usually will sustain me at a certain point but it almost never calms me down. It usually takes hours and hours for me to calm down.

C: After the panic attack is over, do you do something to prevent panic attacks from happening again?

P: Yes, I avoid anything that I think might come close to causing it. Like getting into the shower. I've had to develop ways for getting into the shower because it used to trigger an attack. Like instead of hot water, use cold water and splash it on your feet first and then take a cloth and clean yourself and rinse off without the fear of suffocation. I take every avenue to try to prevent that avenue from starting because once it starts it won't stop. I avoid coffee altogether because I know the sugar and coffee won't kill me, but it's hard to tell my brain that.

C: What other symptoms, other than difficulty breathing, do you have during a panic attack?

P: The largest is the breathing. It feels like someone has placed a heavy rock on my chest and throat. Besides that, I'm assuming because of the oxygen level, but my fingers, hands, toes, stomach, and chest will start to get tingly and go numb. I'll start almost convulsing. I was trying to get out of the restraints in the ambulance. I think that's probably attributed to the lack of oxygen.

C: Do you feel like you're choking?

P: Yes.

C: Do you sometimes feel dizzy?

P: Yes. Sometimes feel like the room is spinning. I'll feel confused. Like maybe forgetting, it seems like hours go by but it's only been 10 minutes.

C: Any nausea or vomiting?

P: Just once but it's not regular.

C: What about sweating?

P: Yes.

C: When you have a panic attack, do you feel like you're going to die?

P: Yes. I'm almost sure that I'm going to die.

C: Do you sometimes feel afraid of going crazy?

P: Yes. That's something I've dealt with not just within the panic attack, but with the anxiety that's been leading up over the past year and a half. I've thought that I'm going crazy and that it's why this is happening. Going into a panic attack, it feels like there are so many things that could be wrong with me. You start to lose sense of reality. You can tell someone the sky is blue all you want, but in my world the sky is purple.

C: You mentioned that you also have some anxiety for hours and hours during the day. Describe for me your anxiety. Do you worry too much about things?

P: Somebody asked me more than several times if it's something in my life that's causing it, like finances. It's nothing like that. It's a general anxious, nervousness. Kind of like frightened of something. A constant state of that.

C: And you think it's more than most people?

P: Yes. This is something that is wrong with me that I've been medicated for. This isn't typical, everyday anxiety.

C: When you feel anxious, do you feel restless and keyed up?

P: I feel very flared up. Almost like getting ready for a fight.

C: Your muscles feel tense?

P: My muscles don't tense, but I will get tense which causes my chest and throat to get tense because I worry about my breathing.

C: Do you feel tired and exhausted when anxious?

P: Yes. It's draining.

C: When you are anxious, do you have trouble concentrating?

P: Yes, because all I can focus on is why am I so anxious?

C: When you are anxious, do you feel irritable?

P: I would say yes.

C: When you are anxious, does it affect your sleep? Do you have trouble falling asleep?

P: Absolutely. I have a fear that I will stop breathing when I fall asleep.

C: Any other anxiety symptoms that we haven't talked about?

P: No, I think that about covered it.

C: Now I just have some questions about depression. You mentioned in the past you've been depressed. When was the last time you felt that way?

P: I would say there was a time when I felt very sad and depressed, currently right now because of all the anxiety issues. I don't think it's a medical depression, more the fact of a state of going through sadness. The only other time I've experienced that was from a wrongful medication that made me feel more depressed than normal.

C: *Think about the past month. Would you describe yourself as feeling sad and depressed?*

P: *I would say sad but not depressed.*

C: *Some sadness, but not really the severe level of depression where you would see a doctor.*

P: *Yes, just a general sadness that there is something wrong with me, but I can't control it. But nothing that was depression that led me to see a doctor.*

C: *When you have time, what do you like to do for fun?*

P: *I enjoy reading. I really enjoy it. I study theology. That's about it.*

C: *What about sports?*

P: *I used to run. Got out of shape when I got in college, but I enjoy that every now and then, and then I really feel like I can't breathe.*

C: *What about watching TV?*

P: *Occasionally my wife and I do. With the two kids now it makes it a bit harder.*

C: *In the past when you felt sad and depressed, were you able to enjoy your activities?*

P: *No, I really wasn't. Not if it got bad enough because obviously that had consumed my life. Even though I have had general sadness from anxiety, it still takes over your mind because the anxiety takes over your mind and the sadness takes over your mind and you can't enjoy the everyday parts of life.*

C: *So when you are feeling very sad and depressed, you don't enjoy anything?*

P: *I wouldn't say anything, but it affects everything and there are a few things I may still enjoy.*

C: *So you still enjoy some things?*

P: *Yes.*

Video #8 Ratings

PAN1. Panic attacks (without phobias)	***Score***
Have you gotten suddenly anxious and frightened for a short period of time (up to 60 minutes)? ***During that time, did you feel that your heart was racing or pounding, or did you start shaking or sweating, or did you feel you were choking?*** 0 Patient had no panic attacks. 1 Patient had panic attacks. . Not sure or not applicable or missing.	*1*
PAN3. Worry about having another panic attack	
After a panic attack, did you worry about having another attack? ***Did you worry about its effects* (e.g., *losing control, having a heart attack, or going crazy)?*** 0 After a panic attack, patient did not worry about having another one. 1 After a panic attack, patient worried about having another one or its effects. . Not sure *or* not applicable *or* missing.	*1*

PAN4. Action to end or prevent panic attacks	
Did you have to do something to end the attack, like leaving a store, calling someone, or taking deep breaths? ***Do you do anything to prevent the attacks (like avoiding places that trigger the panic attacks)?*** 0 After a panic attack, patient does nothing to end or prevent another panic attack. 1 After a panic attack, patient does something to end or prevent another panic attack. . Not sure *or* not applicable *or* missing.	*1*
PAN5. Autonomic symptoms with panic attacks **(enter the number of positive symptoms)** **1 Patient cannot catch breath and has feeling of being smothered.** **2 Patient has chest pain or discomfort.** **3 Patient has feeling of choking.** **4 Patient feels heart is pounding, missing beats, or beating faster.** **5 Patient feels dizzy, unsteady, light-headed, or faint.** **6 Patient has numbness or tingling sensations in face or fingers.** 7 Patient has dry mouth or difficulty swallowing. 8 Patient has nausea or abdominal distress. 9 Patient has trembling or shaking of hands or limbs. 10 Patient has sweating, e.g., palms. 11 Patient feels very cold. 12 Patient has hot flushes. **13 Patient has fear of dying.** **14 Patient has fear of going crazy or fear of losing emotional control.** **15 Patient feels that things are not real.** 16 Patient feels that people are not real.	*9*

GAD1. Generalized anxiety	*Score*
Have you had excessive worry and anxiety for long periods of time (e.g., for hours each day lasting several months), <u>not</u> just during panic attacks? Is it difficult to control the anxiety? 0 Patient has no generalized anxiety or non-significant. 1 Patient has generalized anxiety. . Not sure *or* not applicable *or* missing.	*1*
GAD2. Restlessness with anxiety	
Did you feel restless, keyed up, or on edge? 0 No. 1 Yes. . Not sure *or* not applicable *or* missing.	*1*
GAD3. Tension with anxiety	
Did you feel tense in your muscles? 0 No. 1 Yes. . Not sure *or* not applicable *or* missing.	*0*
GAD4. Exhaustion with anxiety	
Did you feel tired or easily exhausted even without work? 0 No. 1 Yes. . Not sure *or* not applicable *or* missing.	*1*

GAD5. Poor concentration with anxiety	
Did you have difficulty concentrating when anxious? 0 No. 1 Yes. . Not sure *or* not applicable *or* missing.	*1*
GAD6. Irritability with anxiety	
Did you feel irritable when anxious? 0 No. 1 Yes. . Not sure *or* not applicable *or* missing.	*1*
GAD7. Insomnia with anxiety	
Did you have difficulty falling asleep or staying asleep when anxious? 0 No. 1 Yes. . Not sure *or* not applicable *or* missing.	*1*
Generalized anxiety score = 6 (severe)	

Video #9: Narcotic Use and Depression

Transcription of Interview #9 (C = Clinician; P = Patient)

C: *So, I want to thank you again for joining us. I am a resident physician here. I'd like to ask if you could tell me about yourself and where you're from.*

P: *I'm from Wheeling, WV. I am a mom of two little girls. I came to Morgantown when I was 18 and got my Bachelor's in Psychology from here. Then I went to Fairmont State and got my associate degree in Nursing. I then went on and worked in the field as a drug and alcohol counselor for several years. I raised a family, had a marriage, and during all that time, was also in the closet battling a very bad drug addiction.*

C: *Wow. So you have a lot of direct experience in this field itself.*

P: *Absolutely, yes.*

C: *That really raises my curiosity as to what got you here in the hospital.*

P: *About…I mean, my drug addiction had gotten worse throughout the years, of course. My husband and I used together and we were very codependent. Last October, a couple months before that, I quit my job. I was using while I was working there, so that guilt was eating me alive on top of the normal guilt. I got caught with a gram of methamphetamine. I went to jail for the first time in my life with possession. I got bailed out and went directly to detox. I then got out of there, went on house arrest at my parents' house. On New Year's Eve, someone stopped by with methamphetamine, I used it, I got drug tested the next day, I went to jail this time for 90 days, and that was an eye-opener for me. That was not my life and not anything I had dreamed of. When I got out, I found out that my husband had moved a girl into our house while I was in jail and got her pregnant. We were very much married. So that was a shocker for me when I got out, I thought I was going home and my home wasn't there anymore. So then I relapsed again on methamphetamine. My thought then was to, I was in so much emotional pain, I was going to do the biggest shot of heroin I could. I wasn't necessarily suicidal but I just didn't want to feel the pain anymore. That's how I got here.*

C: *Wow. So you've had a very difficult sequent of events. I'm very glad that you decided to get some help. Now, because it sounds like drugs have played a pivotal role in what got you here, tell me a bit about what drugs you've struggled with.*

P: *It started out with pain pills and that escalated to heroin. I graduated nursing school a full-on IV heroin user and was very addicted to heroin. My husband had overdosed. I had to give him CPR, he was in the ICU, it was a horrible mess. I quit heroin and was clean for 3 years and had my youngest daughter. Then slowly at some point, I slipped back into pain pills; he was bringing them around; he went to the Subutex clinic, started getting on Subutex. And then, Xanax came around and I was taking large amounts of Xanax, and then meth came around, and that was it.*

C: *So it started with the opioids, gradually transitioned to the benzos, and then finally the stimulants. Then we kind of fast-forward to now. Which of all of these substances do you identify as the biggest problem nowadays?*

P: *Meth and heroin. Heroin definitely is the physical killer. I think meth is a killer in its own sneaky way. I think people are doing it and not coming back from it. Like I've seen fairly normal people lose their mind and it's not like only when they're using. It's like they went and never went back. Like full-onset schizophrenia occurred. I think we're just learning about meth and its really bad consequences the more widespread it gets. In my town, literally, I can walk out and there's not hardly anyone I know who's not on meth at this point. That's how widespread it is.*

C: *It's everywhere. How long have you been using opioids for?*

P: *They started when I was about 22. And then it got really bad until I was 27. That was with the heroin. So the opioids have been the constant, really.*

C: *So, on that note, what I'll do is focus more on the opioids and we can jump into these stimulants at a later time.*

P: *Okay.*

C: *Over the course of the past year, how often do you feel you've been using the opioids including heroin?*

P: *I haven't used heroin in the past year. It's been Subutex that I've used and that's been on a daily basis.*

C: *Exclusively.*

P: *Yes.*

C: *And no narcotic pain pills on the side?*

P: *No, I guess that's not true. If someone were to have, say a Percocet 30 or a, you know, actually, I'm lying. I did do heroin once in the last year. So it's like if it was there, you would do it. But the basis of it, to not get sick, I had to have Subutex or some type of opiate.*

C: *Virtually every day.*

P: *Yes, if not every day, then I was very sick.*

C: *That's something we commonly hear. Now over the timeframe that you've been using, do you feel that it takes more and more to achieve the same effect?*

P: *Absolutely with heroin and Subutex. There is a ceiling effect, though. Like you definitely have to, you, whereas at the beginning a quarter of one might have made you feel well, eventually you need a whole one.*

C: *Have you made attempts to cut back?*

P: *Only a million times.*

C: *That's what I imagined. And when you tried to stop, or when you did stop, I imagine you felt a lot of withdrawal symptoms. Tell me about that.*

P: *Body aches, tremors, lack of concentration, tearfulness, digestive issues, sometimes vomiting, sneezing, watery eyes. Just generally malaise. Didn't want to get out of bed, a lack of energy that was astounding.*

C: *And you already touched on some of this, but do you feel like in the peak when you were using every day, do you feel like you started to fail to fulfill obligations?*

P: *Absolutely. Especially funding it. The financial obligation. You get to where your whole day is, if you're not getting prescribed the Subutex, you have to start buying it off the streets and find people to sell them to you. And it comes down to you have to find this because otherwise you won't be able to get up the next day and go to work or take care of your kids. It becomes a top priority of finding, obtaining, finding the money to obtain. Everything else takes a backseat to that.*

C: *And this is always on your mind.*

P: *Yes. Even if you have them, you're thinking how 3 days out you're not going to have them. Or God forbid someone steal them and then you'll be sick the next day. It's a constant horrible feeling.*

C: *You certainly painted the picture well. Give me a sense as to whether you feel your substance abuse impacted your social relationships?*

P: *I've lost every good friend that I've had throughout my life. Even if I would deny there was a problem, they could see my life slipping away. It wasn't that they didn't love me, but I was losing my friends, my family, my sister. Everyone.*

C: *So a really significant impact on your support system. Do you feel like when you were going through all of this and recognizing these social changes, do you feel as though you were able to rationally assess the impact?*

P: *It was their fault at the time. I had to perceive it that way instead of being honest about my drug abuse.*

C: *Was there ever a moment where you said, "maybe I need to change my behavior or recognize the fact that I'm continuing to use despite the fact that all of this is taking place?"*

P: *Oh there were several times when I would break down and cry and say "what am I doing? Why am I doing this?" And my husband and I would talk about making a change and it was just so many talks and empty promises. The want was there, I don't think we wanted to become these people. But it was the, definitely being in a codependent relationship made it more difficult. It would just, all in all, you say all that and the sickness would win over and someone would stop by. And when you have the worst flu in the world and you have the one antidote to help it, you do it, and it's a constant pushing back, and before long, you look around and your life has fallen apart.*

C: *Did you ever, during all this, find yourself using in dangerous situations? Like right before driving?*

P: *All the time.*

C: *Did that ever stop you?*

P: *There were times that I knew I had used too much and I wouldn't drive. But looking back I thought I always knew when I wasn't okay to drive. But looking back there were so many times when I shouldn't have and I did.*

C: *Sounds like you have a lot of insight. And looking back and therapy helps that. Are there other problems you can identify that drugs caused you?*

P: *Just about every problem to date has been because of drugs. The lack of trust in my family, my marriage falling apart, the fact that I went to jail and embarrassed my family and children. The fact that my career, just everything. I no longer can walk around in my town with my head held up high. I have to walk around knowing that they look at me as a "druggie." I never felt like that person. I was valedictorian in my high school class. I know it doesn't discriminate, but I let it get so far because I was able to function with it. I kept a job, so even though everything was getting worse, it didn't completely implode. It took 15 years for it to get to rock bottom. People saw me and knew something was wrong but they weren't quite sure. I was able to hide behind my husband's addiction. It took a long time to admit I needed help.*

C: *It takes a lot of strength to talk about this. We appreciate your openness and honesty. I want to talk about the impact of substance abuse on your mood. This being the Dual Diagnosis Unit, we know there is a comorbidity between depression and substance abuse. When was the last time you remember going 2–3 months of complete sobriety?*

P: *When my 7-year-old was born. I was sober 2 years after her birth.*

C: *During those 2 years, or during past periods of sobriety, was depression an issue for you?*

P: *It was always an issue.*

C: *Okay. So even in high school you struggled with depression.*

P: *Yes, I struggled with anorexia and depression in high school. There was a lot of depression in my family history too.*

C: *How's your depression been over the past month?*

P: *Not good. It's probably the most depressed I've been. Finding out about my husband, finding out that he got a girl pregnant. It was like being hit by a truck. I thought there were some days that it would physically kill me. It was like drowning, but you don't die.*

C: *When you reflect on those periods, when you were sober, were there also struggles with enjoying activities? Did you feel like you lost sources of pleasure?*

P: *Yes. I would go through the motions and feel guilty, not feeling as happy as I felt like I should watch my children play sports. That's been a constant in my life, feeling like I should feel happy and not.*

C: *Is there anything you enjoy these days?*

P: *I'm trying to build that back up. My rock bottom, I just got out of jail and just found out about my husband, so lately I've been in such a crisis mode that it's been a lot just to walk across the room or hold a conversation. But I'm really hoping that inside me there's this spark of hope that I can get through this and live a clean and sober lifestyle. I can go back to school, teach yoga again, and do things that bring me joy.*

C: *I think you're holding it together very well. Do you feel, like when you reflect on the future, feeling how you feel right now, do you feel hopelessness?*

P: *I have been feeling hopeless for a long time. I'm just now trying to get back. Like I said, in all the hopelessness, I'm finally, just in the last couple days, I got in the 28-day rehab, I'm at least, I can see this little flicker back there of something. I guess that's hope.*

C: *Sometimes that's all it takes to get us through. I'm really glad to hear that. Tell me about your concentration over the last month.*

P: *It's been very poor. I can't read a book, watch a TV show, trying to read to my daughter. Even focus on what people are saying. I have a really hard time.*

C: *I presume that's been the case most of the past month.*

P: *Yes.*

C: *Along with feeling depressed, do you ever feel that your body movements are slowed down.*

P: *Oh yeah, everything is slowed down. I feel sluggish.*

C: *Is that how you feel right now?*

P: *Yeah.*

C: *Do you feel like, along with hopelessness, do you feel worthless at all?*

P: *Worthlessness has never been a real…I've had times when I felt worthless about letting addiction consume my life and my family, but I've still been able to maintain some sense of self-worth. I feel that in the future there's something I'll be able to offer society, a future partner, a friend. I do feel that I still have something to offer.*

C: *And when you like in the last 30 days, has it been less than half the past month that you felt worthless?*

P: *I would say it's encompassed the majority of the past 30 days. I felt I had nothing to offer. All I did was cry. But I also understood that that won't be forever.*

C: *Do you feel like you're excessively guilty?*

P: *I feel like a lot of it is my fault because in all reality it is. The choices I've made that have directly impacted. The circumstances I'm in right now, it is my fault. I really struggle with guilt for hurting others and my children.*

C: *And that's pretty constant?*

P: *Yes.*

C: *Are there any other symptoms of depression that we've left out?*

P: *I would say, just the loss of interest in activities, the helplessness. As in you want to change but you don't know who or how or when or why. I walk around feeling lost and just not good enough. A lot of that comes with my husband and the affair. Like why I wasn't enough to make this work, even though logically I know it's not my fault. But I do feel that rejection and that, a lot of self-pity too. I caused a lot of this, but still sitting around in that poor me kind of thing.*

C: *When you allow yourself to dwell on some of those thoughts, do you feel as though your depression has escalated to the point where you've thought about hurting yourself or ending your life?*

P: *The week before I came here, it wasn't a thought with a plan or intent or means, but it was a thought in that here is this pain and it's so great that I don't know what to do, how on earth can I make this pain stop. Death was the only thing I could think of and that was as far as it went. I knew I wouldn't do that. That would be the easy way out and it wouldn't be fair to anyone involved. That's when I knew I needed help.*

C: *So it never escalated to where you had a plan or intent. Has it ever been like that in the past?*

P: *A couple times, I thought I would just get enough drugs and overdose. But something always stopped me. I think it was my kids. In all reality, I don't want to die and say that I let another person cause me to lose my own life.*

C: *So it never got to an actual attempt?*

P: *No.*

C: *The last few questions are with regard to other symptoms sometimes seen as a result of depression. Oftentimes with depression, when people start to feel really low or down, or hit "rock bottom" as you mentioned, they start to see things or hear voices that others can't hear or see. And again, we would have to look back to a period of time when you weren't using substances. Are hallucinations something you've experienced?*

P: *I can't answer that question honestly because I don't know that I've had them without substances being involved. I have had them after being up too many days, with stimulants being involved, and depression was also a factor. I wouldn't ever be able to know if that was independent of the drugs or not.*

C: *On a similar note, have you ever experienced delusions when you've been similarly depressed?*

P: *In the last month, I've gotten so depressed that I could tell the paranoia was starting to get increased. I would think I was having to stay at my parents' house and thought they were talking about me. That's when I really started being like okay, they're not talking about you 24/7. Like it's time. I knew things were getting bad.*

C: *So clearly it's impacted you in more ways than one. It's not just a matter of low mood. At times it's impacted your sense of reality. Is there anything else you want to tell us today about your mood or substance use or what you hope to get out of being here?*

P: *I just really want to get myself back. I know it's going to be a long journey, but just to be able to get started here and get the right tools. I've already made the first steppingstone to a 28-day program and that's really the goal I wanted to achieve.*

Video #9 Ratings

DRUG1. Tolerance	***Score***
Did you use a lot more of the drug than you previously used to get the same effect (compared when you first started to use the drug)? ***Did you notice that the same amount of the drug you take now has less effect than before (compared when you first started to use the drug)?*** 0 Patient had no tolerance to the drug. 1 Patient had tolerance to the drug. . Not sure *or* not applicable *or* missing.	*1*
DRUG2. Withdrawal	
When you stopped or cut down on the drug use, did you have withdrawal symptoms? (interviewer gives examples of the drug withdrawal symptoms) 0 Patient had no withdrawal symptoms from the drug. 1 Patient had withdrawal symptoms from the drug. . Not sure *or* not applicable *or* missing.	*1*
DRUG3. Failure to fulfill major obligations	
Did the drug use result in failure to fulfill major role obligations at work, school, or home? 0 Drug use had no effect on work, school, or social obligations. 1 Drug use had a negative effect on work, school, or social obligations. . Not sure *or* not applicable *or* missing.	*1*
DRUG4. Social, interpersonal problems due to drug	
Did the drug cause any social or interpersonal problems (e.g., work problems, school problems, relationship problems, family problems, legal problems, physical fights)? 0 Drug caused no social or interpersonal problems. 1 Drug caused social or interpersonal problems. . Not sure *or* not applicable *or* missing.	*1*
DRUG5. Drug use in spite of problems	
Did you continue to use the drug even though you had problems? 0 Patient had no problems from the drug use. 1 Patient continued to use the drug even though the drug caused problems. . Not sure *or* not applicable *or* missing.	*1*

DRUG6. Drug use in hazardous situations	
Did you use the drug in a situation, in which it was physically hazardous (e.g., driving a car or operating machinery)? 0 Patient did not use the drug in hazardous situations. 1 Patient used the drug in hazardous situations. . Not sure *or* not applicable *or* missing.	*1*
DRUG7. Other DRUG problems	
Did you have any other problems due to drug use? 0 No. 1 Yes (specify). . Not sure *or* not applicable *or* missing.	*1*
Drug use score = 7 (severe)	

D1. Depressed mood	*Score*
Have you been feeling sad, depressed, or in low spirits? 0 Patient has no depressed mood. 1 Patient has depressed mood less than half the time. 2 Patient has depressed mood more than half the time. . Not sure *or* not applicable *or* missing.	*2*
D2. Anhedonia (loss of pleasure and interest)	
Have you been unable to experience pleasure and enjoy things that you used to enjoy like exercising, enjoying your hobbies, or socializing with friends? 0 Patient has no anhedonia. 1 Patient has anhedonia less than half the time. 2 Patient has anhedonia more than half the time. . Not sure *or* not applicable *or* missing.	*1*
D3. Hopelessness	
Have you felt hopeless about your future? 0 Patient is not hopeless. 1 Patient feels hopeless less than half the time. 2 Patient feels hopeless more than half the time. . Not sure *or* not applicable *or* missing.	*2*

D4. Attention impairment/poor concentration	
Have you found that your concentration has decreased and you are unable to complete a task (e.g., at work, reading an article, reading a book, or watching a movie), even though you were able to do that before? 0 Patient has no concentration problems. 1 Patient has difficulty concentrating less than half the time. 2 Patient has difficulty concentrating more than half the time. . Not sure *or* not applicable *or* missing.	2
D5. Psychomotor slowing/retardation	
Have you felt as though you were talking or moving more slowly than normal for you when depressed? 0 Patient has normal activity. 1 Patient has psychomotor retardation less than half the time. 2 Patient has psychomotor retardation more than half the time. . Not sure *or* not applicable *or* missing.	2
D6. Worthlessness (low self-esteem)	
Have you felt that you are a worthless person in the society or a failure? 0 Patient has no feeling of worthlessness. 1 Patient feels worthless less than half the time. 2 Patient feels worthless more than half the time. . Not sure *or* not applicable *or* missing.	*1*
D7. Excessive guilt	
Have you felt guilty or ashamed of yourself for something you have done or thought? 0 Patient has no feeling of guilt. 1 Patient feels guilty less than half the time. 2 Patient feels guilty more than half the time. . Not sure *or* not applicable *or* missing.	2
D8. Other depressive symptoms	

0 Absent. 1 Present (specify). . Not sure *or* not applicable *or* missing.	***1***

D9. Suicidal ideation during the past month	
Have you had thoughts about harming or killing yourself? 0 Patient had no suicidal ideation. 1 Patient had suicidal ideation. . Not sure *or* not applicable *or* missing.	***1***
D10. Suicidal intention during the past month	
Have you had the intention to carry out the suicidal thoughts? 0 Patient had no suicidal intention. 1 Patient had suicidal intention. . Not sure *or* not applicable *or* missing.	***0***
D11. Suicidal plans during the past month	
Have you had specific suicidal plans? 0 Patient had no suicidal plans. 1 Patient had suicidal plans. . Not sure *or* not applicable *or* missing.	***0***
D12. Suicidal attempt during the past month	
Have you made a suicide attempt during the past month? 0 Patient made no suicide attempt during the past month. 1 Patient made one recent suicide attempt during the past month. 2 Patient made two or more recent suicide attempts during the past month. . Not sure *or* not applicable *or* missing.	***0***
D13. Delusions associated mainly with depressed mood	
0 Absent. 1 Present. . Not sure *or* not applicable *or* missing.	***0***
D14. Hallucinations associated mainly with depressed mood	
0 Absent. 1 Present. . Not sure *or* not applicable *or* missing.	***0***
Depression score = 14 (severe)	

Video #10: Full Interview 1

Dr. Hill

Identification: Patient is a 27-year-old male admitted for worsening depression over the past 2 weeks, including suicidal ideation and a plan to overdose.

Chief complaints: Depression worsening over the past 2 weeks and suicidal ideation.

History of present illness: Patient has a history of depression since he was a teenager. He overdosed on pain killers in November 2011 and was admitted to the hospital for 11 days, where he was treated with Cymbalta. Depression has worsened over the past 2 weeks, including suicidal ideation and a plan to overdose.

Review of psychiatric symptoms was positive for depression, anhedonia, suicidality, alcohol, and THC use disorder.

Review of symptoms was negative for panic, OCD, PTSD, mania, delusions, hallucinations, disorganized behavior, disorganized thoughts, or conduct disorder.

Initial diagnosis: Major depressive disorder
Rule out alcohol and THC use disorders.

Transcription of Interview #10 (C = Clinician; P = Patient)

C: My name is Dr. Hill. I am a psychiatrist and I'll be asking you some questions to try to figure out what's going on.
P: Okay.
C: So let's start off with just tell me a little bit about why you ended up in the hospital.
P: From depression. Back in November I was arrested for a suicide attempt, sent to Hagerstown. I signed myself in this time in Morgantown.
C: So back in November this happened. So explain to me what happened.
P: I've had depression forever, but it just got to be too much. I was stressed out.
C: Was there anything in particular back in November stressing you out?
P: Just pretty much the same patterns.
C: So sort of like something getting you down, nothing particular. Tell me exactly what you did.
P: I took a bunch of painkillers.
C: Where were you when you took them?
P: At home.
C: Who was there with you?
P: My wife.
C: Your wife. And when you took the painkillers was she in the room?
P: Yes.
C: So she saw you take them?
P: Yes.
C: And what did she do?
P: Called the cops.
C: Okay. And what did the cops do?
P: They took me out of the car after I left, took me to the ER.
C: So you took off after you took the painkillers?
P: Right.
C: You took off driving?
P: Yes.
C: What happened when you got to the ER?

P: Checked me over, took all my clothes, watched me until they could find someplace to send me.
C: And where did they send you?
P: Brooklean.
C: How long were you there for?
P: Eleven days.
C: What did they do for you there?
P: They started me on antidepressants.
C: What did they start you on?
P: Cymbalta.
C: What happened when you left Brooklean?
P: Started outpatient with a therapist and a psychologist.
C: And you stayed on the Cymbalta?
P: Yes.
C: And how did that work out?
P: I don't think the medicine has done anything.
C: Did therapy help?
P: A little bit.
C: So take me now from November until today.
P: I've still been off work since November because I work around heavy equipment.
C: What made you decide to come back to the hospital?
P: The past couple weeks have been pretty rough for me. I was actually scared of myself and my thoughts.
C: What have your thoughts been?
P: Constant thoughts of suicide that I have no control over.
C: So they're there all the time.
P: Sometimes they're there almost all day, and other times they just pop in there for no reason and ruin my whole day.
C: Okay. Those thoughts of suicide, were they thoughts of actual ways to kill yourself or thoughts of "I wish I was dead"?
P: Both.
C: Okay. And what sorts of ways of killing yourself were you thinking of?
P: Crashing my car, overdosing, cutting my wrists.
C: Since that suicide attempt in November, did you try and kill yourself again?
P: No.
C: Okay. So take me back to where this started. The depression…
P: I can remember having it forever.
C: And how old are you?
P: 27.
C: So you remember having this when you were a little kid?
P: Definitely since I was a teenager.
C: Help me understand the depression. What is that like? What is different when your depressed versus *not depressed?*

P: Well if I'm just sad about things in my life, the depression is more on a personal basis. Not happy with who I am or anything about me. It's like being stuck in a room with someone you can't stand.

C: So a lot of this is not liking yourself. Do you feel worthless?

P: A lot of the times feel worthless.

C: Does the depression affect other parts of your life?

P: It affects everything.

C: Give me some examples.

P: My mood, how I act towards others.

C: How do you act?

P: When I'm depressed I'm not very sociable.

C: So you isolate yourself?

P: Yes.

C: Does it every affect your concentration or energy?

P: Yes. I feel lower energy. Concentration is horrible.

C: What kinds of things can't you concentrate on?

P: Simple things. I'll forget to listen to people when they are talking to me.

C: And how does it affect other parts of your life? Does it affect your appetite?

P: Sometimes I'll go days and just eat a little bit. My sleep is never the same. Sometimes I'm real tired, other times I can't sleep.

C: How does depression affect the fun things in life that you enjoy?

P: It takes away from it.

C: Okay. What are some things you enjoy?

P: Photography helps me a lot.

C: And normally, when you were still working, what would you do for fun?

P: I never really had time when I was working.

C: But you feel like when you're depressed you don't feel like doing things.

P: Yes.

C: Some people with depression have periods where their mood is very high. Have you experienced that?

P: Yeah, but they're not very long. They're short.

C: Explain what you're like on one of those highs.

P: Happy, cracking jokes.

C: During those times would you say that's normal for most people? Or do you get way over hyper?

P: I would say over hyper but I'm not bouncing around. I don't get over happy or too much energy.

C: And during those periods, would I notice anything different?

P: I would have expression in my face, I would have color.

C: Anything else?

P: I don't know.

C: And when you say these periods of feeling high don't last long is it like days, weeks?

P: It lasts a day if I'm lucky.

C: And during those times are you able to sleep?

P: A little bit better.

C: Do people ever say that you're talking too fast or you're having bizarre thoughts?

P: No.

C: And along with the depression some people get anxiety. Have you ever been anxious? Do you over worry?

P: Yes. Even just going to Walmart gets me really anxious. I don't like being around other people, wondering what they're thinking about as far as me. They're probably not paying attention.

C: So you're worried they're thinking about you or saying things about you. Have you ever had a panic attack?

P: No.

C: How do you know what a panic attack is?

P: I watched a video, but I've never had one.

C: It seems like this depression started when you were very young. What was it like for you growing up? Was it a pretty rough childhood?

P: No, it wasn't bad.

C: Who raised you?

P: My mom and grandma mostly. Dad was always at work.

C: Was there ever any abuse at home?

P: No.

C: Ever a time when you were afraid to go home?

P: Only when I got in trouble.

C: What did you get in trouble for?

P: Anything. I was always into something.

C: What was the discipline like?

P: Normally just get grounded.

C: What is the scariest thing that's happened to you?

P: I can't think of anything.

C: So you've never had an experience that's really affected your life.

P: No.

C: Do you use drugs or alcohol?

P: I used to.

C: Tell me about that.

P: I started smoking marijuana and drinking when I was 13.

C: How much would you smoke and drink? Like every day?

P: Yes.

C: How much could you drink?

P: A lot.

C: What would get you drunk?

P: Back then it was a lot.

C: What was the most you could drink?

P: We could finish two fifths of vodka between a few of us.

C: Okay, that's a lot. Do you think you were an alcoholic then?

P: Yes.

C: What problems did the alcohol cause in your life?

P: I quit going to school. I never finished school because of that.
C: Okay. Did you ever have any legal problems?
P: Only once I got caught with some marijuana, but I never really got into trouble.
C: If you weren't able to drink for a few days would you get withdrawal?
P: No, nothing noticeable.
C: Okay. And you started at 13? How long did you go on drinking?
P: Until I was 20.
C: And then what happened?
P: I was in a car accident.
C: Because you were drinking?
P: Yes.
C: Okay. And what happened?
P: I had been drinking after work, and I got into a ditch with my Jeep and it rolled and threw me out, broke my back and neck, my collarbone, shoulder blade.
C: So a bad wreck. Did you feel like you almost died in that wreck?
P: Yes.
C: Were you unconscious?
P: I don't remember.
C: What do you remember?
P: I remember the helicopter taking off and that was it.
C: How long were you in the hospital for?
P: Eleven days.
C: How has that experience affected your life?
P: I got a lot of pain.
C: Do you ever relive that experience?
P: No, only once I had a flashback but that was years ago.
C: So you haven't had nightmares?
P: No.
C: So was it at that point you decided to quit drinking?
P: I still drank, but I never drank and drove again.
C: Okay. Was there a time when you sought treatment for alcoholism?
P: No.
C: So you continued to drink after the wreck. Do you still drink?
P: Very rarely.
C: How long did you smoke marijuana?
P: Until 21.
C: Why did you quit?
P: I got my CDL.
C: What about other drugs?
P: I've done most of everything else. Nothing for a long period.
C: What about right now?
P: I started smoking again a bit. That helps with my depression.
C: Over the years, have there been times when the depression has gotten to the point where you see or hear things that aren't real?
P: No.

C: Ever times where you get paranoid?
P: No.
C: Ever have times where you've thought for a period that you've had special powers?
P: No.
C: Ever thought the TV is talking to you or anything like that?
P: No.
C: Ever had things you do over and over again even though you don't want to do them? Like checking, counting…
P: No.
C: What about your thoughts? Any other intrusive thoughts?
P: Just negative thoughts about myself.
C: Tell me about those.
P: If I think about trying something new, I always talk myself out of it.
C: Why is that?
P: It's how I've always been. I figure I won't be able to do it anyway.
C: Where did that come from?
P: I have no clue.
C: Do you feel like that was a message you got from your family?
P: No, they're supportive.
C: How far did you go in school.
P: Tenth grade.
C: How did you do in school?
P: I did okay.
C: Were you in special?
P: No, regular.
C: Were you a hyper kid?
P: No, I was always sleeping.
C: Why?
P: I was always up drinking.
C: What about before you started drinking, how were you in school?
P: I was average.
C: Did you get into trouble at school ever?
P: Not a whole lot.
C: Ever do illegal things at school?
P: Smoke cigarettes.
C: Ever steal anything?
P: No
C: Ever bully kids?
P: No.
C: Did you have pets growing up?
P: A few here and there.
C: Let's talk about the depression. When was it worst?
P: This past year.
C: When did you first get treatment.

P: In November.
C: Do you know why you didn't seek treatment sooner?
P: I just figured that was how I was.
C: Okay. Did the cops force you to go to the hospital in November?
P: Yes.
C: So the first time you didn't really want to be there.
P: Right.
C: You said you end in Cymbalta back then that did not help much.
P: I do not think so.
C: What other medications have you been on?
P: Depakote.
C: What has that done?
P: Helped me keep my moods in check from going high and low so they're not flipping like a switch.
C: Tell me about flipping like a switch.
P: I get upset sometimes at things that can change in an instant.
C: What do you change into?
P: Sometimes it's depression, sometimes it's just anger.
C: Has anger been a big problem?
P: Not really. I've been able to control it.
C: Any other medications?
P: Xanax.
C: What does that do for you?
P: It helps me be less anxious, like when going to Walmart.
C: So is that something you take every day?
P: Just take it when I need it. Sometimes I go days without it. Other times I take a lot.
C: Ever taken way too many to get high?
P: No.
C: Other medications?
P: Adderall.
C: What did that do?
P: It helps me concentrate a bit.
C: Concentration issues are usually when you're depressed right?
P: Pretty much all the time but worse with the depression.
C: Any other medications?
P: Seroquel.
C: What does that do?
P: About the same as the Xanax.
C: What are you on right now?
P: Just Depakote and Seroquel.
C: What have they diagnosed you with?
P: They haven't said yet.
C: When did you come in the hospital?
P: Monday night.
C: Are you still suicidal?

P: The thoughts are still there.
C: Do you feel like you'd act on those thoughts if you left the hospital?
P: It does worry me, maybe if I got too stressed out.
C: Do you have guns at home?
P: No.
C: Did you ever think of shooting yourself? Could you get a gun if you wanted?
P: Yes.
C: So that's something you've thought about?
P: Yes.
C: Ever had a gun in your hand with the thought of killing yourself?
P: No.
C: Where would you get the gun?
P: I could find one somewhere. I have friends with guns.
C: Ever a time where you've gotten so angry that you've though about killing someone?
P: I've had the thought.
C: Tell me about that.
P: Nobody in particular who I would get that upset with. I don't like having the thought run through my head.
C: Have you ever tried to hurt someone in the past?
P: No.
C: You were working until November. What was your job?
P: I work on a surface mine.
C: Did you do well at work?
P: Yes, I got along with everyone.
C: What about any girlfriend, boyfriend?
P: I'm married.
C: What's your wife's name?
P: Brittany.
C: How do you get along?
P: Okay.
C: Any kids?
P: We have one. She has another one from before.
C: Does your depression affect that relationship?
P: Yes.
C: Since you've been in the hospital have you been getting therapy?
P: A little bit.
C: Sometimes talking through things is helpful. Did you find it helpful before?
P: A little bit.
C: Any depression in your family?
P: No.
C: Any brothers or sisters?
P: Older and younger sister. They haven't been depressed.
C: That's about all my questions. Do you have any for me?
P: No.

Video #10 Ratings of Mood Symptoms

(Positive Symptoms Only)

D1. Depressed mood	***Score***
Have you been feeling sad, depressed, or in low spirits? 0 Patient has no depressed mood. 1 Patient has depressed mood less than half the time. 2 Patient has depressed mood more than half the time. . Not sure *or* not applicable *or* missing.	*2*
D2. Anhedonia (loss of pleasure and interest)	
Have you been unable to experience pleasure and enjoy things that you used to enjoy like exercising, enjoying your hobbies, or socializing with friends? 0 Patient has no anhedonia. 1 Patient has anhedonia less than half the time. 2 Patient has anhedonia more than half the time. . Not sure *or* not applicable *or* missing.	*2*
D4. Attention impairment/poor concentration	
Have you found that your concentration has decreased and you are unable to complete a task* (e.g., *at work, reading an article, reading a book, or watching a movie), even though you were able to do that before? 0 Patient has no concentration problems. 1 Patient has difficulty concentrating less than half the time. 2 Patient has difficulty concentrating more than half the time. . Not sure *or* not applicable *or* missing.	*2*
D5. Psychomotor slowing/retardation	
Have you felt as though you were talking or moving more slowly than normal for you when depressed? 0 Patient has normal activity. 1 Patient has psychomotor retardation less than half the time. 2 Patient has psychomotor retardation more than half the time. . Not sure *or* not applicable *or* missing.	2
D6. Worthlessness (low self-esteem)	
Have you felt that you are a worthless person in the society or a failure? 0 Patient has no feeling of worthlessness. 1 Patient feels worthless less than half the time. 2 Patient feels worthless more than half the time. . Not sure *or* not applicable *or* missing.	*2*

D8. Other depressive symptoms	
0 Absent. 1 Present (specify). . Not sure *or* not applicable *or* missing.	*1*
D9. Suicidal ideation during the past month	

Have you had thoughts about harming or killing yourself? 0 Patient had no suicidal ideation. 1 Patient had suicidal ideation. . Not sure *or* not applicable *or* missing.	*1*
D10. Suicidal intention during the past month	
Have you had the intention to carry out the suicidal thoughts? 0 Patient had no suicidal intention. 1 Patient had suicidal intention. . Not sure *or* not applicable *or* missing.	*1*
D11. Suicidal plans during the past month	
Have you had specific suicidal plans? 0 Patient had no suicidal plans. 1 Patient had suicidal plans. . Not sure *or* not applicable *or* missing.	*1*
Depression score = 14 (severe)	

M2. Irritable mood	
Have you sometimes felt that you were easily irritated without reason? ***Have you found yourself so irritable that you shout at people or start arguments or actually become aggressive?*** 0 Patient has no irritable mood. 1 Patient has irritable mood less than half the time. 2 Patient has irritable mood more than half the time. . Not sure *or* not applicable *or* missing.	*1*
M3. Mixed mood (mood lability)	
Have you had mixed mood swings: periods of depression and elation or irritability on the same day? 0 Patient has no mixed mood swings. 1 Patient has mixed mood less than half the time. 2 Patient has mixed mood more than half the time. . Not sure *or* not applicable *or* missing.	*1*

Video #11: Full Interview 2

Dr. Chandran

Transcription of Interview #11 (C = Clinician; P = Patient)

C: Thank you so much for being here and letting me ask you a bunch of questions. We'll kind of start with having you tell us your story in your own words as best you can.

P: My story of how I ended up here at Chestnut Ridge Hospital? So pretty much, I had a feeling…or a friend who was in desperate need, so I decided to drive over to his house, but I actually couldn't find his house exactly, and then I saw a cat on the side of the road in the neighborhood and I felt like I had to follow the cat, so I followed the cat. The cat was leading me somewhere; I knew it was important. It led me to a house with someone working on it and it stopped right there. I pretty much knew then this was where I needed to go. So, I you know made small chat with the guy who was working on the house, and I asked him very politely if he needed help on this house, and he declined no. Well then, I was going to go but then I had a feeling I had to stay for something; I talked to him a little bit more and said, "Hey we could all use a little bit of help and everything," and then he got kind of angry and he pulled up this shirt at his waist band and had a gun and said, "Hey you better go away, I'm packing heat." Once again, I was about to leave on my merry way but now, I felt something was leading me to him. I felt like God was leading me to go up the steps and to pray for him, so I started going up the steps, and I got to the top step and the gentlemen pulled his gun, had the gun straight to my forehead and said, "Do not take one more step or I'm going to use it." And believe me I was very afraid, but I could see him and he was also very afraid, and I remember thinking why is he so afraid? Why is he shaking? All I'm trying to do is help him. And I don't know something didn't seem right. But at that moment I was thinking, I think we've all heard if someone had a gun to your head and said do you believe in God. What would you do? Would you answer yes or no. And right then that was my question, so I took that one more step, and I got on my hands and knees and I prayed for him. And here I still am.

C: Okay, now when did this happen?

P: This was I think Friday.

C: Friday. So, this recent Friday?

P: Yup.

C: So that was 5 days ago or so. So, you followed the cat. Now where do you live right now?

P: I live in Morgantown.

C: Do you live in an apartment or a house?

P: Yup, I got my own house.

C: How far was this neighbor from you?

P: About 45 minutes away from me.

C: So, you walked and followed this cat?

P: No, no.

C: Tell me how that happened because I want to get the story right.

P: So, I have a I have a friend in Clarksburg.

C: Clarksburg, okay.

P: I felt like he needed help, uhm I don't know, I just wanted to check on him. I felt like there's something that wasn't quite right with him, so I was just gonna drive to his house, and I actually didn't know exactly where his house was, but you know I needed to check on my buddy and see how he's doing, but then the mission wasn't him. It was a gentleman I had never met before.

C: Okay, so how do you know your buddy?

P: Just old-time friends.

C: Old-time friends okay. So, I'm getting the story connected right now—so you're in Clarksburg, you met this guy who you know brandished a weapon against you…how did he not use it? What happened?

P: I don't know how he didn't use it, as soon as I got on the steps, I got on my hands and knees and I prayed for him.

C: And when was this on Friday, Friday night or Friday during the day?

P: During the day, evening, or afternoon.

C: Okay, so you're here at this person's place, what happens then? Like what were the next steps after that?

P: After then, I got off the steps and he called the police, and I waited for the police to come. I told him that this man needed to be saved and that God brought us here to help him.

C: And then what happened?

P: We took a little bit time, we talked and everything. I ended up going to the hospital, and this is when things get pretty fuzzy, but then you know I ended up…they didn't want to take me to jail or anything.

C: Okay.

P: They just wanted me to see someone…go to like Chestnut Ridge or somewhere to get medical help.

C: So, did you come to Ruby Memorial Hospital or Clarksburg?

P: I went to Clarksburg hospital first.

C: And then who did you see there?

P: I'm not too sure who I saw; I swear this is when things get pretty fuzzy.

C: Okay and how did they convince you to consider coming in the hospital?

P: Oh, they didn't have to convince me, I understand how sometimes things seem strange to other people. I just wanna you know make everyone happy, so yeah, I can go, that's fine to me.

C: So, I'm kind of looking at the bigger picture, what were you trying to get from going to the hospital, like what were you thinking that could be helped?

P: Everyone, you know, is telling me that they're concerned for me, so I want to lessen their concerns by going to the hospital getting checked out.

C: Okay, and how were they concerned?

P: How were they concerned? Um 'cause these behaviors don't seem normal.

C: Okay.

P: For most people, I mean even then I was really scared, and I was kind of like all right like why am I doing this? But I definitely felt like I was being tested.

C: Okay, how long have you had these kind of symptoms—or feelings, that's a better way to put it.

P: So, this was probably the second time something like this has ever happened. The first time being last year.

C: First time last year.

P: Yeah, ever since I turned 30.
C: Ever since you turned 30.
P: Yeah, and I'm 31 now.
C: So, prior to that time, have you had any other concern?
P: Never like this at all.
C: At all. As far as anything in your past, nothing that made you concerned about these kinds of feelings or symptoms?
P: Correct.
C: So, a little more detail with the symptoms now. So, you were feeling a calling and how important is that calling to you?
P: Pretty important. I want to blow it off, but I feel too guilty if I do blow it off. Yeah so, we all have our purpose in life.
C: Yeah, that's a great thing you're saying. So, you're in Clarksburg, and they're telling you you're going to go to Chestnut Ridge, what did they tell you there at the hospital? Did they tell you which unit you're going to come into?
P: At this point I'm pretty much blacked out.
C: Okay, yeah and then when did you come to?
P: Pretty much here. And every day, every hour it's becoming more and more clear.
C: What day did do you remember it being a little clearer?
P: So, I'm not even sure exactly what day it is today.
C: Okay, you have an idea what month it is?
P: Oh, I know I know it's June, so I think it's June 29th.
C: Very close.
P: 30th?
C: 30th. What year?
P: 2021.
C: So, every day is getting a little more clear? So, when you're saying you're fuzzy, do you think anything could have contributed to that as far as you feeling fuzzy?
P: Uhm I know they've given me medication.
C: Okay, well prior to them giving medications, were you using any substances of any sort?
P: No substances. No alcohol, no drugs.
C: No alcohol, no drugs. Any marijuana or any synthetic marijuana?
P: No. Not even alcohol. Alcohol is especially bad because a lot of people think they can do a little bit and get away with it, but that's not the case.
C: Right. So what unit are you on now?
P: What unit am I on now?
C: Yeah, which unit at Chestnut Ridge?
P: Uh I'm not sure.
C: So, when you're talking to the team over the last few days, what kind of symptoms were they concerned about or have you talked about with them?
P: So, they were concerned about manic episodes.
C: Manic episodes. And when you say manic, what do you feel that means?
P: They said it's like when I feel high.
C: Okay.

P: I feel like I'm on a mission.

C: Okay. Yeah, and this is a similar kind of thing from a year ago when you said you had that episode?

P: Yes.

C: So, prior to a year ago, right, how was your growing up time and childhood history?

P: Pretty rough.

C: Pretty rough. Okay, we'll talk more about that as we get to know you a little more.

P: Okay.

C: Okay, so with this manic episode, this mission, how long did it last? How many days?

P: Well, that manic episode right there, it was just that timeframe.

C: Timeframe meaning?

P: Few hours. So, it didn't last more than 3 days, 4 days, 5 days, a week?

C: No.

P: So, you were feeling like this calling with a mission. Were you feeling an elevated mood?

C: Yes. How high were you feeling? On a scale from one to 10, 10 being…

P: Probably 10.

C: 10. So really up—that you're on top of the world kind of thing?

P: Yeah, not so much my body but my mind.

C: Your mind. Were you feeling invincible?

P: No definitely not invincible. But I felt like I knew what to do.

C: Okay. It takes a lot of courage to keep going on your mission and talking to someone especially when they have a gun right? Were you feeling afraid at all?

P: Oh, I was very afraid.

C: Very afraid.

P: Petrified. Very, very scared.

C: And we'll talk about that last episode too, but this time it lasted a few hours, right? And then you pretty much were in Clarksburg and the police were encouraging you to get help, right? Any other symptoms associated with that that you remember or that anyone told you that you had? Were you feeling elevated? Were you feeling that you were talking a lot?

P: No.

C: Any like speech that was pressured?

P: No.

C: Any racing thoughts of any sort?

P: No.

C: Were you feeling like you were going to do things without thinking?

P: No.

C: Any impulsive kind of events?

P: No.

C: And during that time, it lasted a few hours, right? Did you find yourself doing anything where you're spending a lot of money?

P: No.

C: Or engaging in any kind of risky behaviors?

P: No.

C: And you did tell me no drugs, no alcohol, no substances of any sort, correct?

P: Correct.

C: Are you on any kind of medications in general before this time?

P: Before this time? Yeah, they had me on my...I mean by previous medications which they've changed a little bit since I've been here.

C: Yeah, that's going to be helpful for us to hear about that story too. So, you came in on Friday night, Saturday morning whatever time it was. And you've been here about 4 days now, right? Friday, Saturday, Sunday, Monday. Yup, 4 full days. How have you been feeling every day?

P: Every day I feel a little bit more clear in the mind.

C: Any concern with your thoughts at all?

P: No.

C: How has your appetite been?

P: It's good.

C: And your sleep?

P: The beds are pretty comfy.

C: Okay, so during this time, I know it was a short period, just a few hours. When you first came in, did it feel like you didn't need sleep?

P: No, I slept. I wanted to sleep; I was very tired.

C: Okay. Had you found yourself before that in the last week or two, not needing sleep?

P: I was really busy before I came in, so I, I needed sleep. But I know I did kind of skip on—I think two nights of sleep, I skipped out on.

C: Okay. When you said you're really busy, what kind of work do you do, I'm sorry I didn't ask you that before.

P: Construction work.

C: So how many hours do you put in a day?

P: A day—at least 12, at least. Well sometimes more per week like 60.

C: Sixty per week, wow. Do you find yourself pretty busy all time? Do you work on your own company or do you work for somebody?

P: It's a family company.

C: So, over the week or two prior to all this happening, you found yourself being really busy...any other stressors that could have triggered this time?

P: Um that's the only one I can think of because this was before everything happened, like a few nights before I was hospitalized. So, I would say its number one.

C: Any family stressors?

P: No.

C: Any losses of any sort?

P: No.

C: Any time where you've been feeling physically ill? Cough, cold?

P: No.

C: So, when you kind of compare to the last episode, that was a year or so ago you said, what happened then?

P: *Um what I do remember—I found myself kind of in a hospital waking up and not really sure what happened, but it was like I was being born again. The most painful moment in my life ever.*

C: *Literally like being born again?*

P: *Like literally being born again.*

C: *This was about a year ago you said?*

P: *A year in January, so like a year and 6 months.*

C: *Okay.*

P: *I did wind up in another facility like Chestnut Ridge and not remembering anything, but little by little grasping pieces and coming to. It took like a week before I was fully conscious. Yeah, that was pretty bad, but kind of like this time, like this time was kind of similar to that time.*

C: *Okay but you knew something was going on this time comparatively because you had been through this before?*

P: *Yes.*

C: *So, that lasted, you said, about a week before you came to, then?*

P: *Yeah.*

C: *So, who encouraged you to get help then?*

P: *I was working…I also deliver medicine, and I was at the hospital and again I was up all night no sleep. And I took a break in the waiting room and then one of the nurses who worked at the hospital noticed I didn't look right, and she asked if she could check me out and I said alright. So, you know I went through everything and she said oh let's get you to get you a bed and have you looked at more thoroughly. I got worse and worse until I was in a hospital bed and at that point I was completely like not in my mind. The only thing I really remember is pain.*

C: *So, with these symptoms, you felt a lot. It's hard to compare two different times and everyone's different obviously, but you've had these callings and missions, have you felt that other people are out to get you during these times? Or any kind of things where you hear voices or see things that aren't supposed to be there? Or have any other sensations that don't seem right, like bugs crawling your skin or anything like that? Or different smells or anything like that?*

P: *No.*

C: *When you had the first hospitalization, what did they diagnose you with?*

P: *I think it was bipolar depression.*

C: *Bipolar depression. And where was that at, do you remember?*

P: *This was at Trinity Hospital, Steubenville, Ohio.*

C: *Steubenville. And they put you on medicines then?*

P: *Yes.*

C: *And you remember the medicines they put you on?*

P: *Depakote and Abilify.*

C: *And how long did you stay on that?*

P: *I was on those for 9 months.*

C: *Nine months, and then what happened?*

P: *Then I kind of just stopped taking them. I didn't feel anything from them.*

C: So, during that 9-month period, did you have any symptoms that you noticed, any kind of symptoms of any sort, like being sad or down or anxious, angry, or moody or anything?

P: No.

C: So, then you stopped the medicines. Then about 3 months later, this happened.

P: Mhhm.

C: Looking back in hindsight, anything that you noticed in the last month or two that seemed different?

P: Last month or two, no.

C: Last week or two?

P: No.

C: Kind of happened very suddenly, huh?

P: Very sudden.

C: I know you mentioned your childhood, we'll kind of talk about that in a bit, but any family history of these kind of conditions or any conditions at all that you know of?

P: I'm pretty sure my late brother had mental illness.

C: You say late brother, how did he die?

P: He was murdered.

C: Oh, I'm sorry.

P: About 10 years ago.

C: Wow. He had some type of mental illness that you're not really sure…

P: Yeah, he had mental disease, depression. He had a lot of stuff. I believe my mother, she has mental illness, but she doesn't talk about it or admit it, or tries to cope with it.

C: Yeah…wow. And we'll talk about more specific questions, but kind of generally your story of growing up and all. Where did you grow up?

P: I grew up here in Morgantown.

C: In Morgantown. And what was your family size like?

P: My family size? So, it was me, my two parents, my late brother, and my sister.

C: And where do you fall?

P: I'm in the middle.

C: In the middle. And you went to school?

P: I went to North Elementary, across the street, Suncrest Middle School, Morgantown High, and WVU.

C: Okay, how long did you go to WVU?

P: Four years.

C: Four years. What did you study?

P: Finance.

C: Finance, wow. So, you went through all the school and you said you had a pretty rough childhood. Tell me about what you describe by that?

P: Just that uh my dad was always working, and then my mom was…I guess she was always sick, so she didn't really do much for taking care of us. Didn't really cook or clean the house, didn't really take us anywhere, like anytime we were like being babysat by like my grandmother, my mom would never pick us up, we just kind of like left with our friends or with other family members.

C: *Did you have extended family or support of any sorts?*

P: *Yeah, I have my aunt's here and my grandmother.*

C: *So, your dad was working a bunch. Was that in the family business?*

P: *Yeah, and then he had a full-time job teaching also, so he was trying to juggle that.*

C: *Where did he teach?*

P: *UHS.*

C: *So, he taught, and he did construction, wow. So, growing up would you feel that you were hurt in any way physically or emotionally or in any way like sexually?*

P: *Not sexually. I would say abused by my mother.*

C: *How so?*

P: *Cause if we would nag her too much, she would kind of snap.*

C: *When she snapped what happened?*

P: *Her favorite thing was she would break glass and try to throw it at us.*

C: *Oh boy.*

P: *That was her favorite thing.*

C: *Do you still have memories of those things?*

P: *Yeah, I do.*

C: *Okay. Did anything ever happen where it extended into anyone being cut or hurt?*

P: *Yeah, we got cut and hurt. We were investigated by CPS, uh nothing happened.*

C: *And how old were you at the time?*

P: *I was 8, my sister was 4.*

C: *How much older is your brother than you?*

P: *My brother is 7 years older than me.*

C: *And how old are you now?*

P: *I am 31.*

C: *You're 31. And your brother's been gone 10 years now.*

P: *Yeah.*

C: *So, a really tough time growing up. So, we always ask those questions because a lot of people are resilient and they survive and they go through life, but do you ever feel that your past is present in your life now?*

P: *Not really.*

C: *Like do you have nightmares?*

P: *No.*

C: *Were you reexperiencing the bad things or any flashbacks of the events?*

P: *No.*

C: *A lot of people were very strong obviously because they survived a lot of things you know, but sometimes we worry about people having post-traumatic stress and so forth. Throughout your life, did you ever feel sad or down at any point that you can kind of pinpoint?*

P: *Looking back I mean I did go through a period of depression I would say.*

C: *When would that be?*

P: This was probably all throughout my 20s. It would come and go because sometimes stuff doesn't go perfectly as planned.

C: Right, the expectations of life and so forth.

P: Yeah.

C: Growing up though, you went through all of the schooling; what kind of activities did you get into?

P: I played sports, football, basketball, music.

C: Did you play in the HS band?

P: Not in high school band.

C: What did you play?

P: Clarinet.

C: Nice! Did you ever perform clarinet?

P: Yeah.

C: Where did you perform?

P: At school, Suncrest Middle School.

C: Okay. Did you notice any sadness as you were growing up because you went through a lot growing up did you notice any sadness or feelings?

P: Looking back on it now, I mean I feel like yeah it was normal stuff I felt. Like it wasn't until I graduated though, and then I was like okay well I did all these steps—I should be happy now and then I wasn't.

C: Graduated what, like college?

P: Yeah.

C: So, you did finance and everything, and then you got to that point and then you started noticing some sadness and so forth. Now comparing that time to what you just went through last couple years, had you had any of those episodes before—where you felt this energized feeling or kind of a calling or any type of religious feelings?

P: No. The funny thing is that kind of got rid of all my sadness once I started having those feelings.

C: That's always an important question for me to ask, as far as one's belief system and how important it is to you. Did you find that you got into religion later?

P: So, I was very religious like in high school and then into college, but then like later in college and early adulthood, you know I kind of lost my way a little bit, and that's probably when I was like my most depressed.

C: Okay and you know whenever we hear people having symptoms like you're talking, we also want to make sure about substances, but you said it pretty clearly that you haven't used any marijuana and no dragging, no other synthetic substances. Any prescriptions that you've used otherwise, any Klonopin, Abilify, Ativan?

P: I don't know what those are.

C: Yeah, we always want to ask because sometimes substance withdrawal can cause all these kinds of symptoms, too, like if you take certain pills and so forth. So, you go through your life and you get to this point, how do you keep yourself occupied—you're really busy with work obviously.

P: Busy with work, yes.

C: Anything important to you like relationships and things like that that are important to you.

P: I mean I would say yeah but I think definitely I focus more on work.

C: Had you had any long-term relationships with anyone at that point?

P: I have but my last long-term relationship was when I was 25.

C: 25, and you're 31 now, right?

P: Yeah.

C: And how did that end?

P: Well, uh so I was more in love with my girlfriend's daughter than I was with my girlfriend, and so when we broke up, it was just really hard because like I never wanted to go through that again, losing someone.

C: Okay, so I'm presuming that you start dating her and had a little daughter.

P: Yes.

C: How old was her daughter?

P: So, when I got into the relationship, she was 3 and then when we got apart, she was like 8.

C: Wow, so that was about 5 years ago?

P: Mhhm.

C: Have you run into them at all?

P: The mother, yes. The daughter, no.

C: Ah well of course, you know as well as I do that Morgantown is not that small.

P: Yeah.

C: And how are you feeling today, like right now?

P: Well right now I'm still a little loopy just from this whole experience that just happened.

C: Yeah, did they put you on any medicines in the hospital?

P: Yeah.

C: What did they put you on?

P: I'm not completely sure what, but I know it is like close to the Depakote and Abilify.

C: Okay and they'll definitely go over all of that before you leave.

P: They did, I kind of just forget.

C: Have you been going to the groups and everything?

P: Yes.

C: Anything you've enjoyed as far as being in hospital as far as clarity-wise anything?

P: It's a good time to relax.

C: You don't get much time doing that do you?

P: No. It's a nice time just to not worry about anything.

C: So, you said you're eating okay, you've slept well here the whole time?

P: Yeah.

C: Any other medical concerns in your lifetime? Any medical issues as far as heart, kidney, diabetes, anything like that? Thyroid illness? Have they checked your thyroid before?

P: Yes, they have.

C: Have they told you how it was?

P: I think they said I have like a low inactive thyroid.

C: Okay. It's something I'm sure the team is looking into to make sure your thyroids are okay. Any questions for me about anything right now? I'm asking a bunch of questions about all the different conditions because this is the part of the interviews where we want to kind of go through all the categories. Whenever we meet people and we hear their story, for example, you've had two episodes like this…

P: Yes.

C: Right. And it's really hard to predict how that goes throughout time. Usually when people have more than one episode, there's a much higher chance it will happen again if you don't stay with treatment, and usually when we're having episodes like where it's not influenced by substances, you know it could be like 75% chance you are having another episode, so we're going to recommend medicines. But we always worry about all the different symptoms right, so as far as depression goes, have you had any feelings of not enjoying things?

P: Not recently, no.

C: When was the last time you think you felt that?

P: Like in my 20s.

C: In your 20s but nothing recently. Okay, so how about any feelings of guilt?

P: Guilt. I feel guilty I didn't study the Bible more when I was younger, that I didn't try harder in that sense.

C: Okay, and then any feelings of worthlessness in general?

P: No.

C: Any feelings of hopelessness now?

P: No.

C: Okay. Any current feelings of suicidal thoughts?

P: No.

C: Or any plans?

P: No.

C: And I didn't ask you, but have you had any attempts in the past of trying to end your life?

P: Kind of, but not really.

C: Tell me about that.

P: So, the reason why I don't use alcohol is because alcohol can make you pretty stupid, but you know I would when I was younger, get drunk and then try to find some stupid way to end my life. Yeah, like I jumped off a cliff before.

C: When was that?

P: Oh, this was a while ago.

C: A while ago meaning?

P: Years.

C: Five years, 10 years?

P: Four years ago, yeah.

C: Okay and were you drinking then?

P: Oh yeah. And I fell, but then like I went through branches, and I hit the snow, and there's a whole bunch of leaves, so definitely it was a lot softer.

C: This was a wintertime thing?

P: This was a winter time thing.

C: How high was the cliff off the ground?

P: It was pretty high.

C: Where at?

P: It was in Morgantown, but like Pierpont Rd, turns into something going towards Pennsylvania.

C: Okay yeah, just trying to get an idea of where you were. What prevented you from getting hurt?

P: Well, I did get hurt, but the branches, the snowpack, and then there's still a whole bunch of leaves and like twigs and stuff underneath it too, plus I had a jacket on yeah. That was more not like trying, but just being careless like I don't care if I die. Then I felt like okay well this is it, I'm dead now. But then it was like, oh wait I lived.

C: How many times do you think you've done stuff like that?

P: Over ten times.

C: Okay.

P: Like I had a motorcycle, or I would be driving recklessly and not really care and do stupid stuff.

C: Yeah, that's why I kept asking about substances, because a lot of times with alcohol and substances, people can tend to do more impulsive and reckless things like you mentioned. Do you have any access to guns?

P: No, I don't like guns.

C: Okay, we always ask that question as far as safety. Now we talked about this episode, which is the opposite of depression, they call it a manic episode.

P: Yeah.

C: So, you had this episode where you felt energized and had this mission, but right now are you feeling any energized feelings?

P: Nope.

C: Any distractibility where you can't feel like you can concentrate?

P: Nope.

C: Any flight of ideas, meaning like where you're thinking of things a lot in your brain?

P: No.

C: Your speech seems pretty straightforward right now, but has anyone talked about you being more talkative?

P: No.

C: Okay, and we talked about questions about engaging in risky behaviors and stuff. How about anxiety wise, tell me about any anxiety?

P: I don't feel like I'm anxious.

C: Any worried feeling? Tense, restless, having problems sleeping because you're worried a bunch?

P: Nope.

C: Okay, any concentration issues because you're feeling really worried? Anything like panic attacks before where you feel like short of breath and overwhelmed because of anxiety or feel like you're dying from worrying?

P: No.

C: Any physical symptoms at all like that?

P: No.

C: Anything where you've ever felt, like that you think about things over and over again in your head? We use the word obsessions, anything that you worry about over and over again?

P: No.

C: Or any kind of behaviors when you find yourself trying to do more and more to leave those worries, like checking on doors, checking on locks, washing your hands a bunch, and counting methods.

P: No.

C: Okay, and the substances we talked about…nothing now, but you had been drinking before, so tell me about that. What did you engage in over the years?

P: Pretty much I dabbled a little bit of…

C: Yeah, we never judge by the way, we know people can use and escape in different ways.

P: I think alcohol—I used to use I mean definitely that like mostly more than anything. Definitely maybe when I was like nervous or shy or have you known like a good time.

C: Did you ever feel like you had a problem with alcohol?

P: No. I never know I never felt like I had a problem, but maybe that was the problem. It was always one drink which turns into two, which turns into more.

C: Did you ever find yourself wanting to cut down?

P: I did yeah.

C: Did you ever find yourself getting angry when you were drinking?

P: Yes.

C: Or other people told you were getting angry or irritable?

P: Yes, emotions are much more pronounced with drinking, like anger and sadness.

C: Yes, you ever find yourself getting guilty about your drinking?

P: Yeah, when doing something stupid.

C: Did you ever first wake up in the morning and drink because you had to deal with shakes and stuff like that?

P: No.

C: Now did you ever have any kind of withdrawal feelings, like you stop drinking and you get really shaky?

P: No, the only thing is it would be like oh it's you know it's a Saturday, it's a holiday, I'm not drinking, I better be drinking 'cause everyone else is doing it. But that's like a mental withdrawal.

C: Did you have any complications from not drinking, like any episodes that they call seizures or times we got confused and had bad shakes?

P: No.

C: Any accidents or injuries other than the events that you mentioned earlier, jumping off the cliff. Any accidents like car accidents or bike accidents?
P: No, not unless I was just trying to kind of try and do stuff.
C: Any illegal consequences from drinking? DUIs?
P: I could have, I could have definitely.
C: Public intoxication charges?
P: No.
C: So, then we talked about…any other substances in the past that were paramount in your life?
P: No.
C: Okay and going back to some of these thoughts, we talked about you having these feelings of callings and religious kind of feelings, but have you ever felt like any feelings of people out to get you kind of feelings—paranoia?
P: No.
C: Are you feeling that now or ever? Or any feelings of hearing voices or seeing things?
P: No.
C: Okay, and then any post-traumatic stress symptoms. We talked about that earlier with childhood, but right now you're not feeling any current flashbacks or reexperiencing any past events?
P: No.
C: Any other symptoms you've ever had, like any concerns with eating any uh restricting of your eating in the past?
P: I did do a fast.
C: Tell me about that.
P: So, uh pretty much I went as long as I could without eating.
C: When was this this?
P: This was in October.
C: October of this past year? Why did you do that?
P: Um pretty much to see if I could…religious reasons.
C: Okay, religious reasons. Okay, and how long did that last?
P: It was just under 40 days.
C: Forty days. Were you trying to get to that 40-day symbolism?
P: Yeah.
C: Okay and how did you do during that time?
P: I did pretty well—I lost a lot of weight. I went from like well, I was 210, and then I was trying to cut down a little bit, but then I started my fast and then I cut it all way down to 159.
C: Tell me more about the fast, it's kind of interesting. Did you just not eat at all?
P: So, at first, I didn't eat or drink or anything, and then I started drinking,
C: Okay.
P: And then I uh just casually supplemented like nonfood-food like liquid-diet stuff.
C: Anything where you felt that your eating habits were problematic in any way where you felt your body image was not intact?
P: Nothing with my body image, no.

C: Or anything like where you felt the need to eat a lot and throw up or make yourself throw up?

P: No.

C: Be on any specific like pills to lose weight or anything like that?

P: No.

C: Okay, anything else you want to ask me about anything, because there are lots of things really actually fascinating that we talked about for a while, and we never want to judge what people believe because when you leave here, Chestnut Ridge, we want to make sure we help support you.

P: Yeah.

C: You know making sure your feelings of guilt aren't there, you know what I mean? And making sure your safety is intact, that's a big thing. Anything else? Actually, just one more category. Any ADHD symptoms over the years like any attention problems?

P: I think so yeah.

C: Okay, how so?

P: Oh, just sometimes I have a hard time paying attention.

C: In what context like where would you find yourself?

P: Reading.

C: Reading, okay.

P: It was hard for me to read for a long time.

C: Okay, did you notice that when you were growing up as a kid?

P: Yeah.

C: Did anyone say you were hyperactive or too active growing up.

P: Yeah, but I don't know like my mom always said, oh that's very normal like all kids have had it. But I definitely think I'm worse than others, yeah. But I definitely think there's a scale, like I might not be the worst, but I think I'm worse than average.

C: Do you ever find yourself not completing a lot of tasks?

P: No, I completed them, just because I hated not getting homework done, so I got it done.

C: How about your jobs over the years? You've done construction for a long time, but after you finish graduation from college did you work anywhere?

P: I worked for a few places selling cars, then I delivered medicine. I still do that. Then mainly construction.

C: Do you find yourself ever finding it difficult with completing all your work tasks?

P: Sometimes but I feel like it's just because I'm overloaded with work.

C: That's also a great point because that's something we always tell people—if you had too much on your plate, all of us can have problems with completing tasks. Any other things you want to talk about?

P: No, I don't think so.

C: So, you're feeling safe overall, as far as currently. Any thoughts where you want to harm yourself or harm anyone else?

P: No.

C: Any other concerns at all in any way? So, the team's really going to take care of you as far as the meds and then really help you with the follow-up plans and so forth. Okay, awesome.

Okay, nothing else really, just basically want to make sure that you stick with the treatment. Okay, like I was mentioning earlier you know we worry about if people have episodes and you kind of described that thing, that fuzziness that I think is pretty classic. That you lost track of time and what happened with all the events. Did anyone witness all the symptoms, or all the events that you had.

P: Not one person witnessed everything, but my dad witnessed a lot.

C: Yeah, have our team members called him?

P: Yeah.

C: Have they told you anything about what he said?

P: No.

C: It's always nice to hear from people that witness it to see what's going on, so we have a better way to prepare for the next time. To prevent the next time, you know it's a big thing we tell everybody to really help you with balancing things, so thank you so much. I'll ask our team if there's anything else we want to ask. Cool.

I really appreciate you doing this.

It really helps us kind of you know get a good feel of what people go through. Because if you ask me what I think there's a lot of potential things obviously we would never want to rule anything out, you know what I mean. But just like you mentioned, if you have a lot of work on your plate and a lot of things from your upbringing, right, can lead to this, just how you cope with everything. I'm very glad you're not using substances, because that risky behavior stuff that we want to prevent. But this is very, very treatable, and I see a lot of people do well over time that are on whatever medicine combinations they are on. And counseling. Have you had counseling?

P: Yes.

C: When did you first start doing counseling/therapy?

P: It was probably right after my first episode, so yeah like a year and a half ago.

C: Have you kept up with that pretty much the whole time?

P: I have except the last time I tried to get an appointment it was like 3 months.

C: We'll have to make sure our team gets you on that, right away.

P: Yes, so my appointment was actually supposed to be yesterday, but I'm already here.

C: They'll make sure they rescheduled that.

P: Actually, yeah, I think I'm gonna be seeing her tomorrow.

C: Beautiful, so any questions for us about anything? We really appreciate you taking time out.

Video #12: Full Interview 3

Dr. Parks

Transcription of Interview # (C = Clinician; P = Patient)

C: Hi, I'm Dr. Parks. I'm just going to talk with you and figure out a little bit about what brought you in and what's been going on and find a little bit out about your history and what not if that's alright?

P: That's fine.

C: Okay and you signed the consents and everything?

P: Yes, I have.

C: Excellent. Okay so tell me a little bit about what was going on before you came into the hospital.

P: Well, I'm in a homeless shelter.

C: Okay.

P: I guess I didn't follow a rule. I try to follow all the rules, but I was 5 minutes early or something, so they called the police and had me medically cleared because I have panic attacks and then I can't breathe, and they medically cleared me from any drugs, and I asked to see Dr. Zheng at Chestnut Ridge, but I had to go through the ER and that's how I'm here today.

C: Okay and so did you come to the emergency department here or somewhere else?

P: Yes, at Ruby (Memorial Hospital) and I told him I wanted to go through WVU Medicine.

C: Okay, and so what kind of things were going on at that time that they decided for you to come into the hospital?

P: Well, I talk out of my mind sometimes. I have bipolar 1 and I get manic then I can't breathe. I have anxiety attacks and I'm diagnosed also with PTSD, so I don't know what makes me…go off; I mean I know what makes me go off, but I don't know how to control it without my medicine, and I had taken my last pill. I had to come back because I don't have a family physician to write it in this county.

C: So, when you say "taken your last pill" how long was that before you came to the hospital?

P: Oh, not quite 12 hours. When they kicked me out, I would have had to walk the streets of Morgantown all day long from 6:30 AM all the way to 8:00 PM that night or the next night without any medication, thyroid pills, anything…it was all locked in my trunk at the homeless shelter. Anything I had around my neck was my key and my identification. So, I could've walked to the hospital or I could have left in an ambulance and maybe I was in the ER 40, at least 41 hours, but I knew eventually that I would come to Chestnut Ridge.

C: Okay and kinds of problems were having at that time?

P: When I was in there?

C: *Whenever you were in the emergency department.*

P: *Well, I felt paranoid. I thought people were talking about me. I felt manic and then I was depressed. So, I've run through all different moods, I'm not sure what is what.*

C: *So, kind of a combination of different things?*

P: *Mhhm, and I figured that might be the bipolar, and I asked the nurse and he said "Yes, you may be depressed, you may be manic and paranoid," but he said that's all part of bipolar. He was an RN at the ER.*

C: *So, is this the first time you're in the hospital or have you been in the hospital before?*

P: *Oh no, this is the fourth or fifth time in a very short period of time. So, right now I think my mental health is a lot of the problem of why I can't get a job. Because I talk too much or I have legal problems, too, that I didn't cause—I think I had a complete mental break when they arrested me.*

C: *Okay and so had you been working in the past?*

P: *Yes, I was a college student at DevRy University, and I have about 4 to 6 months and I'll graduate and do very well, but my mental health is number one right now.*

C: *Gotcha and so do you know as far as what kind of medications that are treating you with currently?*

P: *Zyprexa should be 5 mg.*

C: *Okay.*

P: *And Ativan for nerves or panic attacks, I think its 1 mg. I take thyroid medication because I don't have one, I had a thyroidectomy. And I take bumetanide 1 mg once a day and potassium 20 mEqs once a day.*

C: *Gotcha and so how was your sleep doing before you came to the hospital?*

P: *It was horrible. Three to four days I wouldn't have any sleep; I'd be starting into mania. I was so afraid. They had me on a shot, but I can't get it because of the time and the distance of where I'd have to go to get it.*

C: *Do you know what shot it was?*

P: *It was Invega.*

C: *Invega, gotcha.*

P: *So, I'm doing fine on the Zyprexa without it, maybe I do need it, maybe I don't.*

C: *Gotcha, and show so hadn't been sleeping for 3 or 4 days? How would your energy have been during that time?*

P: *Way up over the top, my mind wasn't right, but my energy was just crazy, like I'm on something.*

C: *Okay, and was your mind racing a fair amount?*

P: *Oh, terribly.*

C: *Talking faster?*

P: *Yes, sometimes nasty. I would get nasty with people and I'm not a mean person.*

C: *Okay so getting more irritable at that time?*

P: *Yes, exactly.*

C: *How would you say that your mood was then whenever you were having the more energy not sleeping as much?*

P: My mood was fine as long as nobody cornered me, then I would get angry. I feel smothered when people get too close to me and I think that's a panic attack of some kind.

C: Is this distance ok for you?

P: Yep.

C: Excellent.

P: Yeah, you're safe.

C: So, do other people notice the difference that are around you whenever you're having those break downs?

P: My family does, and I'm sure other people do too.

C: What have they said to you?

P: Do you really want me to tell you? "Shut the hell up." They're cruel to me. And then I'm either alone or I'm able to be around people and be medicated.

C: Any changes in terms of being more impulsive or doing things you otherwise wouldn't during those times?

P: Oh yeah, years ago I used to shoplift. I was compulsive then I believe, but I think that's quite kleptomania or compulsiveness, I'm not sure. But I mean that was oh, 10, 12, or 14 years ago at least.

C: Would there be any changes in terms of spending during those times?

P: Yeah, I spend it all and then I had no money.

C: So, when you say spending it all how much are we talking?

P: Whatever I made.

C: Okay.

P: And now I don't have a job, but I hang on to our money very tightly, so I am much better than I used to be.

C: Okay.

P: But I used to drink alcohol as well and I wouldn't touch it—I can't stand the smell of it now. But I'm the one who broke that cycle; I didn't go and get help for it—maybe I drank because I've always had a mental issue; I'm not sure.

C: How long has it been since your last alcoholic beverage?

P: A while.

C: A while as in weeks, months, years, decades?

P: Years.

C: Years, okay.

P: Like 5. And I have no interest in it, like I don't even want to be around it—that or illegal drugs; I don't want around anything like that.

C: Outside of the alcohol, had there been any other substances that you used?

P: I've tried marijuana—it didn't work for me, I didn't like. It made me do stupid things like…and I even was honest with my doctor and told him, and he said well maybe it's the drug itself, "when it makes you strip your clothes off and stop traffic because you feel you can't breathe you shouldn't be smoking it." But I always was honest with my medical doctor.

C: And so, with the marijuana was that a one-time thing, a couple times?

P: Two times. I was like 20 and maybe 26 and then I did one hit. I was the one-hit wonder, and then never again.

C: Okay.

P: I'd rather come to a doctor, and if they have to medicate me, I'd rather be on something that's not a narcotic that works.

C: So, going back to the alcohol what had ultimately happened to make you decide to stop drinking?

P: Well because I felt I needed it to function through day-to-day life and you don't. It's just really…they say that the hardest substance to get off of is alcohol, if you're an alcoholic. Well, it runs in my family, I don't want to be…I don't want to die from alcoholism, I wanna die of old age, healthy, and have a healthy life and mind, as healthy as I can.

C: And so back then, had it been daily when you were drinking alcohol?

P: Oh yeah.

C: How much could you drink in a day?

P: At least a pint a day or a fifth, depending on if I worked or not.

C: What kind of a pint or a fifth was it usually?

P: Usually it was a pint every day.

C: Whiskey, vodka?

P: Whiskey, and now if someone is drinking, I couldn't even stand the smell of it.

C: Gotcha, Okay, did it cause any problems in your life?

P: Well, if I let it, it would have. But I tried not to let it get that bad. I'd stay home and drink it, and I just pass out on the bed or in the chair and then I wake up, drink a little more. I usually drink it in a cup of hot tea, but I don't drink anymore; I have no desire.

C: Gotcha.

P: And I did that on my own. I didn't go to a rehab, maybe I should have. I don't know, but I don't think I need that now. But I do need like a psychiatric unit or doctor to help me, but I wouldn't lie. I'm a Christian so I don't lie anymore.

C: Any tobacco use?

P: Oh yeah, I do smoke, but I don't even have them with me and I'm wearing a patch as we speak. Oh no, I'm not; I took it off and they're supposed to give me another one; I'm sorry, I thought I had it on.

C: Alright, and is it a pack a day? Two packs a day, half a pack?

P: Well, no. It's about a half a pack or maybe five of those little cigars that look like cigarettes. I don't smoke cigarettes anymore.

C: Okay.

P: They're too expensive and they smell horrible and little cigars don't smell as bad, I don't think. But I think they're kind of a crutch for me more so than a need.

C: Alright and so you had mentioned in terms of before coming into the hospital having some thoughts that people were meaning you harm, has that pretty consistently happened when you're having those periods and not sleeping, or have you noticed feeling that way other times?

P: No, I feel like that off and on my whole life, but my mother was mean to me. She abused me, and I'll be honest, she used to beat me over the back and tell me I was fat, and it's just been my whole life now.

C: Sorry to hear that—how often do thoughts about that come up for you?

P: *All the time, well not all the time, but whenever people ask me about it. I kind of bottle it up. And then my dad left when I was 15, well on my Sweet 16 birthday party. And he said horrible things to me and now he's dying, and I forgive him for never speaking to me for 20 years since my mother died. I've seen him, and he says horrible things about me like, you know that I'm no good, I'll never be anything, same thing. So, he disappeared for a long time and then now we appear.*

C: *So, he disappeared for a long time and then when he reappeared, he's still negative?*

P: *Now he's living in my childhood home with his new wife and I've forgiven him through prayer. And through prayer I've forgiven myself for every bad thing I've done, and God takes care of the rest, you know.*

C: *Do those memories ever feel like you're back in those moments?*

P: *When I'm at Bartlett house, I feel that way. I don't like it there. I'm not saying it's a bad place, but it's not good for me; I know that much.*

C: *Does it impact your sleep?*

P: *Very much so. And impacts a lot of things for me and I mean yes, I'm homeless, but I'm still a person with feelings and I don't like the way that things are ran, so I'd rather leave and find a better place.*

C: *Do you get nightmares?*

P: *Sometimes.*

C: *Is it about what's happened or is it about other things?*

P: *It's when I'm there. If I'm asleep, I can have weird dreams, or if there's certain people around me, I'll sit up and fight sleep. So, or maybe I won't take my medicine and then I won't sleep, you know? That's not good, it's just a bad environment.*

C: *Gotcha, has there been anything in your adult life as far as bad things that have happened or was it mostly in your youth?*

P: *I've been raped.*

C: *I'm sorry to hear that.*

P: *And uh my husband that I loved shot himself. So yes, there's been a lot of bad thing. My niece that I love shot herself, so it's been suicides, rapes. I'm used to being without money. Now if I get money, I stretch it until it snaps and bad things happen to good people, you know. Everybody has problems; you just have to work them out or try to do better.*

C: *How have you coped with everything that has happened in your life?*

P: *Because I just always believe someone has it worse off than me and it's hard. This is the worst. This is the hardest thing I've ever been through.*

C: *I'd offer you a tissue, but I don't think there's any around…and so have you been through therapy to help with things?*

P: *No, I was there once through Appalachian mental health, but they said you just need someone to listen. You need maybe psych, but you need someone to listen. That was almost 4 years ago that I was there, just one time 'cause I thought I couldn't cry, just everything got real tight, I was having panic attacks. She said all you need is for someone to listen; you need therapy, you can come back here. But I never went back.*

C: *Gotcha.*

P: *Well, it seems like when I'm working, I can put my everything into my work. But I don't know—I don't know the answers yet.*

C: *And so thus far, it's been more so on the medication end as far as treatment.*

P: *Yeah.*

C: *And what have you found helpful as far as medication wise?*

P: *Ativan, Zyprexa, and then just knowing that there's people around that care and will help me, you know. And they may not be the answer. But the Invega helped, but I can't get the shot. And I could do the Zyprexa, and I believe as long as I can…I do certain herbal things for anxiety like lavender teas, and celery has tryptophan which naturally will calm me, but I can't be in an environment that makes me nervous, you know without medicine. So right now, I think the Ativan works. And I can control it on the outside as long as I'm not around a bunch of people, I could lock it up in a box or a safe you know, and never have it with me and still be able to stop and pick up some lavender tea and drink it. The smell plugs me, it's allergy, but I can drink it and it doesn't bother me.*

C: *Any other over-the-counters or herbals that you use outside of the lavender tea and tryptophan?*

P: *No, just gummy vitamins, which we all need.*

C: *So, you've mentioned the Invega, Zyprexa, Ativan. Had you been on other medications before?*

P: *Yeah, I've been on Klonopin. When Eric died, they started me on Xanax, and they took me off because all I did was sleep, but they never cut me back. I know my sister takes 1/4 milligram and so does my sister-in-law for bipolar, she's bipolar. And trust me she needs something, she makes me…I have to leave her house, I want to hurt her, and I don't hurt anybody. But she just she gets in my face and she's a more…I don't know how to explain it, but she's bipolar and she takes 1/4 milligram of Xanax instead of Ativan. That's what her regular doctor prescribes her after she's had four nervous breakdowns—I think I might have had one. But mine started when my husband shot himself and I loved him, and he was my best friend but he was sick.*

C: *How long ago was that?*

P: *Twelve years ago this June.*

C: *Did you have any psychiatric treatment back before then?*

P: *No, not even for my rape, I just got through it myself.*

C: *And so, you've mentioned as far as the hospitalizations that you had several over a somewhat short span of time. Had you had them in the past, or has it all been pretty recent?*

P: *Oh, it's all been pretty recent, especially the hospitalization. I've never been hospitalized for it.*

C: *When's the first time you went into the hospital for psychiatric reasons?*

P: *To be honest I went into Ruby and my brother and his wife brought me back. I can't remember, I think…I can't remember who took me the first time. Oh, I remember, the ambulance brought me from Elkins WV into Ruby. I got a room and my niece…or I got a room in 9E, or I got a room anyway, and they brought me back and I was able to stay with Jeff and Lisa. And Lisa came up to the home-*

less shelter in Elkins and picked me up, and I went to their house in Maryland and I refused to take my meds. I was really, really hard on them, and now they say they can't believe the difference in me how I can speak and actively listen. But it's because of WVU Medicine, they brought me back and I don't know if she called Dr. Zheng, but he was there for me. He was there the last time, and the last time, and he's here for me this time. I'm happy to be his patient because I know now…cause I think how did I get back here? And I always know why, it's because I asked for him.

C: *Okay and so were you living up in that other area or where do you live?*

P: *I was living in Chrisville, but normally I had a house in Elkins, well Beverly. But they already rented it because I wouldn't stay there. Ultimately, I was homeless and the homeless shelter in Elkins was good for me, but now I'd rather go somewhere and just get better. Other than Bartlett house, I don't want to go back there, only for my things. They owe me a paycheck, for the other Bartlett House because I went there, worked in the kitchen, but I'd rather just get my things and move on to a better shelter for women or more doctors or clinics.*

C: *So, were all the hospitalizations through WVU at Chestnut Ridge or had you been admitted anywhere else?*

P: *Never. I was admitted one time in my life and that was in Elkins. But I didn't understand what was going on, but they sent me up here to WVU medicine from that hospital.*

C: *How did those admissions compare to what was going on this time?*

P: *I don't know, to be honest; they would laugh, and I'd think they were making fun of me. Alright so it wasn't that I was hearing voices, I could hear them tentatively laughing and I thought they should help me right away. Now I'm more patient, I know people laugh and they're laughing at other things, not just me.*

C: *And so before you went into the hospital the other times, was it similar to not sleeping and having a lot of energy?*

P: *Yup, I've always been like that and my mother brought me to WVU, and they would check my adrenal glands, my pituitary, everything. But they didn't see anything wrong, so maybe I've had this since I was little. I thought maybe I was ADHD; I don't know what's wrong. But I know that whatever they're treating me for now, bipolar and PTSD, and anxiety I think is what my paper is saying, I believe that.*

C: *What's the longest period of time you've gone as far as having lots of energy, not sleeping, and doing things outside of your character?*

P: *At least 11 days. I could just stay at my house and not leave. But one day I walked on foot and I'm glad my family came and got my dog, or she would have died in that house because I thought it had been a day or two, but it was more like 9 1/2 days.*

C: *Gotcha.*

P: *I didn't do that though. I had all this stuff…people stealing stuff at my house and I couldn't get them to leave, couldn't get any help. Usually, I'm good, it's just me and my dog and my medicine, but I had people in my house stealing my medicine, so I just threw it all away and I didn't take my thyroid pills for a couple months. It about killed me. And I don't have a thyroid so it messed me up big time.*

C: Any thoughts of not wanting to be alive recently or in the past?

P: No, no I like myself too good now, I don't wanna die. I wanna get better.

C: Ever tried to take your life or any self-harm?

P: When I was, I think I was 9 or 12 in that area, my mom would torture me so bad I took a bottle of those Mini Thins, but that was the only time. My sister she was a nurse, she took warm milk and just a little and scrapped black toast and made charcoal; she called it charcoal, and everything would come out. But I ripped my hair out until my scalp bled from my mother the way she used to talk to me.

C: Gotcha, okay. And so, the Mini Thins, that was to take your life?

P: Well that's what I thought, pills ya know? But I don't feel that way anymore.

C: Was there just the once or was it there more than one?

P: Just one time.

C: Okay. Ever any cutting, burning yourself?

P: No. No. My scars are usually from a doctor cutting me (laughs) or a burn from...I love to bake and cook, but I always just give it away to friends or family.

C: Any particular dishes that are your specialty?

P: Well, lasagna. I make grape pies. Breads. I can make anything pretty much. My mom, she was a chef, but she was…she was hard on me.

C: Gotcha. And so, you mentioned as far as depression and feeling depressed as well as manic at the same time when you were in the emergency department, can you tell more about that?

P: Well, I just thought I was depressed because I knew it had been more than 30 hours and I wanted a bigger room with bigger space that was all. But I got… I'm over it, I'm not depressed now.

C: How would you say that your mood is today?

P: Good. My mood is good today.

C: Okay. And so, have you had periods of time where you kind of stay depressed for days?

P: A couple of days, usually in the winter, when it's 15 degrees outside because my joints and stuff hurt. I don't know if it's depression, but I feel better just laying in a recliner watching television, and there's days that the roads are too bad, and they tell ya don't go out on the roads. So yeah, it's not really depression, and maybe it's just being smart thinking well today I'm not going out, I'll go outside in the yard with my dog or to check my mail, but I could just grab a blanket and curl up and watch TV all day so.

C: In any extended periods of time for weeks where you're not really enjoying things? Don't maybe want to get out of bed? Not having energy?

P: No, just whenever it's cold out. And it's not weeks, just a couple of days. Because I'm…I need to go out and do things. I can't just sit around and wait around for long periods of time.

C: So, doesn't really stick around for you?

P: No, not the depression.

C: Okay.

P: The hyper-like does. It sticks around. I have medicine to bring me out of it.

C: Ever any hearing or seeing things?

P: Nu-uh.

C: Never?

P: I never hear anything. I can lay in bed and I think oh my I could be a vacuum and I could be doing this, and then I'm up cleaning. Well, my dogs are used to other people ya know? They sleep ya know. So I just don't do well living with other people. But on my own place, I'm fine.

C: Okay. Ever feeling particularly talented?

P: Oh yeah, but I am talented. Singing and cooking, but I don't feel like granier or grandeur if that's…I'm not sure how to say it but…no I don't think I'm the president of the United States sometimes, no.

C: Okay. So just kinda having that self-confidence in your abilities?

P: I need to have more self-confidence, I think. To make it from where I am now.

C: Okay, but not feeling like that it's ever above the norm?

P: No power trip or anything no.

C: Okay. And ever feeling like the radio or the news giving messages specifically for you?

P: Oh, no. Not that I can remember.

C: Okay. Ever hearing other people's thoughts or feeling like they can hear yours?

*P: No. No but like I said if they're laughing and I hear "yes she's going to Sharp's" I've said to em please, don't, I know what the 302 means *chuckles* because I used to work at Hopemont State Hospital, in the behavior department, and I know what 302 means and I thought they meant me. But I don't know, it's not a television but it's people close to my door, people I can hear…so.*

C: Okay.

P: But I don't…when it's quiet, I don't hear anything, I could be alone with my thoughts and not be afraid of my thoughts, if I am, I would come straight to the ER.

C: Okay. And you'd mentioned sometimes you'd get more irritable when you haven't got much sleeping. Have you ever kinda lashed out at anyone or gotten in fights?

P: I got, yeah, yes, I have.

C: Can you tell me more about that?

P: Just when someone gets in my face and corners me and I feel threatened, that's whenever I can lash out. But I don't…I try not to hurt people ever. I warn 'em, just don't get in my face, and be an adult. I can be an adult and still be sick, you know, so I've been raped, and I've been cornered, and I've been beat in the corner, and just that will bring it on for me.

C: Gotcha. So, kind of those similar settings bring you back to those times.

P: Well, I will black out and then I wake up hurt. I've broke my tail bone, I've broken ribs. I don't want to do that anymore. I know what causes it. It's bad, bad panic attacks from people that you know if I lash out on the street and tell people, please don't get close to me because I still, you know the rape thing. He beat me half to death and he lived in my home. So, if I'm out in public, why do I have to have someone put me in a corner if I'm minding my own business. Especially if it's a male doing it. It's just not a good thing for me.

C: Does it ever get to the point where you want to kill someone.

P: Oh no, nobody ever worth going to jail over and nobody's life is worth me taking, you know? I don't have that right.

C: Okay, and so you mentioned legal problems, can you tell me more about that?

P: I went into a church because I was hungry and cold. And had a big light above me that said "Hey you" and I thought there was somebody inside because they opened the door freely by security and I walked in. I had went in and pooped myself in a church, and I tried to get out. There was lights and whistles going off and it confused me and I tried to get out the back, and they came and handcuffed me. They said I entered a vessel, which was a church. And I knew it was a church. It's the summit church. I didn't steal anything, I didn't break anything, I just sanitized my hands trying to be clean because I had poop in my pants and lots of it. And I think I had a complete mental break and I just wanted to go and get a bath and something to eat. That's it. And I might have a bad check in Randolph County I've got to make right when I can.

C: Are any of those legal charges active?

P: They're active.

C: Okay, gotcha.

P: But I got to get my family member. He will take off work to take me. But I got to get a phone so I can call him, or he can call me and say hey do you have a ride to Randolph County. I don't have to even go to court is what I'm hearing; I just have to go into court with my attorney. But I have to get there. I don't know how I'm going to get there so that's it.

C: And so, you mentioned that person. Who all do you have that supportive in your life?

P: Just two brothers and one sister-in-law. The rest of 'em, they all think I'm on meth and I'm not on meth, believe me. I used to get so mad about it, but now I just think they're crazy because I'm not on meth. And I was never on meth.

C: Mhhm.

P: But I was having this, I don't know it was like this "ta ta ta uh uh uh" and I couldn't speak. And I don't know what caused that if that was some kind of a mental break down. That's what I was doing. I don't know if it was some kind of a seizure. But I would have to write down, and they thought I was on meth.

C: Were you on any medications at that time?

P: None, I wasn't even taking my thyroid pill.

C: Gotcha. And so had you ever been on anything like lithium or Depakote.

P: No, but they might have given me a shot of Deb…deb. I thought it was debradoe.

C: Depo?

P: No, no isn't that for pregnancy?

C: Well, they kind of use Depo.

P: This was given to me in the Med G room at Ruby, this was in the ER. And someone said Depakote, I thought it was Debradoe or something, but they might have said Depakote.

C: Okay. And so were you seeing someone in the outpatient setting before being in the hospital?

P: No, not for psych, no.

C: Had you ever or had it all just been medications from the hospital?

P: Well my family doctor said "Have you ever tried Paxil" and I said no. And he said, "Well, have you ever been diagnosed bipolar" and I said no. Him and a couple of doctors have asked me have I been diagnosed as bipolar. And I say no because I had never been diagnosed. Now that I've seen Dr. Zheng, I am diagnosed bipolar 1.

C: And so, had they put you on Paxil and then you had ended up in the hospital?

P: No, they put me on Ativan.

C: Okay.

P: And then what I had left, someone had stolen. So, I threw all my medicine away in my trash can in my bedroom, and I refused to take medicine and that's when everything fell apart.

C: Mhhm, Okay. And is anxiety a problem for you?

P: Yes, it is.

C: What kinds of things do you find worry you?

P: Money, stress, you know the day-to-day, really.

C: Do you feel like your worries are more than other people worry? Or do you feel like it's pretty similar?

P: I think that everybody has worry and stress just how you deal with it that's all.

C: Growing up did you have problems with anxiety?

P: Yes, and it was from being verbally abused and physically abused by my mother. She loved me but she was mean to me, I don't know how else to explain it. I was never good enough, I was fat, I was ugly—you know she beat me with her fist.

C: What's been helpful for the worry or anxiety of those memories in the past?

P: Drinking.

C: Do you feel like that's what kind of led to the drinking?

P: Absolutely I do.

C: How old were you when you started drinking?

P: 21–22. I didn't drink though and lay drunk, I used to be a singer—well I still sing—but on a stage, I would sing for God, not in a bar and drink. That's the difference. My dad didn't want me to do it. My mom, she said I could be famous, but I was never good enough till she heard me sing. Now I don't sing, but I will again. In fact, I sang up on the unit today and one of the patients said, "Oh my gosh you're awesome singer." I don't have to feel bad about myself—I know what I can do good and what I can't. But I think we all have a chance to prove it now.

C: Are there any things in terms of checking locks, checking you phone, checking on people, counting any types of things like that that you find that you do or have done in the past?

P: I used to, and now I don't want to think about it. It just boggles my mind, but I don't have anything really. My lock that I have where my medicine and money is at you know where I'm staying I would like to get that stuff back, but I don't want to stay there anymore. I hope they saved my purse and things that I didn't lock up yet. Because the last time I was here, they threw everything I owned away, all the junk I brought with me. This time I don't I didn't bring too much.

C: Any excessive hand washing or worrying about germs?

P: Yeah, oh yes. And I always thought it was like obsessive-compulsive disorder. I don't know what it really is, but yes, I've had that.

C: How much time would you spend as far as focusing on…

P: Hours. Not on my hands, but on the house. But mine I did clean it before all this happened, and I could really seriously do the whole house in 6 hours, and it was done you know and do it right like a deep clean because maybe I'd work the next 6 days.

C: So, would that happen just kind of in general or would that happen when you were having the not sleeping episodes?

P: Not sleeping.

C: Okay, and is the same as far as you've mentioned some theft or taking items, was that when you weren't sleeping as well?

P: Yes.

C: Okay, not outside of that?

P: No.

C: Okay and then as far as outside of the marijuana and alcohol, ever used more benzos than prescribed?

P: No actually, I had more left and people would steal them from me. I've had people hold me at gunpoint in the city for them.

C: Oh jeez.

P: Yes, and that's truth, because in the city they can shoot up with what I used to take—Klonopin. Or they can trade it for heroin which I didn't know, and someone said they're banging your pills and I said what do you mean they're banging them? So, I even asked my doctor I said, "Why do people wanna kill me for a Klonopin if they don't make me high?" He said because they're therapeutic to your brain, you need them, but they like them. Because they can get really high really easy. That's why I said I didn't want them, but I told the doctor in the ER if that's what it takes for me to get better, I'll try them again. But I was on them for 10 or 11 years and I weaned myself off, and my doctor said, "Why didn't you get your pills filled it's the beginning of July and you didn't fill them at all in June?" I said because I don't want to take them anymore, I don't have these blackout episodes and that's been almost 5 years ago. So, I weaned myself off in a month and a half because I had extra, I didn't need to refill it and I should have called and told him. He shouldn't have to ask, you know.

C: So, time wise you were on the Klonopin around the time that you were drinking around daily and then stopped, both of those around the same time?

P: Yes, yes ma'am.

C: Okay. And never any inhalants, pain pills, anything like that?

P: Pain pills, yup. But I don't even ask for pain pills any more. Tylenol is good enough for me. Nothing injected, no.

C: Had pain pills ever become a problem for you?

P: No, but I've taken them. But they make me itch so bad I can't sleep when I take a Percocet, I'm on the opposite.

It's so bad. And I get more hyper, why would I want that? So they're on my list of allergies and maybe I am allergic to them, I don't know.

C: And anything like mushrooms, LSD, cocaine?

P: Cocaine one time I tried it and that's been...well it was right after my husband blew his head off. I thought I'll get you! Someone offered me and I took a little spot of it, just a little spot, and I said I don't want it. I just don't want it.

C: Any other substances?

P: No, no. So, I don't think cocaine hurt me one time, I think it was this side of my nose. I'm honest.

C: So, going back, you been inpatient at Chestnut Ridge a number of times and then you said outpatient, you haven't seen a psychiatrist but had followed with your family doctor for the Klonopin, I believe. But nothing beyond that as far as psych meds?

P: No...oh Cymbalta. But I don't believe it works for me anymore, I know it's not a narcotic. If I thought Cymbalta would help, I would take it. But I don't think it works anymore.

C: And so, you mentioned your sister having bipolar, anyone else have bipolar?

P: I think my mother had it now that I know I have it. Grandma always called Mom her "special child," she wouldn't let my grandfather correct her because he was mean. He would get mean and I think maybe I reminded my mother too much of herself.

C: Anyone in the family with schizophrenia, schizoaffective, anxiety, depression?

P: Anxiety.

C: Okay.

P: But I'm not sure if my sister Sharon...she takes Celexa, I believe is what it's called. She says, "Oh my nerves," but I don't know if that's for anxiety or what it's for, but she takes Celexa.

C: And then you mentioned that your husband had passed from suicide and I think a niece?

P: Yes, my sister Sharon, that was her daughter, her baby.

C: Anyone else in the family?

P: No.

C: Okay and then you mentioned alcohol, who all in the family has problem with alcohol?

P: Oh my, my uncles, my brother—both brothers. I have a little problem with, well a lot. But like I have a brother right now that's drank his self to death over his wife's death, and I know because he's swollen and purple and he looks awful. My father drank moonshine, my uncles made it. Their father died when my dad was 17, I never got to meet him. He was an alcoholic. He died from an alcoholic seizure and he swallowed his tongue and died.

C: Anyone in the family have problems with other drugs?

P: Just a nephew. And a niece...well I call her a niece, but she's not a blood relative. She's grew up since she was two around...she's an actual heroin addict that takes her son's Adderall. So, there you have it. And her brother Dylan, which is my nephew, he went off heroin, drank beer, smoked marijuana, and now I heard he's back on heroin. I just try not be around it and pray for them.

C: *Did your mother use any substances?*

P: *Cigarettes and coffee.*

C: *No alcohol or drugs?*

P: *No, she hated it.*

C: *And so, you mentioned that you used to live in Elkins but more recently living at the Bartlett House. How long have you been at the Bartlett House?*

P: *Oh, my goodness, probably since sometime in May. I know it's been at least 2 months. And that's 2 months too long for me, truly.*

C: *And so, who all had you been living with prior to living at the Bartlett House?*

P: *Where did I live prior to there? I had my own house.*

C: *Were you living by yourself or were you living with anybody.*

P: *I was living with Mark; his name was Mark, and he was stealing everything I own. He even locked up my bank account and now it's 43 in the red. Yes, I worry about it. But I don't care what he does anymore, he can fly away for all I care.*

C: *Okay, and was that a former friend or a family member?*

P: *Well, no he was a boyfriend.*

C: *Any significant others currently?*

P: *Yeah, a husband that lives in Ohio, but he won't help me with even $5. He's been gone 7 years. All I want to do is divorce him. But I have to find a place that doesn't cost me money, or I have to get a job. But that's on my list of to-dos.*

C: *Okay, and do you have any kids? Just the fur baby?*

P: *Just the fur baby.*

C: *Okay. Alrighty. And then you mentioned some college, is it a bachelor's you're working on?*

P: *No, it's an associate.*

C: *Okay and what is that in?*

P: *Medical coding specialties, which pays very well, I could work from home if I had to, it depends on who you work for.*

C: *And then with thyroid, did they remove that did you say?*

P: *Yeah, at first, I had a goiter and then they went in and they had to remove it all. But it was removed here at Ruby.*

C: *Any other medical problems?*

P: *Just allergies and my heart and lungs are supposedly good. And I get on a lot of fluid; they said that I had ureteral stricture. I had a KUB scan done and they saw that I had ureteral strictures as a birth defect or something.*

C: *Okay. Any history of any seizures?*

P: *Well that's why they gave me Klonopin, they said that I had seizure activity but it was brought up by anxiety. That's why I had the Klonopin, they told me it was therapeutic to my brain, that's all I know.*

C: And any history of concussions, hitting your head and passing out, strokes?

P: I had an ischemic episode when I was throat punched by a man at work and got hit in the head and I woke up in the hospital. And I've had headaches, but yes they said ischemic episode.

C: Any problems with blood pressure?

P: It's always low, usually.

C: And any diabetes, high cholesterol, anything like that?

P: No, not that I know of.

C: Okay, and any other surgeries outside of what you mentioned before?

P: No.

C: Okay. Can you tell me what 7 from a 100 is?

P: 93.

C: Can you do it again?

P: 93.

C: Seven from that?

P: Is uh, well give me a minute is 80...no...70...you caught me, so wait a minute 93–7...is 86.

C: And seven from that?

P: Is 78...or 9...79.

C: Seven from that...

P: is 67.

C: Alright, and what does it mean when people say "don't throw rocks in glass houses"?

P: It means keep your mouth shut about other people because maybe they have the same problems you do. Or I shouldn't because I live in a glass house. I'm not sure exactly what it means.

C: Okay.

P: But I've heard it said.

C: What about "all that glitters isn't golden"?

P: It means that not everything is what you think it is, it's not perfect.

C: Do you have any questions for me? Is there anything that I haven't asked about that you feel like would be helpful for me to ask about?

P: No, I feel fine.

C: Well, I appreciate you taking the time to talk with me.

P: Oh, not a problem.

C: Hope everything gets sorted out.

P: Oh, it will, it will.

Video # 13: Extra Practice 1

Transcription of Interview #13 (C = Clinician; P = Patient)

C: I'm going to ask you some questions about what brings you into the hospital today. First, what do you like to be referred to as?

P: Dee.

C: Okay, Dee. Tell me what brings you to the hospital.

P: Alcohol. To the point of wanting to harm myself.

C: Really. Okay. Can we talk a little about alcohol? Tell me what was going on that made you decide now was the time to come into the hospital?

P: Because I was drinking the alcohol and I had a fear that I would, if I didn't get help, I would harm myself.

C: So that became even more of a fear for you, that it could become actually reality.

P: Yes.

C: Okay.

P: Yes. Because there was no fear.

C: It was the fact that you didn't have fear.

P: Yes. I thought I would be in a better place. And being sick with the alcohol in a cycle.

C: Can you tell me some of the problems alcohol has created for you?

P: Not to where I've, you know, broken the law or anything. It's uh…relationships. With some family, you know. Not to where I was drinking, spending money, not paying rent, losing, getting my utilities shut off, things like that.

C: So alcohol was harming relationships.

P: Yes, fighting with significant others, too.

C: And not only that, but because of your drinking you were neglecting bills that you had to pay.

P: I was not paying attention to my bank account. Drinking and not checking if I had enough to pay this bill or that. I got behind in my rent.

C: Was a lot of money going towards the alcohol?

P: It was for other persons who was buying it. My boyfriend, he was working and his paycheck was going towards alcohol. You know, you're talking about 30 packs a day.

C: Give me an idea of the amount of alcohol you've been drinking.

P: There would be some bad days I would get up in the morning, and as soon as he left for work, I would start drinking at 6:00 in the morning.

C: So you'd start drinking pretty soon after you got up.

P: Yep.

C: Would you get shaky before you had a drink?

P: I would get sick.

C: Sick in what ways?

P: Sick to my stomach, shaky. I was depressed, anxiety, scared.

C: Would you feel upset in your stomach?

P: Yes.

C: On an average day how much would you drink?

P: Before he got home, maybe I'd drink 8 or 9. And then he'd bring some more beer home and I'd finish off another 10. And I didn't eat. I neglected eating to where I was about, it affected my brain. Irreversible. Like in a dementia state.

C: Did that worry you?

P: Yes. When the doctor brought it to my attention because I didn't know who I was or where I was, I didn't know what was going on around me.

C: So not only some of these physical problems, it was also causing mental problems. Were you losing track of time?

P: Yes. Days, things that, maybe appointments, stuff like that. Losing track of important things, papers I needed to fill out. My son would call me and listen to me and it affected him.

C: How so?

P: To hear his mother had started drinking that early in the day and talking and crying. So he came and took me to his house and with a counselor, up at Summit. She arranged to get me in the hospital. They said it could have been a lot worse because I stayed at my son's and he tried to get me to eat. It hurt him to hear me opening a beer at 6 AM.

C: Your son was really worried about you.

P: Yes. I'd drink all day and all night.

C: How long have you been drinking?

P: I started drinking late. Never was early. My first drink was 30 years old. I wasn't a teenager. My heaviest drinking started in my 50s. Before I would socially drink. I could go have a couple drinks with friends or out to dinner.

C: Did you find with time that you needed more alcohol to make you feel a certain way?

P: Yes, it got to the point where I wasn't even getting drunk. I needed a lot more. I wasn't even feeling drunk. It took more and more to the point, and then I wasn't drunk, I'd just pass out. There was also always a lot of fighting, arguing. That was getting out of hand because we were blaming one another for not paying bills. We were both drinking the alcohol. It was his place to pay the bills, you know. He had my bank card and I did not realize how we drank so much.

C: So you lost track of your bank account too?

P: I was over drafted $800 in a month. I couldn't figure out how that happened.

C: Over the past year, it sounds like you've been drinking regularly. Has there been a time when you stopped drinking for a while?

P: I would go like I'd say, I'll try to cut back. I had some advice from a neighbor. He said to try to cut back and each day count your beers.

C: How did that work?

P: They started tasting good and I'd drink some more.

C: Did you find that you were able to not drink for a couple days or more?

P: Yes.

C: Would you get irritable?

P: Sometimes. But I'd start eating and it would help. I was shaking a lot though. I wasn't eating when I was drinking. And that concerned my son. The drinking and not nourishing my body. I was malnourished. He said "Mom, your hair is falling out." I was weak. I wasn't eating. I just, I would stay in bed and get up and go to the refrigerator.

C: So most of your time was spent drinking?

P: I wouldn't even go out. I was ashamed that I looked terrible.

C: Would other people say anything to you? Besides your son?

P: Yes, my neighbor, Mary. She mentioned it to me. And thank God. She has an alcoholic son, I guess. So she's been through it. She was concerned.

C: So she's witnessed it firsthand and was seeing these same things happening in your life and trying to help.

P: And not nicely.

C: How did you respond?

P: It wasn't a nice, dignified.

C: Would you get annoyed?

P: Yes. She didn't put it real nice. It was real stern. To the point it hurts your feelings. I kind of resented that.

C: Did you feel like your sleep was affected by drinking?

P: Oh yeah. I'd wake up drinking and the anxiety hit me.

C: Would you have another drink at that time?

P; Sometimes I would. My mind, racing racing racing. It wouldn't shut off. I'd get up at 3, 4 o'clock in the morning and sneak to the refrigerator and have a beer. Then go back to bed. Just to shut my mind off.

C: Do you have hope that things can get better?

P: Yes. Most of my drinking started, related to anxiety. I'm an anxious person. I have been all my life. When the doctor took me off the anxiety medicine, I was able to control my drinking. I didn't want to drink on the anxiety medicine. When she took me off, I just went straight downhill. I was having panic attacks, I was drinking, too. I started picking up the drink to stop the anxiety. So there is mostly my drinking, related to the anxiety. After I was taken off the medicine, that's when I started the heavy drinking. I drank for the anxiety, anxiousness, panic. For me to go to the store, I would go into a horrible panic attack. I would be scared to go out. Panic and anxiety started after the abuse I suffered from my son's father.

C: So you drank to cope with these anxious feelings?

P: Yes. That panic and anxiety. If I had to go somewhere, I got scared and panicky. I wanted to take a drink to stop it. I would panic and feel like running. Just couldn't sit still. I couldn't answer questions.

C: Must have been frustrating.

P: And scary. If I was alone, it was worse. The anxiety and panic were worse. I get really panicked and scared. Fear.

C: Anything else you think I should know regarding your drinking?

P: Just, uh…anything in my past?

C: Not necessarily. I'm wondering if there's been any other problems. You mentioned worrying about your physical and psychological health. The problems with your relationships, with feeling guilty.

P: I've always, um. After my mother died. I cared for my mother; she had Parkinson's. I cared for her the last few years at home until she died. So that was hard. And then there was, as we all feel, after we lose a loved one, guilt. Feeling like I could have done more, said more. I did not deal with my grief. So that's when it started.

C: So the fact that you didn't deal with it.

P: It was terrible. The family was fighting. It was terrible. It shouldn't have been. She had a hard life, and she should have had more peace.

C: And you picked up the alcohol more after that?

P: Yes. That's when I started. Then the doctor put me on anxiety medicine because I wasn't sleeping. Feeling that panic and anxiety. I should have gone to a support group. Hospice asked me to.

C: You feel like you would have been better off with that?

P: Yes. The family wasn't supportive, either. The family was separating. It was very ugly. I think it was a sin. The family separated and was fighting and it was…I don't…It's something my mother wouldn't have wanted. She was a good person, a giving and religious person. I don't think she would have liked that.

C: Sounds like you're still wrestling with guilt surrounding that.

P: I don't think the family…they should have come together at a time like that. Should have been together. I mean…they were fighting before they carried my mom out on a gurney. I could never deal with that. I was screaming, crying. And she was concerned about me. I never got over her death.

C: So you still struggle with that. And that's probably something we could work on.

P: Yes. She was my best friend. She died in 2003.

C: Okay.

P: They say time will heal, but it hasn't healed me.

C: What did you like about your mom?

P: She was very intelligent. She had good advice. Very knowledgeable. Very common sense. She'd always give you the best advice. She'd see you pick up a can of beer and she'd say "you better leave that stuff alone."

C: So she didn't like you drinking?

P: No. She was scared. She told me not to fool with it too much. She said it would get you. She had a lot of good advice. Any type of problem I had, she was. I would feel better because she would solve it for me.

C: Sounds like she was a real rock in your life.

P: Yes. I wasn't close to my father. He was abusive to my mother.

C: Was your mother your closest relationship?

P: Not at the beginning. But as I grew. I ran away from home at 17. I wasn't around my mother as much. It bothered her when I did that.

C: Did mom or dad have a drinking problem?

P: My father did. He drank all his life. He started when he was 12 years old.

C: So you may have come about your alcohol problems naturally.

P: He was very anxious too. To the point where if you got him upset, he got too anxious—he'd be dangerous. He could hurt you. I went to see him before he died.

C: What did he die from?

P: Wasn't his liver. His lungs. He was 83 years old.

C: Did he drink throughout his whole life?

P: Yes. Not a day went by. If he couldn't buy it, he'd make it.

C: I'm going to finish up the interview right now, but before I finish, have you ever had a seizure before?

P: I believe I have.

C: Did you remember what was happening during that time?

P: It was after she took me off the anxiety pill. I fell forward into the bathtub. It was Clozapine. I just stood there and just shook and fell forward.

C: Did your whole-body shake?

P: Yes.

C: Did you lose bowel or bladder control?

P: Yes.

C: Did you hit your head?

P: No.

C: Was that the only time you had a seizure?

P: I think I had another before when I got up and started walking. Like someone with Parkinson's.

C: Were you aware of what was happening at that time?

P: Yes. I could feel myself.

C: What brought you out of it? How did it stop?

P: I sat down and I laid down and relaxed myself. Kind of meditated and brought myself down slowly. And I grabbed a beer.

C: Did you feel better after that?

P: Yes.

C: Had you not had a beer for a while before that? How long had it been?

P: Maybe 2 days, day and a half. I was visiting somewhere, some elderly sick person. Wanted to be respectful and I went without it.

C: Thank you so much for spending the time today with the interview.

Video #13 Ratings

ALC1. Tolerance	***Score***
Did you use a lot more alcohol than you previously used to get the same effect (compared when you first started to drink)? ***Did you notice that the same amount of alcohol you take now has less effect than before (compared when you first started to drink)?*** 0 Patient had no tolerance to alcohol. 1 Patient had tolerance to alcohol. . Not sure *or* not applicable *or* missing.	*1*
ALC2. Withdrawal	

When you stopped or cut down on alcohol use, did you have withdrawal symptoms? (interviewer gives examples of alcohol withdrawal symptoms) 0 Patient had no withdrawal symptoms from alcohol. 1 Patient had withdrawal symptoms from alcohol. . Not sure *or* not applicable *or* missing.	*1*
ALC3. Failure to fulfill major obligations	
Did alcohol use result in failure to fulfill major role obligations (work, school, or home)? 0 Alcohol had no effect on work, school, or social obligations. 1 Alcohol had negative effect on work, school, or social obligations. . Not sure *or* not applicable *or* missing.	*1*
ALC4. Social, interpersonal problems due to alcohol	
Did alcohol cause any social or interpersonal problems (e.g., work problems, school problems, relationship problems, family problems, legal problems, physical fights)? 0 Alcohol caused no social or interpersonal problems. 1 Alcohol caused social or interpersonal problems. . Not sure *or* not applicable *or* missing.	*1*
ALC5. Alcohol use in spite of problems	
Did you continue to use alcohol even though you had problems? 0 Patient had no alcohol problems. 1 Patient continued to use alcohol even though alcohol caused problems. . Not sure *or* not applicable *or* missing.	*1*
ALC6. Alcohol use in hazardous situations	
Did you use alcohol in a situation, in which it was physically hazardous (e.g., driving a car or operating machinery)? 0 Patient did not use alcohol in hazardous situations. 1 Patient used alcohol in hazardous situations. . Not sure *or* not applicable *or* missing.	*Missing*

ALC7. Alcohol blackout	
Did you have a blackout after drinking so much alcohol that the next day you could not remember what you said or did? 0 Patient had no blackout. 1 Patient had blackout. . Not sure *or* not applicable *or* missing.	*Missing*
ALC8. Other alcohol problems	
Did you have any other problems due to alcohol use? 0 No. 1 Yes (specify). . Not sure *or* not applicable *or* missing.	*1*
Alcohol use score = 6 (severe)	

Video # 14: Extra Practice 2

Identification: Patient is a 33-year-old White male who has been engaged for 3 months. Patient is divorced and has two sons, 9 and 11 years old. Patient finished high school and works. Patient moved from Oklahoma to WV 4.5 months ago.

Chief complaints: Mood swings, anger, and no medications.

History of present illness: Patient has experienced mood swings for most of his life and was diagnosed with bipolar disorder at age 15. Patient has only participated in outpatient treatment and took lithium for about 4 years. He reported that he responded well to these interventions. Patient's psychiatrist passed away and the patient did not take lithium for the past 3.5–4 years. Patient moved from Oklahoma to WV about 4 months ago. Patient has had mixed mood swings (same-day mood changes) and depressive symptoms for the past couple years, during which he was not taking lithium. Three weeks ago, the patient had suicidal ideation and held a knife to his chest, but he did not actively attempt suicide. The fiancé took the patient to UHC hospital and he was released. Patient continued to have racing thoughts and was taken to UHC 2 days ago and he was released again. Patient went home, had suicidal thoughts, and planned to overdose. Patient was admitted to Chestnut Ridge Center yesterday.

Review of psychiatric symptoms was positive for anxiety, panic, agoraphobia, PTSD, depression, suicidality, irritability, and mixed mood swings. Generalized anxiety, agoraphobia, and specific phobia are present, but not to a significant degree as they do not interfere with overall functioning. Review of psychiatric symptoms was negative for conduct disorder, gambling, social phobia, OCD, delusions, hallucinations, violence, or disorganized thoughts.

Initial diagnosis: Bipolar disorder, unspecified.
Anxiety disorder, unspecified.

Transcription of Interview #14 (C = Clinician; P = Patient)

C: Tell me where you're from?
P: Clarksburg.
C: How old are you?
P: 33.
C: From Clarksburg originally?
P: No, I'm from Oklahoma.
C: How long have you been in Clarksburg?
P: 4.5 months.
C: Okay, so relatively new to the area.
P: Yeah, just getting used to learning where all the main places are.

C: *Alright, well I know you've probably talked to some of the folks in our treatment unit but if you'd let me know just a brief background of what's been going on and what brought you to the hospital.*

P: *I was diagnosed with bipolar quite a few years back. I quit taking my meds because the doctor I was seeing is what we call an "old-school doctor" and he had a private practice, but he passed away. I hadn't found another doctor to go back to until I came out here. And that's been 3.5–4 years. Just recently I've been telling my fiancé that I've been feeling like I need help with getting back on my meds. My mood swings, being able to control my anger…*

C: *So you've had some anger and some mood swings and irritability. Can you tell me a little bit more about that, what types of things have been happening?*

P: *I get aggravated over the simplest little things. She, my fiancé, and numerous other people tell me that I have an attitude that I don't realize I have, and it makes them not want to be anywhere close to me. They want to separate and have distance from me.*

C: *How long have you been engaged?*

P: *Going on 3 months now.*

C: *Okay. And how long have you been with your fiancé?*

P: *We started out talking online and then we called each other, and it's been about 3 years that we've been talking online.*

C: *And you've been engaged for just 3 months?*

P: *Right.*

C: *For the duration she's known you she's noticed this irritability?*

P: *Yes.*

C: *And you've noticed it as well?*

P: *Yes.*

C: *Okay. So there's mood swings, do you damage or break things at home?*

P: *No. I walk off before I get to that point or I listen to music.*

C: *So you do things to help. Okay. Now, does this stuff last for long durations or does it come and go through the day?*

P: *Sometimes it'll last 15–20 minutes, then it'll go away, then a couple hours later, it comes back. Sometimes it's worse than others.*

C: *Do you feel like the medication you were taking was helpful for you? What was that medication?*

P: *It was lithium.*

C: *How long have you been off of it for?*

P: *3.5–4 years.*

C: *Okay. How long did you take it previously?*

P: *About 3, almost 4 years.*

C: *When did you first start having these spells?*

P: *When I was 15.*

C: *It was mood swings back then?*

P: *Oh yeah, when I was playing high school football, they'd know when I was aggravated. I'd go after the other team pretty bad.*

C: *Did you get into trouble back then a lot?*

P: No.

C: Did you start fires or hit someone?

P: No. I hit somebody when they deserved it.

C: Okay, so when something prompted it. Any history of legal problems?

P: No.

C: Since age 15 until your most recent treatment, have there been periods where you've been not just irritable, but sort of revved up?

P: It's hard to explain. Um. I've had the irritable spells that have gone further down, almost suicidal. I've had suicidal tendencies. I've wanted to hurt myself a couple times.

C: Have you ever followed through with that?

P: I was close about 2–3 weeks ago. Had a real bad spell. Held a knife against my chest in the kitchen until my fiancé said something that made me laugh, say it ain't worth it, and put the knife back.

C: And that's the closest you've ever been to hurting yourself?

P: Yes, and 2 days prior, matter of fact the same day they brought me up here, I went to UHC down there and they released me to go back home. A few hours after that I had a real bad spell. I was real upset, had racing thoughts. Fiancé called the summit center crisis line and they moved me back up to UHC, back up there.

C: Do you have outpatient care with Summit Center right now?

P: I've started to. They said they wouldn't be able to get me in until October 20th. It wouldn't have helped.

C: So just to be clear, you had your provider, he was retiring…

P: He passed away.

C: Passed away, sorry. And you subsequently moved here to West Virginia, and they have plugged you in for outpatient care; then things got worse, then about 2 weeks ago.

P: The deal with UHC was the day before yesterday.

C: And that just happened again then.

P: Yes. Twice in the same day I was up there. That's when they sent me home and I got upset and it kind of snowballed from there. Had a real bad spell. I made the comment to my fiancé that I was going to take my bottle of pills and down that with alcohol. And the crisis center then shipped me up here. I've been here since Monday.

C: Okay, so just a couple days here at the hospital. Do you have any firearms in your home?

P: No.

C: Does your fiancé help with your medications and things like that?

P: We just got started on it. I took one pill before I came up here and it just, everything, my anxiety and depression, just snowballed and went downhill.

C: That's the first time you've mentioned feeling depressed. Now, have you felt depressed?

P: Yes, I've felt depressed for the last couple years.

C: Has there been relief from the depression over that time?

P: No.

C: So you've had persistent depression and depressed mood.

P: Bad attitude, yes. The mood swings that I don't realize I get. People shy away from me because they're afraid if they say something wrong I'll yell at them or scream.

C: How's your sleep?

P: It hasn't been real good for the last 3 weeks. I'm lucky to get 3 hours at most.

C: And during these times when you're not sleeping, I assume they've happened before?

P: Yes.

C: And during that time, you want to sleep?

P: Yes.

C: So you don't feel like when you're not sleeping, you're getting work done or being creative.

P: Since I've been up here, I've done to help bide my time with my anxiety and stuff I've been doing a lot of drawing.

C: What do you like to draw?

P: Anything that comes to mind. I've been working on a brick wall.

C: And that's helping you?

P: Yes. Helping keep me from getting depressed and stuff.

C: Let's talk a bit about your depression. Do you have hobbies and things you like to do?

P: I like riding my four-wheeler.

C: Have you been able to do that lately?

P: No, I haven't been able to get my four-wheeler out for a while.

C: How about spending time with your fiancé? Do you still enjoy that?

P: Yes. Me, her, and her daughter, we go out to Tygart Lake and go swimming. I do enjoy that.

C: Do you have crying spells frequently?

P: Not very often. The other day when I told my fiancé what I was planning on doing, when I had racing thoughts, I did cry.

C: Do you feel guilty about things?

P: No, not all the time. I had something happen to me when I was younger. I've held it in for numerous years and I've always believed it was my fault.

C: This was a traumatic experience for you?

P: Yes. It happened to me and three of my best friends. The person that did it, they gave him 80 years in prison. I normally check on the website for his parole hearings. I saw he had a discharge date a few days prior to me calling. I called and they said no he's not discharged, he passed away. It took a bit off my chest but I've never been able to do a whole lot of talking about it.

C: So you've never been allowed to sort of process it with a therapist or anyone.

P: Yes. I've told my fiancé about it and she said it's not your fault.

C: Okay. We don't necessarily get into the nature of the trauma at this point, but there are some questions that are very important with that. Do you have a lot of nightmares about what happened?

P: No, I had one since I've been out here, 2 days after I found out about that. It scared me and woke my fiancé up.

C: So that's not something that happens frequently. Do you ever feel like you're back experiencing that trauma?

P: The last time when I had that dream, yes.

C: But no flashbacks?

P: No. That's one thing I try to block it, but it sits on my mind.

C: It sounds like this is a safe place for you to discuss that and you have some therapists upstairs that you're going to be working with. Let's talk a bit more about some of your symptoms. I'll go through a couple things. For the most part, these are questions about things that tend to cause problems in your everyday life. Do you have rituals that you do?

P: No.

C: Any intrusive thoughts or feelings that your hands are dirty?

P: No.

C: And do you have any problems with really having specific things you're afraid of?

P: It might sound funny but I'm deadly afraid of clowns.

C: I think that's pretty common.

P: That and being in enclosed areas. Not claustrophobic, it's just being trapped in a spot.

C: Do any of those fears interfere with your daily routine or life?

P: No.

C: How about being in social situations or in public?

P: Sometimes when my anxiety is really bad, when there are a whole bunch of people crowding around me, I feel like everything is closing in. It just makes me want to hide.

C: If you need to go to the store, would you go at a quieter time or avoid going?

P: If I'm having a bad spell, I'll try to find one that's not busy and just do what I have to do to get in and get out.

C: Do you have a fear of eating in public?

P: No.

C: Any history of hallucinations?

P: No.

C: Do you ever feel like people are causing specific trouble just for you?

P: When I was younger, people that knew my past, stuff that had happened, they'd torture me with it and hold it over my head. It bugged me for a while, but it finally got to the point where I just gave up on trying to reason with them and just ignored them.

C: Any history of feeling paranoid into your adult life?

P: No.

C: Do you feel like the TV, radio, or newspaper have messages specifically for you?

P: No.

C: And no history of any situations like that?

P: No.

C: Any history of, you've described anxiety, can you tell me a little more about that piece?

P: I've had that ever since I was little.

C: In general, let's say like in the last couple months, do you feel anxious in general every day?

P: Seems to come and go every couple of days. When it goes away, I feel like I'm ready to venture out and stuff doesn't bother me. When it comes back, it's real quick and I don't want to be around a lot of people.

C: Do you worry about lots of things at one time?

P: I was afraid that I wasn't going to be getting help until October, and my fiancé and I were arguing about it, saying that if I didn't get help that we were going to be going our separate ways. And I told her when I called her yesterday that I was getting help.

C: How about when you have spells of getting anxious and it gets real bad, is it within 5–10 minutes?

P: Oh yeah.

C: And do you have any chest pain with that?

P: It feels like everything is pressed against my chest.

C: Short of breath? Sweaty?

P: Yes. It's almost like having an asthma attack.

C: Do you worry about having another one of those spells?

P: Not now, not since I'm in a safe place.

C: At home, would you spend time worrying about having another spell?

P: No. Once I've had it, it drains the energy out of me.

C: Does it happen a couple times a week, a couple times a day?

P: My last big one was a month and a half ago. I try to avoid situations that lead up to that.

C: How has your memory and concentration been?

P: Alright. I just try to avoid a lot of things that happened back when it was worse. There're things I try to block out.

C: Do you use substances at all?

P: No.

C: Any past substances?

P: No.

C: Any alcohol? Tobacco?

P: No.

C: Any medical problems?

P: Besides being bipolar? Nothing.

C: Before you came to the hospital were you taking any medications?

P: No.

C: And have they since put you on new medicine?

P: I'm back on lithium. They started me with a higher dose. They also prescribed Trazadone for sleep.

C: Is it helping you sleep?

P: I haven't taken it yet today.

C: So you're still having sleep problems here.

P: Yes. I was up until 4:00 this morning.

C: Are you allergic to any medicines?

P: No.

C: Normally I ask about a lot of different medical things. I'll just ask a few. You were a high school football player, any bad head injuries?

P: No, just have a scar where my helmet came off.

C: Were you ever concussed or lost consciousness?

P: No. It aggravated me.

C: No seizures or major surgeries?

P: No. I went through a barbed wire fence once and had stitches.

C: How old were you then?

P: 19.

C: Anything run in your family of importance?

P: No.

C: Any family history of depression?

P: No.

C: So you've told us a little bit about yourself. You have known your fiancé of about 3 years. Any previous marriages or relationships?

P: I was married prior but my ex-wife is hard-headed.

C: Any children?

P: Two boys, 9 and 11.

C: Do you still keep contact with them?

P: Yes. Every couple of days when I'm at home.

C: Are you working?

P: Yes. The golf course in Bridgeport—maintenance crew.

C: How far did you go in school?

P: I graduated.

C: Any college or vocational training?

P: No.

C: Do you have any spiritual involvements right now?

P: No.

C: I assume your fiancé is your main source of support. Any other sources of support?

P: My mom and stepdad in Oklahoma. I call them if something is bothering me when my fiancé is at work. She drives an ambulance for a living and I can't constantly call her.

C: You guys are both pretty busy it sounds like.

P: Yes. I go to work at 5 in the morning until 2 PM. She goes from 6 until whenever they decide to let her off work.

C: Any siblings?

P: I've got one stepbrother.

C: Do you get along okay?

P: No. We clash.

C: Typically I'd ask you more questions about your mood memory and concentration, but in the interest of time, I'm just going to ask you some brief questions. How about as far as your mood, on a scale of 1–10, where 10 is the best day ever, where would we be today?

P: I'd say a 4.5.

C: So that's pretty low.

P: Yes. My anxiety is not helping. It's making everything feel balled up.

C: So you'd describe your mood as anxious today.

P: Extremely.

C: And you're feeling down because you're anxious. And as you said being around the cameras and light and microphone haven't helped that.

P: Yes.

C: Just to clarify a couple things. You told me you were diagnosed with bipolar at what age?

P: 15.

C: Were you ever hospitalized?

P: No.

C: So you basically saw your physician as an outpatient previously and felt you did good with the lithium. No family history of bipolar?

P: No.

C: So now just a bit more detail. What does bipolar mean to you?

P: Up and down mood swings. Anger control.

C: And those mood swings can happen within the day.

P: Yes.

C: You might feel happy right now but in 10 minutes get angry.

P: I'd say more like a few hours.

C: So, you can stay in a bad mood for a while, but then it can switch.

P: Yes.

C: And you've had extended periods of time with no sleep but you missed the sleep.

P: Yes.

C: You mentioned racing thoughts. Tell me more about that.

P: I couldn't grasp what was going on, everything was going too fast. I couldn't concentrate on it. It made everything ten times worse.

C: With the irritability, have you had persistent irritability for more than a week?

P: Yes. my fiancé would agree.

C: And relief from irritability has been hard lately. You definitely saw relief from that with the lithium before though right?

P: Yes.

C: And you don't have any history of getting in fights, what about driving fast?

P: If I'm aggravated on the road, I'll stop and get out to walk before it gets any worse.

C: How about when you were younger. Would you have more sexual urges or risky behaviors?

P: No. I'd ride my four-wheeler.

C: You wouldn't be super risky?

P: No.

C: No smoking or alcohol?
P: No.
C: What about gambling?
P: Not unless you consider playing video games.
C: Okay, so no betting involved. Do you have any goals to clarify?
P: Just get help and get meds and get my anger under control.
C: You feel like you have a safe environment to work in?
P: Yes. Thank you.

Video #14 Ratings of Panic and Mood Symptoms

(Positive Symptoms Only)

PAN1. Panic attacks (without phobias)	***Score***
Have you gotten suddenly anxious and frightened for a short period of time (up to 60 minutes)? ***During that time, did you feel that your heart was racing or pounding, or did you start shaking or sweating, or did you feel you were choking?*** 0 Patient had no panic attacks. 1 Patient had panic attacks. . Not sure or not applicable or missing.	*1*
PAN3. Worry about having another panic attack	
After a panic attack, did you worry about having another attack? ***Did you worry about its effects* (e.g., *losing control, having a heart attack, or going crazy)?*** 0 After a panic attack, patient did not worry about having another one. 1 After a panic attack, patient worried about having another one or its effects. . Not sure *or* not applicable *or* missing.	*0*
PAN4. Action to end or prevent panic attacks	
Did you have to do something to end the attack, like leaving a store, calling someone, or taking deep breaths? ***Do you do anything to prevent the attacks (like avoiding places that trigger the panic attacks)?*** 0 After a panic attack, patient does nothing to end or prevent another panic attack. 1 After a panic attack, patient does something to end or prevent another panic attack. . Not sure *or* not applicable *or* missing.	*1*

PAN5. Autonomic symptoms with panic attacks	*3*
(enter the number of the positive symptoms) **1 Patient cannot catch breath and has feeling of being smothered.** **2 Patient has chest pain or discomfort.** 3 Patient has feeling of choking. 4 Patient feels heart is pounding, missing beats, or beating faster. 5 Patient feels dizzy, unsteady, light-headed, or faint. 6 Patient has numbness or tingling sensations in face or fingers. 7 Patient has dry mouth or difficulty swallowing. 8 Patient has nausea or abdominal distress. 9 Patient has trembling or shaking of hands or limbs. **10 Patient has sweating, e.g., palms.** 11 Patient feels very cold. 12 Patient has hot flushes. 13 Patient has fear of dying. 14 Patient has fear of going crazy, or fear of losing emotional control. 15 Patient feels that things are not real. 16 Patient feels that people are not real.	

D1. Depressed mood	***Score***
Have you been feeling sad, depressed, or in low spirits? 0 Patient has no depressed mood. 1 Patient has depressed mood less than half the time. 2 Patient has depressed mood more than half the time. . Not sure *or* not applicable *or* missing.	*1*
D7. Excessive guilt	
Have you felt guilty or ashamed of yourself for something you have done or thought? 0 Patient has no feeling of guilt. 1 Patient feels guilty less than half the time. 2 Patient feels guilty more than half the time. . Not sure *or* not applicable *or* missing.	*1*
D8. Other depressive symptoms	
0 Absent. 1 Present (crying spells). . Not sure *or* not applicable *or* missing.	*1*
D9. Suicidal ideation during the past month	
Have you had thoughts about harming or killing yourself? 0 Patient had no suicidal ideation. 1 Patient had suicidal ideation. . Not sure *or* not applicable *or* missing.	*1*
D11. Suicidal plans during the past month	
Have you had specific suicidal plans? 0 Patient had no suicidal plans. 1 Patient had suicidal plans. . Not sure *or* not applicable *or* missing.	*1*
Depression score = 5 (moderate)	

M2. Irritable mood	***Score***
Have you sometimes felt that you were easily irritated without reason? ***Have you found yourself so irritable that you shout at people or start arguments or actually become aggressive?*** 0 Patient has no irritable mood. 1 Patient has irritable mood less than half the time. 2 Patient has irritable mood more than half the time. . Not sure *or* not applicable *or* missing.	*1*
M3. Mixed mood (mood lability)	
Have you had mixed mood swings: periods of <u>depression and elation or irritability on the same day?</u> 0 Patient has no mixed mood swings. 1 Patient has mixed mood less than half the time. 2 Patient has mixed mood more than half the time. . Not sure *or* not applicable *or* missing.	2
M4. Racing thoughts (observed as flight of ideas)	
Have you felt that you had too many different thoughts racing through your mind compared with normal? 0 Patient has no racing thoughts. 1 Patient has racing thoughts less than half the time. 2 Patient has racing thoughts more than half the time. . Not sure *or* not applicable *or* missing.	*1*
M10. Decreased sleep	
Have you needed less sleep than usual and without getting tired? 0 Patient has normal sleep. 1 Patient sleeps 4 hours or less (in a 24-hour period including naps) and feels rested. . Not sure *or* not applicable *or* missing.	*1*
Manic score = 5 (moderate)	

Video # 15: Extra Practice 3

Transcription of Interview #15 (C = Clinician; P = Patient)

C: Thank you for being here with us and thank you for signing the consent forms. My name is Sarah. Essentially we just want to start from the beginning so if you could just tell me a bit about your story and what brought you here.

P: So I've been struggling with depressive and suicidal thoughts for a while now, I'd say about 2 years. Previously I'd struggled with disordered eating. Over the years things have accumulated and escalated to the point where the therapist I was meeting with just had a really strong goal of just keeping me safe and encouraged me to be admitted and that's how I got to where I am today.

C: So what had been happening just in the few weeks before when you were admitted?

P: It was a combination of sleepless nights and excessive sleep, being overwhelmed emotionally, losing my sense of time, losing my ability to remember things or to even learn new things. Things I had known for a while, I just forgot. I wasn't functioning well cognitively, so yeah.

C: *Was there a certain breaking point where something happened that made you feel like this is the day that I feel like I need to come and get help.*

P: *I was really hesitant myself. Even if it was really bad objectively, I myself would probably think that it's fine, I can manage it myself. What happened was on my third night of not being able to sleep, my suicidal thoughts just escalated, right to the point of writing a detailed plan of everything I need to get done. That frightened me as well, I think that was my red flag to say this is out of my control now.*

C: *Did you come here by yourself or did someone take you?*

P: *I had a friend take me to their therapist the same day I was admitted. When I was thinking clear at one point, I said just bring me because I may just pull back and not show up.*

C: *You said there were several days of sleepless nights. Had anything been going on personally or professionally, or have you always struggled with sleep?*

P: *I've always struggled, but not to the point where I'm up and emotionally overwhelmed.*

C: *Any other acute life stresses?*

P: *I've been told coming to graduate school and moving to a new country is a major stressor. I think they're there, but mentally it's hard for me to not downplay them.*

C: *You brought up graduate school and a big move as well. Tell me a bit about yourself, where you come from and what brought you here to Morgantown.*

P: *Six years ago, I moved to the States by myself. I came here for college, came from an underprivileged home, and managed to get a good scholarship. The experience was shortened though because I was so eager to save a year of tuition. So a few months later, I graduated from college and enrolled in graduate school here. It seemed natural for me to dive into the sciences. I always liked science and I didn't really think of anything else. Being in Morgantown at WVU, I had done an internship here, so it was a natural fit for me to come here after college.*

C: *So when did you start to feel, I know you mentioned it was within the last few weeks, but before then, when did you start to feel there was something shifting in you as far as a difference in your mood?*

P: *Knowing the things I know today and having worked with a therapist, I think there was a great shift as soon as I came to college. I realize it's not normal for a college student to wake up hyperventilating, to experience significant heart palpitations and chest tightening. I assumed it was just caffeine or lack of sleep, but I think it was something greater. Struggling with binge eating was also another big indication for me.*

C: *Was that in college as well?*

P: *That started in college.*

C: *And you started college 6 years ago when you moved?*

P: *Yes. I moved from Malaysia.*

C: *How would you describe that transition coming here?*

P: It is probably something I didn't think too much about because I had two other sisters who came to the States for college. It seemed like the right thing to do for us.

C: How soon after did you find yourself feeling down and depressed?

P: That requires me to be able to look and know myself. I am one to suppress emotions so I don't think I can accurately answer that.

C: How many days per week do you find yourself feeling down, depressed, or hopeless?

P: As of most recently, almost every day.

C: Do you find that you're sleeping more, less, or both?

P: I go through phases of not sleeping at all to sleeping a lot, which may be a vicious cycle.

C: As far as your interests, what are you interested in or things that you do in your free time?

P: I don't remember ever having a hobby. I remember struggling to find one because nothing seems worthwhile.

C: Anything that gives you pleasure, like spending time with people, friends, family, pets? Going out?

P: I know what I don't like, and I guess finding things I do like is harder. Mostly stay isolated, and indoors. It seems like that's already a formula for trouble. I think that one thing I have to work on is to find something that actually brings me pleasure.

C: As far as your schoolwork, did you ever find yourself struggling to keep up or stay interested? I know you mentioned you're in a grad program now, which can be difficult. Do you find that your interest in your schoolwork has changed?

P: Absolutely. I think during my first year, even though I was going through something mentally, I wasn't at my optimal state, I was just so eager that now I look back and think I should have saved some of that energy for now because I have none of that. I lose interest. I think I've lost almost all my interest at this point, but that's not because it's school or research, it's because of me.

C: Okay. Is there anything you wake up in the morning and look forward to?

P: I don't know. I think I'd rather not wake up.

C: Any feelings of worthlessness in general?

P: Absolutely. That is pretty much how I define my life.

C: Any changes or fluctuations in your weight?

P: Because of my disordered eating, I avoid weighing myself. I do know that I've gained since I first started around 6 years ago.

C: Does that bother you?

P: It does. I think the voice is softer and quieter than it was, perhaps 3 or 4 years ago, but it's those things a little bit.

C: How about your ability to concentrate on things?

P: Practically nonexistent.

C: How long ago did you notice that starting?

P: I assumed it was just because I was active mentally, that I can't stay focused on one thing. I remember growing up and many people telling me that I just get bored easily. I thought it was part of my nature since childhood.

C: Any family history of ADHD or concerns that you might have ADHD?

P: No, nothing really.

C: Do you ever find yourself feeling guilty about anything?

P: Almost everything. I think I say "I'm sorry" more often than people are comfortable with, but I wish they knew it was actually genuine for me.

C: Yeah. What about your energy levels?

P: Low. I would sleep, but I don't think I feel recharged.

C: Do you ever find yourself waking up feeling tired?

P: Between feeling tired and like a train wreck.

C: Do you feel like you're ever moving slower or at a slower pace? Has anyone else ever told you that?

P: I don't think anyone has ever told me that. I do feel like on a really bad day, I feel like I'm in slow motion. It takes me a lot longer to formulate my thoughts and to decide what I want to do. Simple things like brush my teeth, what do I wear, those become tiring.

C: Tell me about the natural progression of things for the last 6 years. When did you first start feeling like something was getting worse to the point where you had a plan? It's okay if you can't think of an answer.

P: When it hurts and I don't know why. For a while there I couldn't pinpoint a trigger, and then I couldn't explain things to myself. That's when I realized it's above me and it's bad. I think it hit the strongest when my therapist blatantly said "It has gotten this bad." And I replay that line in my head a lot, I'm glad she told me that because my number one question at the time was "how did it get this bad" and "why did it get this bad?" It was just helpful when she said that.

C: How long ago was that?

P: The Friday before I was admitted. It was also the day she had told me to get admitted, but I had negotiated to just pass the weekend to sort things out and think. So I arrived in the ED on Monday.

C: You mentioned earlier that you had started to have suicidal ideation and then developed a plan. What do you think brought you to that point? How long had you been having the ideation for? Was it fairly recent or do you feel like it had been there for a while?

P: The first time I can remember it coming to me was 2 years ago during the summer. I couldn't sleep for nights and I was so tired that I wanted it all to be over. I really wished that when I went to bed that I wouldn't wake up the next day. Rather than playing the guessing game, I just wanted to be sure that I wouldn't wake up.

C: I see. Had you had a plan at that point?

P: I had considered many possibilities but nowhere as detailed as more recently when I considered overdosing or cutting.

C: Have you ever cut before in the past?

P: No. I actually had not made any attempts yet.

C: Any past psychiatric history? How long ago did you start seeing a therapist?

P: I had one in college, just a counselor. I thought I was under stress, simple college stress. I took about a year break because I came to graduate school and I felt pretty okay, and then that first episode hit with the suicidal thoughts and that's when I saw a counselor.

C: So that was this past year?

P: That was 2019.

C: So what year of grad school are you in?

P: I'll be in my fourth year.

C: So you're almost done?

P: I probably could have finished in another year, but because of this and not performing at 100%, I think there will be some pushback.

C: So about 2 years ago, felt like you needed some extra help with stress and sought out a counselor. Ever had any previous hospitalizations like this?

P: No.

C: Ever had feelings this strong before that you felt like you had a plan?

P: No. Even to the extent of family history, I don't know.

C: Would you say most of your symptoms fit with depression? Has anyone ever talked to you about anxiety? Do you feel anxious at all?

P: I think I experience the kind of anxiety where my thoughts are obsessive. But mostly what I can remember are symptoms of depression.

C: Ever any panic attacks?

P: I haven't learned how to identify one myself.

C: So typically we tell people that if you've ever had a sharp quick sensation, like a feeling in your chest, some people describe it as a similar sensation to a heart attack. A lot of people even present to the ER thinking they're having a heart attack, when in fact they're having a panic attack. Some people say they can't catch their breath or their heart is beating fast. It's a full-body reaction to that strong emotion. Ever had anything like that?

P: I think I've come close to one but I don't know if those would qualify as a panic attack.

C: When was that?

P: Most recently during a session with my therapist when she told me to label things, that I was struggling with anxiety, and that in itself triggered a reaction in me. We had to put the session on hold and get me going on diaphragmatic breathing again because it really hurt in my chest, I was struggling to breathe and couldn't hear anything. It was like I was sucked into my own mind. She thought that might be a panic attack, but thankfully she was there.

C: It does sound like a panic attack. And that was the first time you had ever experienced anything like that?

P: She had asked if that was the first time but to me that's usually what I go through when I'm overwhelmed with emotions and can't sleep. That sort of experience.

C: Do you find yourself frequently worried about things?

P: I'm a worrier.

C: What do you worry about?

P: Anything and everything. Especially things that are beyond my control or that are uncertain.

C: Do you have racing thoughts?

P: I spiral very easily. Unfortunately it usually ends up in a dark place.

C. Do you ever find yourself having several days where you can't get any sleep and have any sort of unexplainable behaviors? Tell me a little more about what happens on those days when you can't sleep.

P: Music is my companion when I'm too tired to do anything else.

C: Does your energy feel higher or lower?

P: Lower. It's not so much like a surplus of energy, it's not a manic episode.

C: Do you stay in bed all day?

P: I've had days where I just miss work, sometimes I get up and make it to brushing my teeth because it's a big step if I actually leave the apartment.

C: Do you ever feel like you have a weight on your shoulders?

P: There's an absolute burden.

C: What's the longest period of days that you've stayed awake for?

P: I don't remember. Let's just say for the three nights most recently before I came in.

C: When you're having days where you're staying up, do you ever have increased shopping sprees, gambling, or sexual behavior?

P: No. I don't take part in any risky behaviors during those episodes. I sort of shut everything down to do anything. I feel like a meat bag.

C: What does that mean to you?

P: Everything that my body needs to do autonomously, it does. Anything I need to do voluntarily, I can't.

C: Have you ever had any traumatic experiences?

P: No. I can't think of any and I've been trying to think.

C: Any nightmares?

P: No.

C: Ever find yourself having flashbacks to any major events in your life?

C: No.

C: Do you ever find yourself seeing things that aren't there?

P: Probably close to when I was being admitted. I thought it was just me being weird that day. I was working in a room in the lab, and I thought I saw the lights come on in a neighboring room and thought I felt the ground shake. That was the only time it happened.

C: Did you see or hear any voices?

P: No.

C: Have you ever felt so strongly about a certain, whether it be event or something that happened that felt real to you but someone else could not explain it? We call them delusions.

P: I don't think so.

C: We talked a bit about disordered eating and you mentioned that started in college. How did that start for you?

P: Choosing to skip meals was the easiest one to do. I was so busy and it was easy to stay occupied. That cycled with eating large quantities, whether something happy or sad happened that was a thing I went to, was food. It was also a huge part of my social life. Anytime you wanted to celebrate or talk about something, it would be centered around food. Over time I started being shameful of eating in front of others. I was particular about who I ate with, what I ate, where I ate. I started looking if others ate as much as I did. They would proceed to dessert and if they didn't I felt like I couldn't, so I would eat in secret.

C: When you started skipping the meals, was there ever any thought process about your body image that influenced that choice?

P: Probably thought it was good for me. Probably thought my body could afford to skip a meal here and there. Probably also thought that I was compensating with my binges.

C: Ever had any issues in childhood or your teenage years with body image?

P: I had always been athletic when I was younger. I remember my sisters telling me that they envied my figure compared to theirs. It was never an issue for me. I couldn't care less and was enjoying whatever I did. I remember when my sisters came back from the States the first thing people said when they saw them was that they had gained weight. I remember older family friends coming up to them and pinching them in their arms, their cheeks, and seeing that happen right before I left for college. Maybe that's a traumatic event.

C: Did you feel like maybe they would do that to you if you had returned?

P: I was so ready to make sure that I went home in the exact same shape, if not better.

C: Do you feel like culturally any things from your culture have influenced anything related to your body image or maybe just your images of yourself?

P: I think so. Growing up in an Asian culture that very specifically defines what they consider as beauty, that felt like a high standard for me to try to uphold. It didn't seem like there was any leeway. Maybe not just in Asian cultures but anywhere, as soon as you say "weight gain," that cannot be a good thing.

C: Did you feel like coming here and being away from that home culture, how did you feel like that impacted you?

P: In some ways I was glad to be away and start fresh where no one knew me. In other ways I still missed being home even if it wasn't a good place for me to be in. This is not to say that the house that I was in was abusive, but just being in that form of thinking, that culture, wasn't healthy for me. It was still something I knew the most and it seemed weird to want to go back to that.

C: Do you have a big family?

P: Just two older sisters and my mom and dad.

C: While you were here in college, did you feel like it got to the point where you were eating a lot of food and feeling like you had to retch or vomit to bring it back up?

P: The thought passed my mind. I did purge for a while. For a summer, and it just really hurt so bad that it wasn't working for me.

C: How long ago was that?

P: Summer of 2017.

C: Since then, no purging?

P: No.

C: Are you still doing the restricting or the bingeing?

P: I work with a dietitian. I've been working with her since the start of this year, and it's been helpful to try to get out of that restrictive mindset, but these habits have been building for years, so I know it will take a while before it becomes more intuitive for me.

C: Who set you up with the dietitian?

P: I sought help myself. Initially before all of this unfolded, I thought the only thing I was battling was disordered eating, so I tried to look for a dietitian and it was her who referred me to the therapist that I'm working with today.

C: And that was about a year ago?

P: Yeah.

C: How were things during the pandemic, staying at home, has that influenced your emotions at all or difficulty with school?

P: I loved lockdown, but not in a way that was good for me. Pure isolation, not having to come up with excuses to why I didn't want to leave my apartment, whether it was for work or for pleasure, social hangouts. I could just stay in my own little bubble and be very happy.

C: How were things school wise?

P: I had at most one virtual class but most of what I was doing at that time was research, very much at my own pace. There were some things we couldn't do not being in lab, but I was at liberty to pace myself and decide how much I wanted to work each day.

C: Changing gears a bit, I know you mentioned you had never been previously hospitalized, but had you ever been on any kind of psychiatric medications?

P: No.

C: Are you currently on them now?

P: No, but today should be the first day that I take my first dose of Lexapro, 5 mg.

C: How do you feel about that?

P: I am pessimistic about anything working for me, but I'm in a "simplified stable environment," so I think this is a good time to try something new.

C: Any other past medical history outside of psychiatric problems?

P: No.

C: Healthy otherwise? No issues with blood sugar, blood glucose, cholesterol?

P: No.

C: Any family history?

P: Alcoholism runs on both sides of my family, as does hypertension. High cholesterol runs on my maternal side and breast cancer.

C: I'm sorry to hear that. Are your mother and father still present?

P: Yes.

C: Does your mother have the breast cancer?

P: Yes. Her and a great-aunt.

C: How are they doing?

P: My great-aunt passes, but my mom is in remission.

C: I'm happy to hear that about your mom, but I'm sorry about your great-aunt. Had your mom been undergoing treatments?

P: Yes, she's doing well.

C: Were you around for that?

P: I was when she was first diagnosed before I left for college.

C: That must have been tough.

P: Yeah.

C: Do you feel like that affected you emotionally, having your mom deal with a difficult medical condition while you were away?

P: I think it was overwhelming, but I quickly just reacted by not talking to them at all. I barely contacted them in college. It was easier for me to detach.

C: Had you had a close relationship growing up?

P: Yeah. I was the last one to leave the nest for college.

C: You mentioned two sisters and a brother?

P: Just the two sisters. I'm the youngest.

C: Do you feel like there was a reason you weren't calling home while in college? Did anything happen between you two?

P: It was weird. I just started thinking it was easier to not know much about home, to not communicate, because that would stir up feelings of homesickness. It was easier to be focused on finishing school and get my degree.

C: Your sisters, were they also here with you?

P: We all came for college at different times, so we were different stages. We were in different states, all scattered. Little did I know that was going to resemble us today because we are scattered further apart than ever.

C: Do you see each other or visit?

P: No. It's hard to work out because they're both working in different countries.

C: That can be tough. Would you say that you're close with your sisters?

P: No.

C: Are they healthy?

P: I think so. I don't think I've talked enough to them to know that answer.

C: Any past psychiatric family history that you're aware of?

P: My sister mentioned anxiety in college, but I don't know to what extent she got help.

C: Any previous suicides in the family?

P: Not that I know of.

C: I know we talked about how you ended up here, but did you spend your entire life in Malaysia.

P: Yes.

C: Did you move anywhere before college?

P: No.

C: Who are you living with here?

P: I live by myself.

C: Have you always lived by yourself?

P: Since graduate school. I had roommates in undergrad. I was a resident assistant, supposed to be well socialized.

C: Did you like your roommates?

P: Yeah. We had fun. I miss that dynamic but I don't think I could manage that today.

C: Did you like that having roommates gave you connection to other people?

P: I think that's maybe why I considered that maybe I should get a roommate now in grad school. But then I sort of, since I'm pessimistic by nature, looking at what I'm going through now, I'm not sure I'd be able to express myself. If I had roommates around it would perhaps my mode of coping would be to suppress even more.

C: When you're living at home, do you have any guns or weapons that you'd be concerned about here?

P: Just some over the counter pills and simple household items, but no guns.

C: Any pets?

P: No. I can barely take care of myself.

C: Any social relationships?

P: I spend most of my time alone.

C: Any close friends?

P: I think it's hard to answer that because I've moved so close friends from back home, we're not close anymore. Same for close friends from college. Friends that I work with now, I already view it as a transient friendship.

C: Do you ever hang out outside of the school environment?

P: Rarely. It's hard to bring myself to show up, even if I say yes, I'm likely to cancel.

C: Earlier you mentioned alcoholism in the family. Who has the alcoholism?

P: My paternal side, my uncles, and my maternal side as well.

C: Mom and dad?

P: No.

C: Any alcohol abuse for you?

P: I rarely drink.

C: Any drug use?

P: Never.

C: Ever smoked cigarettes?

P: No.

C: Any marijuana use?

P: No.

C: Stimulants at all?

P: I only take pain relievers.

C: Do you ever feel like you're using them very frequently?

P: It came to the point that I would wake up and just take Advil anyway before the headache could kick in.

C: You suffer from headaches? Always in the morning?

P: They can happen any time of day.

C: And usually just an Advil, does that help?

P: It helps for a while. Then I feel the need to take more.

C: Do you feel any other aches and pains in your body?

P: No.

C: As far as your adolescence and growing up, anything from your history that you feel has impacted you today?

P: I think when I think of my past, only pleasant memories come to mind. Then it just makes me grateful that I experienced those.

C: And when you came here, do you look at college as a positive experience as well?

P: Mostly a blur. Don't remember much from college. I remember short moments of fun, but mostly clouded by a blur.

C: The first few years of college, did you feel overwhelmed at first with getting acclimated?

P: I think it was whether or not I believed it myself. I remember my roommate telling me that I seemed very scared, very intimidated. Afraid to make connections.

C: Have you always felt more on the introverted side? Or is that a change from when you moved here?

P: I think that changed the most from when I turned 15. Growing up I was the extroverted one. I remember my sisters and mom telling me that I didn't want to leave school because I had so much fun and I would ask my mom to wait in the car because I wanted to play with friends for longer.

C: How do you see school now? Is it still fun?

P: I don't think I know fun right now.

C: Anything happen at 15 that felt like it changed for you?

P: The only reason I remember that was because I was in high school and I guess most people thought it was a phase because of puberty, but it started feeling more comfortable for me to stay secluded.

C: Did you struggle in school at all?

P: I was a typical overachiever.

C: Do you ever feel like you were "obsessive" at all about school?

P: Yeah. Even when I got an A, if it was under 100, I would get upset and wonder why I didn't get the last few points. If there was an extra credit question, I had to get above 100.

C: Where do you feel like that pressure came from?

P: I thought it was because I wanted to know everything I could learn. Thought that defined mastery for me to actually master it, not just know it. I thought that was taking the most out of every opportunity.

C: Did you ever have any external factors that made you feel like you had to be at a certain standard?

P: No. My parents never really cared for grades. I don't know if that's their response to us performing well. I felt I had to be a self-motivator. Perhaps I over compensated.

C: Did you ever feel like you had feelings compelling you to do certain behaviors? Like checking locks frequently?

P: No. I have my niche way of doing things in lab where my coworkers would let me know, but I don't think they were quite as you described.

C: Would you describe yourself as a perfectionist?

P: Yes.

C: And always? Schoolwork, otherwise?

P: More recently I started giving myself slack. I don't know if it's the "I don't care mentality" because I lost the ability to realize what the point is.

C: Ever anything you can recall of feeling like you had any sort of abuse?

P: No, we weren't super privileged, but all my basic needs were met and more. My emotional needs were met. At least I thought I had everything in my upbringing to succeed.

C: Coming out here, do you feel like you intentionally lost that support system and wanted to try things on your own?

P: Coming here I got obsessive with the idea of independence. I hate feeling like I owe somebody something. I also think it's easier to not depend on others. I don't think people intentionally try to upset others, but it's easier if I'm depending on myself.

C: Did you ever feel like you had to be there for your parents or feel pressure as far as your siblings?

P: The latest thing I remember feeling like I had to follow was finishing college a year early. I took 18–21 credits. It seemed so natural for them to do that, so first semester I said to my advisor "I'm doing this," and it said it seemed unlikely, and I still wanted to do it. Because I had chosen a science degree and my sisters hadn't, very quickly our paths diverged and I no longer felt like I had to live up to their standards.

C: Staying up and doing that work, did you find yourself relying on caffeine or anything?

P: No caffeine pills, but I started having a strong cup of coffee, green tea first in the morning. By the time it was 10 AM, I probably had four cups. It was all I would sip on. Then I graduated from college and quit cold turkey. It was the worst decision.

C: Did you find yourself more tired?

P: I had the summer to sleep which saved me. In graduate school I thought I might need coffee casually, but I was fearful that my obsessive mentality would take over and it would be easier to avoid as best I can. That was my way of protecting myself.

C: What made you want to stop drinking it?

P: I experienced heart palpitations and thought it was due to the caffeine. I finished college and thought why would I need it, so I quit.

C: As far as the concentration issues, did you notice difficulties remembering things in college?

P: Yes. If I didn't write it down, I wouldn't remember it. I double-check my planners. If I forgot to write it down, it wouldn't happen. I started writing on my hands.

C: When did you start writing things on your hands to remember them?

P: College. I would go and write on either side and could go past the wrist and write ridiculous notes on there. I always rationalized that it was something I could carry with me and never had to worry about losing a paper.

C: Did you lose things often?

P: No, it just seemed more natural to write on my hands.

C: Had you ever felt fidgety or difficulty staying still?

P: Yeah. Being so tired, staying still seems nice.

C: Any trouble maintaining attention on something? How long can you go reading a book?

P: Less than a minute. I hate reading.

C: What about something like watching TV?

P: I try streaming but just for background noise. I can't ever watch a show and sit down without my mind wandering.

C: Is that new?

P: It's always been me. Comes with getting bored easily.

C: You've never been screened for ADHD?

P: No. It became most apparent to my parents when I tried to learn the keyboard and would play whichever tempo I preferred to make the piece end faster. That became an issue because my teacher didn't like that very much. My parents took my off keyboard lessons then.

C: Do you find that the troubles with attention have affected your relationships? Ever have trouble listening to people?

P: Maybe not so much listening to people. In relationships, I fear commitment.

C: Why do you think that is?

P: People change. I don't even dare use the word "best friend" because best is a superlative and I don't think there's such a thing as "best friend."

C: Anyone that you can rely on to talk about your feelings with?

P: No. I think it's not that people aren't there; it's that I can't bring myself to share with them fully and be vulnerable, I guess.

C: Has therapy helped?

P: I think it's helped me learn more about myself. It's helped me to put labels on some things and identify what the issues are and what solutions are. It helps the scientific person within me to define things in my life.

C: I'm going to ask some questions. What day do you think it is?

P: The 11th of August 2021.

C: Who's the president?

P: Joe Biden.

C: Where are you right now?

P: Morgantown, WV.

C: What is 7 from 100?

P: 93.

C: Seven from that?

P: 86.

C: Can you spell "world" backwards?

P: DLROW.

C: Remember three words for me: dog, bird, acorn. Repeat those for me?

P: Dog, bird, acorn.

C: Just remember that for me. What does the phrase "you shouldn't throw rocks at glass houses" mean?

P: That's a phrase?

C: Or "all that glitters isn't gold."

P: Everything isn't as it seems.

C: Good. What does "don't cry over spilled milk" mean?

P: It's past the point of recovery.

C: What were those three words?
P: Dog, bird, acorn.
C: Is there anything else that's important for me to know?
P: No. I think everything has been covered.
C: What have they diagnosed you with since coming here?
P: Depression and anxiety.
C: Do you feel like that's a good fit?
P: I think a part of me cares about terms that are in my diagnosis and a part of me wants it all to be over. I sway back and forth.
C: That's fair. And you're starting the Lexapro today. I know you said you're. not optimistic, but are you hopeful that maybe it can help somewhat? Will you continue taking it after you leave?
P: Once I commit to something, it's a lot easier to help me see it through. Choosing the commitment is difficult. Thankfully I have a scientific background, so I remind myself that I trust the system. Probability wise, something should happen in my favor.
C: I will say I'm hopeful that trying a medication might help, and therapy as well. Do you have any questions for me?
P: No, I think that's all.
C: Thank you again.

Chapter 11
The Standard for Clinicians' Interview in Psychiatry (SCIP) as an Assessment Tool for Personalized Medicine in Psychiatry

The twenty-first century commenced with the emergence of measurement-based care (MBC) as the clinical standard of care (Chap. 6) and personalized medicine in psychiatry (PMP) as a new model for personalized treatment of mental disorders. Personalized medicine utilizes the patient's unique clinical, genetic, and environmental characteristics as the basis for treatment and prevention [1]. Personalized medicine in psychiatry (PMP) is the science of the systematic use of individual characteristics across four domains (biological factors, social and environmental factors, psychopathology assessment, and translational sciences (e.g., biomarkers, brain imaging, pharmacogenomics, endophenotypes, or any newly developed techniques of translational research)) to guide the clinician toward a person-centered diagnosis, a person-centered prognosis, and person-centered therapeutics (e.g., personalized selection and personalized dosing of medications), with the ultimate goal of improving the outcomes of the disease, and eventually the prevention of the disease.

Clinicians have known for centuries of the heterogeneous etiology and symptomatology of mental disorders [2]. Experienced clinicians "personalize" treatments by taking a large array of factors into account when assessing and treating patients, with the ultimate goal of providing care that completely accounts for individual variations in pathophysiological mechanisms [3]. For instance, we know today that childhood trauma increases the risk of many mental disorders, including psychosis, mood, anxiety, posttraumatic stress, and other disorders [4–7]; therefore, one can make a case that psychiatry is the most personalized branch of medicines. Yet, the progress of personalized medicine in psychiatry has been limited and is still in its early phases [8]. Other fields such as oncology and hematology have already implemented personalized medicine in clinical settings [9].

The current Diagnostic and Statistical Manual (DSM) and the International Classification of Diseases (ICD) describe all mental disorders based on polythetic-categorical concepts [10]. Polythetic is defined by multiple symptoms, and not all listed symptoms are necessary to establish a diagnosis. Categorical means that the

A. S. Aboraya, *Manual for the Standard for Clinicians' Interview in Psychiatry (SCIP)*, Advances in Mental Health and Addiction,
https://doi.org/10.1007/978-3-030-94930-3_11

diagnostic process results in a binary outcome: the patient either has the diagnosis or not. The polythetic model allows for different manifestations of the same disorder. For instance, when considering two patients diagnosed with a schizophrenia spectrum disorder, one patient may have paranoid delusions, tangentiality, and aggressive episodes, while the other patient may have auditory hallucinations, bizarre delusions, and a flat affect. Similarly, for two patients diagnosed with a major depressive episode, one may have depressed mood, weight loss, insomnia, psychomotor agitation, and suicidal thoughts, while the other might have anhedonia, fatigue, increased appetite, hypersomnia, and psychomotor retardation [1]. The phenomenological heterogeneity of each diagnosis as described in the DSM and ICD hampers progress in PMP.

A biological marker (biomarker) was defined by the Biomarkers Definitions Working Group as "a characteristic that is objectively measured and evaluated as an indicator of normal biological processes, pathogenic processes, or pharmacologic responses to a therapeutic intervention" [11]. There are three subcategories of biomarkers in psychiatry: molecular markers, genetic markers, and neuroimaging markers. Biomarkers are central to the notion of personalized medicine, yet no single biomarker has been found to be specific for any psychiatric illness [1]. In sum, the existing taxonomy systems of the DSM and ICD hamper the progress of biological markers, which subsequently impedes the progress of PMP.

The dissatisfaction of the DSM and ICD taxonomy led many investigators to call for a new classification of mental disorders based upon advances in neuroscience [12–17]. The National Research Council's report on precision medicine recommended the development of a new taxonomy to improve health care. "Many disease subtypes with distinct molecular causes are still classified as one disease and, conversely, multiple different diseases share a common molecular cause" [15]. In 2009, the National Institute of Mental Health (NIMH) proposed the Research Domain Criteria (RDoC) framework, which focuses on new ways to classify mental disorders based on empirical data from genetics, neuroscience, and dimensions of observable behavior [16, 17]. The RDoC model represents a radical shift in psychiatry and conceptualizes mental disorders as "disorders of brain circuits" [17].

A new taxonomy of mental disorders based on neuroscience advances will take decades to be developed and accepted by the scientific community and will have enormous clinical, legal, societal, and economic implications [18]. In the meantime, the 230 psychopathology items of the SCIP offer a practical alternative to the outdated taxonomy of the DSM and ICD. The following description illustrates the new proposed model of personalized medicine in psychiatry.

The ABCD Model for Personalized Medicine in Psychiatry

The ABCD proposed model for personalized medicine in psychiatry has four stages:

Stage A: Clinical start point (how the patient feels prior to contact with the clinician)

Stage B: Translational sciences
Stage C: Scientific methods to transform translational sciences into clinical outcomes
Stage D: Clinical outcomes

Table 11.1 shows examples of each stage.

Stage A: Clinical Start Point

Patients go to mental health professionals on their own volition, or they are brought by significant others because they suffer from symptoms that affect the quality of their lives and their ability to function, with the hope of symptom remission and improvement in their function. This is the starting point and the core of clinical sciences, including psychiatry. Instead of describing patients with diagnostic labels such as "schizophrenia spectrum" or "a major depressive episode," which do not serve or advance PMP, patients' initial clinical start points can be described by descriptive psychopathology codes (DPCs) and descriptive psychopathology maps (DPMs).

A descriptive psychopathology code (DPC) is a comprehensive psychological assessment (symptoms, signs, and dimensions) of an individual at one point in time using the SCIP 230 items. *A descriptive psychopathology map (DPM)* is two or more descriptive psychopathology codes (DPCs) for the same patient obtained over time, as rated by either the same or different clinicians.

Table 11.1 Stages of Personalized Medicine in a Psychiatry Model

Stage A	Stage B	Stage C	Stage D
Clinical start point	Translational sciences	Scientific methods to transform translational sciences into clinical outcomes	Clinical outcomes
Descriptive Psychopathology Code (DPC) and Descriptive Psychopathology Map (DPM).	Biomarkers (molecular, genetic, neuroimaging) Experimental psychopathology Pharmacogenomics Pharmacogenetics Neurocircuits Neurosciences Newly developed techniques in translational sciences	Research Domain Criteria (RDoC) framework Epistemic iteration (successive iterations) approach Newly developed scientific methods	Clinical endpoint (how patient feels after treatment) Diagnostics outcomes Efficacy outcomes Toxicity outcomes Prognosis Prevention Other outcomes

Table 11.2 shows the PMP codes of the 230 psychopathology items. The 30 screening items' codes range from PS1 to PS30. The 200 psychopathology items' codes start with item #1 panic attacks (P_A1), and the last item #200 is blurt-out answers (P_ADHD200). Out of the 200 psychopathology items, 48 items (24%) have 3 or more categories. Each PMP code has the same number in the measurement-based care (MBC) code, and both codes reflect the same psychopathology item. For example, item # 45 is a depressed mood item, the PMP code is P_DEP45, and the MBC code is 45_DEP. The main purpose of the PMP code is to translate the patient's clinical presentation into a personal code specific to the patient at the time of the evaluation. Psychiatric evaluations and progress notes can be transformed into DPCs and DPMs. For example, a 40-year-old female may present with derailment (P_DIS102), paranoid delusions (P_DEL93), conspiracy delusions (P_DEL94), and bizarre delusions (P_DEL101). The DPC of this patient's episode is *[P_DIS102(2) P_DEL93(2)P_DEL94(2)P_DEL101(1)]*. The number in parenthesis reflects the severity of the symptom and sign as described in the SCIP glossary. By using the DPCs and DPMs, researchers can progress to stage two and explore the relationship between psychopathology as presented by the patient and the findings of translational sciences.

Stage B: Translational Sciences

Translational research in medicine has advanced over the past few decades [19]. In psychiatry, translational studies have grown rapidly since 2004 and include biomarkers, experimental psychopathology, neuroimaging techniques, pharmacogenomics, pharmacogenetics, neurocircuits, and other newly developed techniques in neurosciences [20]. Translational research provides the best hope for individualizing treatment, understanding the causes of mental disorders, and preventing mental disorders. Research findings of translational sciences are enormous and advance daily. The challenge remains as to how to transform translational research findings in order to benefit patients in clinical settings.

Stage C: Scientific Methods to Transform Translational Research into Clinical Outcomes

Researchers' efforts to find ways to use neuroscience findings to benefit patients in clinical settings can be demonstrated by the National Institute of Mental Health (NIMH) Research Domain Criteria (RDoC) framework and the epistemic iteration process [14, 17].

The Research Domain Criteria (RDoC) framework conceptualizes mental disorders as disorders of brain circuits. Critics of the framework argue that it

Table 11.2 Personalized medicine in psychiatry (PMP) codes

Personalized medicine in psychiatry (PMP) code	Item titles	Ratings
Screening items		
PS1	Generalized anxiety	0,1
PS2	Panic attacks	0,1
PS3	Agoraphobia	0,1
PS4	Social phobia	0,1
PS5	Screening for obsessions	0,1
PS6	Screening for compulsions	0,1
PS7	Witness or experience traumatic events	0,1,2
PS8	Re-experience traumatic events	0,1
PS9	Depressed mood	0,1
PS10	Anhedonia	0,1
PS11	Suicidal ideation, intention, and plan	0,1,2,3,4
PS12	Self-mutilation behaviors	0,1
PS13	Elated mood	0,1
PS14	Irritable mood	0,1
PS15	Mixed mood (same day mood changes)	0,1
PS16	Paranoid delusions	0,1
PS17	Other delusions	0,1
PS18	Auditory hallucinations	0,1
PS19	Visual hallucinations	0,1
PS20	Violence	0,1,2,3
PS21	Disorganized behavior	0,1
PS22	Disorganized thoughts	0,1
PS23	Alcohol problems	0,1
PS24	Drug problems	0,1
PS25	Somatic symptoms	0,1
PS26	Pain symptoms	0,1
PS27	Worry about weight gain	0,1
PS28	Binge eating	0,1
PS29	Sustained attention impairment	0,1
PS30	Fidgety	0,1
Psychopathology items		
P_A1	Panic attacks	0,1
P_A2	Worry about having another panic attack	0,1
P_A3	Action to end or prevent panic attacks	0,1
P_A4	Social phobia	0,1
P_A5	Agoraphobia	0,1
P_A6	Generalized anxiety	0,1
P_A7	Restlessness with anxiety	0,1
P_A8	Tension with anxiety	0,1
P_A9	Exhaustion with anxiety	0,1

(continued)

Table 11.2 (continued)

Personalized medicine in psychiatry (PMP) code	Item titles	Ratings
P_A10	Poor concentration with anxiety	0,1
P_A11	Irritability with anxiety	0,1
P_A12	Insomnia with anxiety	0,1
P_OBS13	Obsessions	0,1,2,3
P_OBS14	Aggressive obsessions	0,1
P_OBS15	Contamination obsessions	0,1
P_OBS16	Sexual obsessions	0,1
P_OBS17	Religious obsessions	0,1
P_OBS18	Somatic obsessions	0,1
P_OBS19	Appearance obsessions	0,1
_COM20	Compulsions	0,1,2,3
P_COM21	Checking compulsions	0,1
P_COM22	Cleaning/washing compulsions	0,1
P_COM23	Repeating compulsions	0,1
P_COM24	Ordering/arranging compulsions	0,1
P_COM25	Hoarding/collecting	0,1
P_COM26	Mental compulsions	0,1
P_PTSD27	Witness or experience traumatic events	0,1,2
P_PTSD28	Distressing recollection of events	0,1
P_PTSD29	Bad dreams or nightmares	0,1
P_PTSD30	Flashbacks	0,1
P_PTSD31	Avoidance of thoughts and feelings	0,1
P_PTSD32	Avoidance of people, places, and activities	0,1
P_PTSD33	Amnesia	0,1
P_PTSD34	Diminished social interest (asociality)	0,1
P_PTSD35	Detachment and isolation	0,1
P_PTSD36	Diminished emotional feelings (Diminished experience of emotions)	0,1
P_PTSD37	Insomnia	0,1
P_PTSD38	Anger	0,1
P_PTSD39	Attention impairment (poor concentration)	0,1
P_PTSD40	Hypervigilance	0,1
P_PTSD41	Startle response	0,1
P_PTSD42	Psychological distress due to events	0,1
P_PTSD43	Physical reactions due to events	0,1
P_PTSD44	Daze (feeling out of touch with surroundings)	0,1
P_DEP45	Depressed mood	0,1,2
P_DEP46	Anhedonia (Loss of pleasure and interest)	0,1,2
P_DEP47	Hopelessness	0,1,2

(continued)

Table 11.2 (continued)

Personalized medicine in psychiatry (PMP) code	Item titles	Ratings
P_DEP48	Attention impairment (poor concentration)	0,1,2
P_DEP49	Psychomotor retardation/slowing	0,1,2
P_DEP50	Worthlessness (low self-esteem)	0,1,2
P_DEP51	Guilt	0,1,2
P_DEP52	Suicidality	0,1,2,3
P_DEP53	Crying when depressed	0,1,2
P_DEP54	Fatigue and loss of energy	0,1,2
P_DEP55	Loss of appetite when depressed	0,1,2
P_DEP56	Increased appetite when depressed	0,1,2
P_DEP57	Weight loss	0,1,2
P_DEP58	Weight gain	0,1,2
P_DEP59	Initial insomnia	0,1
P_DEP60	Middle insomnia	0,1
P_DEP61	Late insomnia	0,1
P_DEP62	Hypersomnia	0,1
P_DEP63	Decreased libido	0,1
P_MAN64	Elated (euphoric) mood (Expansive mood)	0,1,2
P_MAN65	Irritable mood	0,1,2
P_MAN66	Mixed mood (mood lability) (same-day mood changes)	0,1,2
P_MAN67	Racing thoughts	0,1,2
P_MAN68	Pressured speech	0,1,2
P_MAN69	Flight of ideas	0,1
P_MAN70	Increase in activities	0,1,2
P_MAN71	Decreased sleep	0,1
P_MAN72	Distraction (attention is distracted by environmental noises)	0,1,2
P_MAN73	Grandiosity	0,1
P_MAN74	Overspending (poor judgment in new activities)	0,1
P_MAN75	Hypersexuality	0,1
P_MAN76	Clanging	0,1,2,3,4
P_HAL77	Auditory hallucinations (hallucination quality)	0,1,2
P_HAL78	Frequency of auditory hallucinations	0,1,2,3
P_HAL79	Hallucination duration	0,1,2,3
P_HAL80	Audible thoughts	0,1
P_HAL81	Voices arguing	0,1
P_HAL82	Voices commenting	0,1
P_HAL83	Internal hallucinations	0,1,2,3

(continued)

Table 11.2 (continued)

Personalized medicine in psychiatry (PMP) code	Item titles	Ratings
P_HAL84	Second/third hallucinations	0,1,2,3
P_HAL85	Observed hallucinations	0,1
P_HAL86	Visual hallucinations	0,1
P_HAL87	Olfactory hallucinations	0,1
P_HAL88	Tactile hallucinations	0,1
P_DEL89	Somatic passivity	0,1
P_DEL90	Thought insertion	0,1
P_DEL91	Thought withdrawal	0,1
P_DEL92	Thought broadcasting	0,1
P_DEL93	Paranoid/ persecutory delusions	0,1,2
P_DEL94	Conspiracy delusions	0,1,2
P_DEL95	Delusions of reference	0,1,2
P_DEL96	Delusions of reading thoughts	0,1
P_DEL97	Religious delusions	0,1,2
P_DEL98	Grandiose delusions	0,1,2
P_DEL99	Delusions of control	0,1
P_DEL100	Other delusions	0,1
P_DEL101	Bizarreness of delusions	0,1
P_DIS102	Derailment (loose associations)	0,1,2
P_DIS103	Tangentiality	0,1,2
P_DIS104	Incoherent speech	0,1
P_DIS105	Illogical speech	0,1
P_DIS106	Other disorganized thoughts (e.g., word salad, clanging)	0,1
P_BEH107	Agitation	0,1,2,3,4
P_BEH108	Violence toward others	0,1,2
P_BEH109	Odd appearance and behavior	0,1
P_BEH110	Inappropriate affect	0,1
P_NEG111	Alogia	0,1,2
P_NEG112	Anhedonia (loss of pleasure and interest)	0,1,2
P_NEG113	Blunted/flat affect (Decrease in affective expression)	0,1,2
P_NEG114	Avolition (Decrease in goal-directed activities)	0,1,2
P_NEG115	Diminished social interest (asociality)	0,1
P_NEG116	Attention impairment (poor concentration)	0,1,2
P_NEG117	Psychomotor retardation/slowing	0,1,2
P_NEG118	Poor self-care	0,1,2
P_ALC119	Alcohol tolerance	0,1

(continued)

Table 11.2 (continued)

Personalized medicine in psychiatry (PMP) code	Item titles	Ratings
P_ALC120	Alcohol withdrawal	0,1
P_ALC121	Drinking alcohol to avoid withdrawal	0,1
P_ALC122	Unable to control alcohol	0,1
P_ALC123	Unable to reduce or stop alcohol	0,1
P_ALC124	Time spent to drink alcohol	0,1
P_ALC125	Failure to fulfil major obligations	0,1
P_ALC126	Giving up social or recreational activities	0,1
P_ALC127	Less time working due to alcohol use	0,1
P_ALC128	Alcohol-related work problems	0,1
P_ALC129	Fighting when intoxicated	0,1
P_ALC130	Alcohol-related family problems	0,1
P_ALC131	Alcohol-related legal problems	0,1
P_ALC132	Alcohol-induced medical problems	0,1
P_ALC133	Alcohol-induced emotional problems	0,1
P_ALC134	Alcohol use in spite of problems	0,1
P_ALC135	Alcohol use in hazardous situations	0,1
P_ALC136	Alcohol binge	0,1
P_ALC137	Alcohol blackout	0,1
P_DRG_138	Drug tolerance	0,1
P_DRG_139	Drug withdrawal	0,1
P_DRG_140	Using drug to avoid withdrawal	0,1
P_DRG_141	Unable to control drug use	0,1
P_DRG_142	Unable to reduce or stop drug use	0,1
P_DRG_143	Time spent to use drug	0,1
P_DRG_144	Failure to fulfil major obligations	0,1
P_DRG_145	Giving up social or recreational activities	0,1
P_DRG_146	Less time working due to drug use	0,1
P_DRG_147	Drug-related work problems	0,1
P_DRG_148	Fighting when using drug	0,1
P_DRG_149	Drug-related family problems	0,1
P_DRG_150	Drug-related legal problems	0,1
P_DRG_151	Drug-induced mood problems	0,1
P_DRG_152	Drug-induced psychosis	0,1
P_DRG_153	Drug use in spite of problems	0,1
P_DRG_154	Drug use in hazardous situations	0,1
P_EAT155	Being underweight	0,1
P_EAT156	Weight affects feelings	0,1
P_EAT157	Fear of weight gain	0,1
P_EAT158	Losing weight by fasting	0,1
P_EAT159	Losing weight by exercise	0,1
P_EAT160	Losing weight by diet pills	0,1

(continued)

Table 11.2 (continued)

Personalized medicine in psychiatry (PMP) code	Item titles	Ratings
P_EAT161	Losing weight by vomiting	0,1
P_EAT162	Losing weight by laxatives	0,1
P_EAT163	Losing weight by other methods	0,1
P_EAT164	Binge eating	0,1
P_EAT165	Binge eating frequency	0,1,2
P_EAT166	Losing control with binge eating	0,1
P_EAT167	Eating fast during binge eating	0,1
P_EAT168	Eating until uncomfortably full during binge eating	0,1
P_EAT169	Eating when not hungry during binge eating	0,1
P_EAT170	Eating alone during binge eating	0,1
P_EAT171	Feeling disgusted and guilty during binge eating	0,1
P_EAT172	Distressed by overeating during binge eating	0,1
P_EAT173	Fasting after binge eating	0,1
P_EAT174	Exercise after binge eating	0,1
P_EAT175	Using diet pills after binge eating	0,1
P_EAT176	Vomiting after binge eating	0,1
P_EAT177	Taking laxatives after binge eating	0,1
P_EAT178	Other losing weight methods after binge eating	0,1
P_EAT179	Binge eating compensatory behavior frequency	0,1,2
P_EAT180	Other eating behaviors	0,1
P_ADHD181	Attention impairment (poor concentration)	0,1
P_ADHD182	Sustained attention impairment	0,1
P_ADHD183	Avoiding sustained attention tasks	0,1
P_ADHD184	Attention when spoken to	0,1
P_ADHD185	Organization and meeting deadlines	0,1
P_ADHD186	Changing activities	0,1
P_ADHD187	Distraction (attention is distracted by environmental noises)	0,1
P_ADHD188	Misplacing things	0,1
P_ADHD189	Forgetting daily activities	0,1
P_ADHD190	Losing track	0,1
P_ADHD191	Fidgety	0,1
P_ADHD192	Leaving seats	0,1
P_ADHD193	Restlessness/moving	0,1

(continued)

Table 11.2 (continued)

Personalized medicine in psychiatry (PMP) code	Item titles	Ratings
P_ADHD194	Hyperactivity	0,1
P_ADHD195	Waiting in line	0,1
P_ADHD196	Talking too much	0,1
P_ADHD197	Loud and noisy	0,1
P_ADHD198	Impulsivity	0,1
P_ADHD199	Disturbing others	0,1
P_ADHD200	Blurt out answers	0,1

overemphasizes biological units and measures [21]. For example, the etiology of PTSD is in one's environment, such as childhood abuse. Researchers using the RDoC model may focus on the brain-based changes in PTSD patients rather than on the principal source of the early abuse experiences. Another criticism is that the RDoC dismisses clinical science, which is based on a competent clinical differential diagnosis of an individual case prior to considering laboratory tests or biomarkers [22]. With large funding currently being directed to RDoC research, time will tell if the RDoC model can successfully classify mental disorders based upon neuroscience and translate neuroscience to benefit patients in clinical settings.

Another proposed scientific model is the *epistemic iteration principle*, previously used by Chang in the science of temperature [23]. *In essence, epistemic iteration is a scientific process with three sequential steps. First*, science is built upon prior research. *Second*, science advances with a bottom-up approach. For example, experimental psychopathology (the correlation between psychopathology and objective measures) starts with one individual item, followed by a sequence of carefully selected groups of items.

1. *One-item experimental psychopathology*: For a case of psychosis, researchers start with patients who present with only one symptom, such as auditory hallucinations, and examine the correlation between auditory hallucinations and brain changes.
2. *Selected two-item experimental psychopathology*: Researchers can select patients who present with two symptoms simultaneously (e.g., auditory hallucination and visual hallucination) and examine their correlations with brain changes.
3. *Selected multiple-item experimental psychopathology*: After performing adequate one-item and two-item experiments, researchers may decide to examine brain changes in patients who present with several symptoms such as tangentiality, delusions, and auditory hallucinations.

Third, as scientific knowledge accumulates, successive iterations and revisions of experiments lead to a better approximation of reality. Kendler proposed using epistemic iteration in scientifically based psychiatric nosology to produce "more accurate approximations of the reality of psychiatric illness" [14]. A similar model termed "successive iterations" proposed by Carroll describes how initial syndromal disorders can be deconstructed into discrete entities by incorporating biomarkers, course, family history, symptoms, and signs into disease definitions [22].

Stage D: Clinical Outcomes

Clinical outcomes include clinical endpoints, more accurate diagnostic tools, more effective and less toxic treatment modalities, prognostic tools, and disease prevention. The clinical endpoints are variables that reflect how the patient "feels, functions, or survives" [11]. Clinical endpoints reflect the success or failure of the treatment provided to the patient. A patient may see the clinician in stage A because he feels sad, hopeless, suicidal, and unable to function. By stage D, the same patient may feel good, hopeful, and function as well as he used to. This scenario would be considered a success that is gratifying for both the patient and the clinician. Whatever methodology the clinician used in stage B and/or stage C was a success, and the outcome was good. On the other hand, if the patient reaches stage D and feels more depressed and more suicidal, the outcome in stage D is considered poor. In this case, the clinician needs to analyze what went wrong over the course of treatment and identify how to improve the patient's outcomes.

Not all patients need to proceed through the four stages. A patient may go to a clinician for grief therapy after the loss of a loved one (stage A). After a few sessions of grief therapy, the patient may feel well, hopeful, and ready to move on with life (stage D). This patient went directly from stage A to a good outcome in stage D, and there is no need for "biological markers" or "pharmacogenomics" in order to reach this outcome. However, many patients with serious mental disorders (schizophrenia spectrum, bipolar, neurocognitive disorders, and others) need stage B and stage C in order to reach good outcomes in stage D. If patients reach stage D with poor outcomes (e.g., medications are not effective or produce negative side effects), clinicians and researchers need to revisit stages A, B, and C and keep researching and innovating until patients reach stage D with good outcomes. Figure 11.1 shows the different pathways of the ABCD model. Hopefully, over time, the ABCD model of personalized medicine in psychiatry will lead to good clinical endpoints, more valid diagnostic and prognostic tools, more effective and less toxic therapeutics, and improved measures for disease prevention.

Concluding Remarks

The author holds great optimism for the future of psychiatry. The improved availability and accessibility of biomarker research will advance translational research. New classification systems based on neuroscience and translational research will

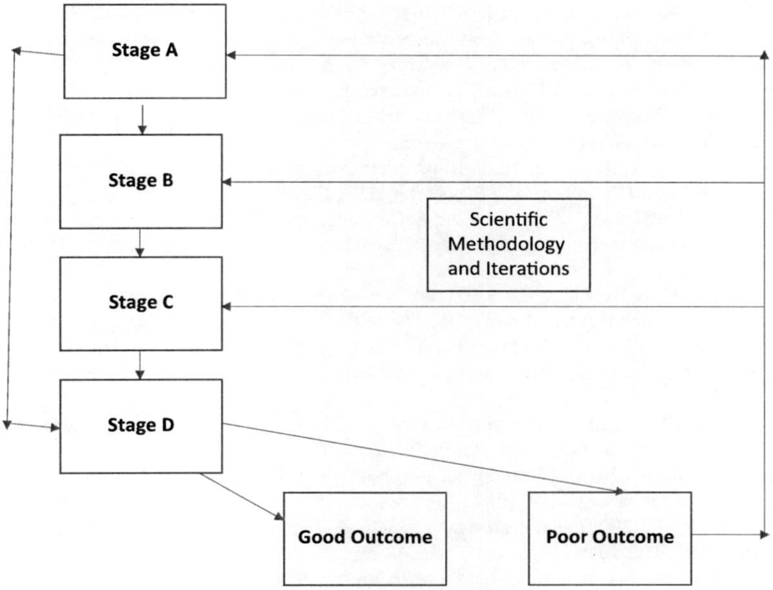

Fig. 11.1 Pathways of the ABCD model of personalized medicine in psychiatry

improve abilities to identify and target high-risk groups of patients. These systems can also lead to more effective and safe treatment modalities and hopefully will aid in advancing our understanding of the etiology and prevention of mental disorders.

References

1. Wium-Andersen, I. K., Vinberg, M., Kessing, L. V., & McIntyre, R. S. (2017). Personalized medicine in psychiatry. *Nordic Journal of Psychiatry, 71*, 12–19.
2. Domschke, K., Muller, D. J., & Serretti, A. (2015). Personalized therapies in psychiatry: Promises, pitfalls and perspectives. *Journal of Neural Transmission, 122*, 1–3.
3. Hong, D. S. (2014). Here/in this issue and there/abstract thinking: Personalized psychiatry: Are we almost there? *Journal of the American Academy of Child and Adolescent Psychiatry, 53*, 263–264.
4. Kessler, R. C., McLaughlin, K. A., Green, J. G., Gruber, M. J., Sampson, N. A., Zaslavsky, A. M., Aguilar-Gaxiola, S., Alhamzawi, A. O., Alonso, J., Angermeyer, M., Benjet, C., Bromet, E., Chatterji, S., de Girolamo, G., Demyttenaere, K., Fayyad, J., Florescu, S., Gal, G., Gureje, O., … Williams, D. R. (2010). Childhood adversities and adult psychopathology in the WHO World Mental Health Surveys. *The British Journal of Psychiatry: The Journal of Mental Science, 197*, 378–385.
5. Varese, F., Smeets, F., Drukker, M., Lieverse, R., Lataster, T., Viechtbauer, W., Read, J., van Os, J., & Bentall, R. P. (2012). Childhood adversities increase the risk of psychosis: A meta-analysis of patient-control, prospective- and cross-sectional cohort studies. *Schizophrenia Bulletin, 38*, 661–671.

6. Sonnby, K., Aslund, C., Leppert, J., & Nilsson, K. W. (2011). Symptoms of ADHD and depression in a large adolescent population: Co-occurring symptoms and associations to experiences of sexual abuse. *Nordic Journal of Psychiatry, 65*, 315–322.
7. Weber, K., Rockstroh, B., Borgelt, J., Awiszus, B., Popov, T., Hoffmann, K., Schonauer, K., Watzl, H., & Propster, K. (2008). Stress load during childhood affects psychopathology in psychiatric patients. *BMC Psychiatry, 8*, 63.
8. Peterson, B. S. (2020). Editorial: Biomarkers in precision medicine for mental illnesses. *Journal of Child Psychology and Psychiatry, 61*, 1279–1281.
9. Manchia, M., Pisanu, C., Squassina, A., & Carpiniello, B. (2020). Challenges and future prospects of precision medicine in psychiatry. *Pharmacogenomics and Personalized Medicine, 13*, 127–140.
10. Krueger, R. F., & Bezdjian, S. (2009). Enhancing research and treatment of mental disorders with dimensional concepts: Toward DSM-V and ICD-11. *World Psychiatry, 8*, 3–6.
11. Biomarkers Definitions Working Group. (2001). Biomarkers and surrogate endpoints: Preferred definitions and conceptual framework. *Clinical Pharmacology & Therapeutics, 69*, 89–95.
12. Keshavan, M. S. (2013). Classification of psychotic disorders: Need to move toward a neuroscience-informed nosology. *Asian Journal of Psychiatry, 6*, 191–192.
13. Keshavan, M. S. (2013). Nosology of psychoses in DSM-5: Inches ahead but miles to go. *Schizophrenia Research, 150*, 40–41.
14. Kendler, K. S. (2009). An historical framework for psychiatric nosology. *Psychological Medicine, 39*, 1935–1941.
15. National Research Council. (2011). *Toward precision medicine: Building a knowledge network for biomedical research and a new taxonomy of disease*. National Research Council.
16. Cuthbert, B. N. (2014). The RDoC framework: Facilitating transition from ICD/DSM to dimensional approaches that integrate neuroscience and psychopathology. *World Psychiatry, 13*, 28–35.
17. Insel, T., Cuthbert, B., Garvey, M., Heinssen, R., Pine, D. S., Quinn, K., Sanislow, C., & Wang, P. (2010). Research domain criteria (RDoC): Toward a new classification framework for research on mental disorders. *The American Journal of Psychiatry, 167*, 748–751.
18. Keshavan, M. S., Tandon, R., & Nasrallah, H. A. (2013). Renaming schizophrenia: Keeping up with the facts. *Schizophrenia Research, 148*, 1–2.
19. Stoyanov, D. S. (2017). Key developments in translational neuroscience: An update. *Balkan Medical Journal, 34*, 485–486.
20. Aragona, M. (2017). The impact of translational neuroscience on revisiting psychiatric diagnosis: State of the art and conceptual analysis. *Balkan Medical Journal, 34*, 487–492.
21. Lilienfeld, S. O. (2014). The Research Domain Criteria (RDoC): An analysis of methodological and conceptual challenges. *Behaviour Research and Therapy, 62*, 129–139.
22. Carroll, B. J. (2015). Clinical science and biomarkers: Against RDoC. *Acta Psychiatrica Scandinavica, 132*, 423–424.
23. Chang, H. (2004). *Inventing temperature: Measurement and scientific progress*. Oxford University Press.

Appendices

Appendix I

SCIP Screening Questionnaire

Screening item #	Screening item question
S1	***Have you felt very anxious and afraid out of proportion to the situation (with or without physical symptoms) for a prolonged period almost every day?*** 0 Absent or nonsignificant 1 Symptom present . Not sure *or* not applicable *or* missing
S2	***Did you have a panic attack, during which you suddenly felt anxious and frightened for a short time (up to 60 minutes) and developed physical symptoms (e.g., fast heart beats, shaking, sweating)?*** 0 Absent or nonsignificant 1 Symptom present . Not sure *or* not applicable *or* missing
S3	***Have you been afraid of being alone (at home or outside of home), traveling in a car, train, or plane, being in an open space (e.g., park), or being in a closed space (e.g., store), or being in crowds?*** 0 Absent or nonsignificant. 1 Symptom present. . Not sure *or* not applicable *or* missing.
S4	***Have you been afraid and anxious when you do things in front of people, such as eating or speaking in public?*** 0 Absent or nonsignificant. 1 Symptom present. . Not sure *or* not applicable *or* missing.

(continued)

A. S. Aboraya, *Manual for the Standard for Clinicians' Interview in Psychiatry (SCIP)*, Advances in Mental Health and Addiction,
https://doi.org/10.1007/978-3-030-94930-3

Appendix I (continued)

Screening item #	Screening item question
S5	***Do you ever have an intrusive thought or image that does not make sense and keeps coming back to your mind even when you try not to have the thought or the image?*** 0 Absent or nonsignificant. 1 Symptom present. . Not sure *or* not applicable *or* missing.
S6	***Do you find that you have to do things over and over, that is, checking things you have done (such as washing your hands even if they are clean, checking doors, or repeating mental acts such as counting or praying)?*** 0 Absent or nonsignificant. 1 Symptom present. . Not sure *or* not applicable *or* missing.
S7	***Have you ever witnessed or experienced a traumatic event that involved actual or threatened death or serious injury to you or someone else (e.g., physical or sexual abuse, terrorist attack, natural disaster, war)?*** ***Did you feel intense fear and helplessness?*** 0 No traumatic events. 1 One traumatic event. 2 More than one traumatic event. . Not sure *or* not applicable *or* missing.
S8	***Over the past month, have you re-experienced the event in a distressing way (e.g., flashbacks, nightmares, bad dreams)?*** 0 Absent or nonsignificant. 1 Symptom present. . Not sure *or* not applicable *or* missing.
S9	***Have you been feeling sad, depressed, or in low spirits?*** 0 Absent or nonsignificant. 1 Symptom present. . Not sure *or* not applicable *or* missing.
S10	***Have you been unable to experience pleasure and enjoy things that you used to enjoy like exercising, enjoying your hobbies, or socializing with friends?*** 0 Absent or nonsignificant. 1 Symptom present. . Not sure *or* not applicable *or* missing.
S11	***Have you had thoughts about harming yourself?*** ***Have you had the intention to carry out the suicidal thoughts?*** ***Have you had suicidal plans?*** ***Have you attempted to harm yourself during the past month?*** ***(multiple choices allowed)*** 0 Absent. 1 Current suicidal ideation. 2 Current suicidal intention. 3 Current suicidal plans. 4 Recent suicide attempts (past month). . Not sure *or* not applicable *or* missing.
S12	***Have you attempted self-mutilation behaviors without intent to die (e.g., burning, cutting, scratching)?*** 0 Absent. 1 Current self-mutilation (past month). . Not sure *or* not applicable *or* missing.

(continued)

Appendix I (continued)

S13	***Have you felt very happy, elated, or on top of the world for no apparent reason?*** 0 Absent or nonsignificant. 1 Symptom present. . Not sure *or* not applicable *or* missing.
S14	***Have you felt easily irritated without reason?*** ***Have you found yourself so irritable that you shout at people or start arguments or actually become aggressive?*** 0 Absent or nonsignificant. 1 Symptom present. . Not sure *or* not applicable *or* missing.
S15	***Have you had mixed mood swings: periods of depression and elation or irritability on the same day?*** 0 Absent or nonsignificant. 1 Symptom present. . Not sure *or* not applicable *or* missing.
S16	***Have you felt that someone is spying on you or trying to harm you or has a plot or conspiracy against you?*** 0 Absent or nonsignificant. 1 Symptom present. . Not sure *or* not applicable *or* missing.
S17	***Do you have strange thoughts such as that you are a prominent person in society, or you yourself are divine or you are God, or you receive special messages from TV or newspapers?*** 0 Absent or nonsignificant. 1 Symptom present. . Not sure *or* not applicable *or* missing.
S18	***Have you had experiences of hearing voices or noises that other people cannot hear?*** 0 Absent or nonsignificant. 1 Symptom present. . Not sure *or* not applicable *or* missing.
S19	***Have you had experiences of seeing things (shadows, objects, people) that other people cannot see?*** 0 Absent or nonsignificant. 1 Symptom present. . Not sure *or* not applicable *or* missing.
S20	***Have you been violent (destructive to objects or violent towards people) in the past (with or without the influence of alcohol or drugs)?*** 0 No history of violence. 1 Yes, due to alcohol and/or drugs. 2 Yes, without use of alcohol or drugs. 3 Both, with and without use of alcohol or drugs. . Not sure *or* not applicable *or* missing.
S21	***There is evidence of disorganized behavior by observation during the interview (agitation, odd appearance, inappropriate social behavior, inappropriate affect).*** 0 Absent or nonsignificant. 1 Symptom present. . Not sure *or* not applicable *or* missing.

(continued)

Appendix I (continued)

S22	***Evidence of disorganized thoughts by observation during the interview (loose associations, tangentiality, incoherent speech).*** 0 Absent or nonsignificant. 1 Symptom present. . Not sure *or* not applicable *or* missing.
S23	***During the past year, did alcohol cause problems for you at work or school, problems with family or friends, legal problems, or other problems such as getting in physical fights?*** 0 Absent or nonsignificant. 1 Symptom present. . Not sure *or* not applicable *or* missing.
S24	***During the past year, did drug use (___________) cause problems for you at work or school, problems with family or friends, legal problems, or other problems such as getting in physical fights?*** 0 Absent or nonsignificant. 1 Symptom present. . Not sure *or* not applicable *or* missing.
S25	***Have you visited doctors due to physical illness and the doctors did the necessary workup and could not find a medical explanation (have patient give examples)?*** 0 Absent or nonsignificant. 1 Symptom present. . Not sure *or* not applicable *or* missing.
S26	***Have you had pain and your doctor did the necessary workup and could not really explain why?*** 0 Absent or nonsignificant. 1 Symptom present. . Not sure *or* not applicable *or* missing.
S27	***Have you worried about gaining weight to the point that you did things such as self-induced vomiting, using diet pills, laxatives, or heavy exercise?*** 0 Absent or nonsignificant. 1 Symptom present. . Not sure *or* not applicable *or* missing.
S28	***Do you have episodes of binge eating (eating within one or two-hour period what most people would consider an unusually large amount of food)?*** 0 Absent or nonsignificant. 1 Symptom present. . Not sure *or* not applicable *or* missing.
S29	***Do you have difficulty concentrating on one thing for a long time (e.g., reading a book, writing a letter)?*** 0 Absent or nonsignificant. 1 Patient has difficulty concentrating for a long period of time. . Not sure *or* not applicable *or* missing.
S30	***Do you have difficulty remaining seated (fidget with hands and feet, squirm, or wiggle in seat) when expected to remain seated (e.g., in a meeting or a church service)?*** 0 Absent or nonsignificant. 1 Patient fidgets with hands and feet, or wiggles in seat. . Not sure *or* not applicable *or* missing.

Appendix II

The SCIP Clinician-Administered (CA) Scales

	Clinician-administered (CA) Scales	Number of items	Reliability	Validity
1	Anxiety	7	Yes	Yes
2	Panic	5	Yes	Yes
3	Phobia	9	Yes	Not studied
4	OCD	18	Yes	Not studied
5	PTSD	16	Yes	Yes
6	Depression	14	Yes	Yes
7	Mania	13	Yes	Yes
8	Hallucinations	9	Yes	Yes
9	Delusions	9	Yes	Yes
10	Disorganization	4	Yes	Yes
11	Aggression	6	Yes	Not applicable
12	Negative symptoms	6	Yes	Not applicable
13	Core schizophrenia	22	Yes	Yes
14	Alcohol	8	Yes	Yes
15	Drug	7	Yes	Yes
16	ADHD	20	Yes	Yes
17	Anorexia nervosa	9	Yes	Not studied
18	Binge and bulimia	15	Yes	Not studied

(continued)

SCIP Generalized Anxiety Scale

Codes for GAD
0 Absent or nonsignificant.
1 Symptom present.
. Not sure *or* not applicable *or* missing.

GAD1. Generalized anxiety:	***Score***
Have you had excessive worry and anxiety for long periods of time (e.g., for hours each day lasting several months), not just during panic attacks? ***Is it difficult to control the anxiety?*** 0 Patient has no generalized anxiety or nonsignificant. *1* Patient has generalized anxiety. . Not sure *or* not applicable *or* missing.	
GAD2. Restlessness with anxiety	
Did you feel restless, keyed up, or on edge? 0 No. 1 Yes. . Not sure *or* not applicable *or* missing.	
GAD3. Tension with anxiety	
Did you feel tense in your muscles? 0 No. 1 Yes. . Not sure *or* not applicable *or* missing.	
GAD4. Exhaustion with anxiety	
Did you feel tired or easily exhausted even without work? 0 No. 1 Yes. . Not sure *or* not applicable *or* missing.	
GAD5. Poor concentration with anxiety	
Did you have difficulty concentrating when anxious? 0 No. 1 Yes. . Not sure *or* not applicable *or* missing.	
GAD6. Irritability with anxiety	
Did you feel irritable when anxious? 0 No. 1 Yes. . Not sure *or* not applicable *or* missing.	
GAD7. Insomnia with anxiety	
Did you have difficulty falling asleep or staying asleep when anxious? 0 No. 1 Yes. . Not sure *or* not applicable *or* missing.	

Generalized anxiety score			
Severity of anxiety	**1**	**Mild**	**1–3**
	2	**Moderate**	**4–5**
	3	**Severe**	**6 or more**

SCIP Panic Scale

<u>**Codes for panic scale**</u>
0 Absent or nonsignificant.
1 Symptom present.
. Not sure *or* not applicable *or* missing.

Questions apply to <u>the present episode, typically the past month,</u> unless otherwise specified by the interviewer.

PAN1. Panic attacks (without phobias)	*Score*
Did you have a panic attack, when you suddenly become anxious and frightened for a short period of time (up to 60 minutes)? ***During that time, did you feel that your heart was racing or pounding, or did you start shaking or sweating, or did you feel you were choking?*** 0 Patient had no panic attacks. 1 Patient had panic attacks. . Not sure *or* not applicable *or* missing.	
PAN2. Frequency of panic attacks <u>per week</u>	
PAN3. Worry about having another panic attack	
After a panic attack, did you worry about having another attack? ***Did you worry about its effects (e.g., losing control, having a heart attack, or going crazy)?*** 0 After a panic attack, patient did not worry about having another one. 1 After a panic attack, patient worried about having another one or its effects. . Not sure *or* not applicable *or* missing.	
PAN4. Action to end or prevent panic attacks	
Did you have to do something to end the attack, like leaving a store, calling someone, or taking deep breaths? ***Do you do anything to prevent the attacks (like avoiding places that trigger the panic attacks)?*** 0 After a panic attack, patient does nothing to end or prevent another panic attack. 1 After a panic attack, patient does something to end or prevent another panic attack. . Not sure *or* not applicable *or* missing.	
PAN5. <u>Autonomic symptoms with panic attacks</u>: **(Enter the number of positive symptoms)** 1. Patient cannot catch breath and has feeling of being smothered. 2. Patient has chest pain or discomfort. 3. Patient has feeling of choking. 4. Patient feels heart is pounding, missing beats, or beating faster. 5. Patient feels dizzy, unsteady, light-headed, or faint. 6. Patient has numbness or tingling sensations in face or fingers. 7. Patient has dry mouth or difficulty swallowing. 8. Patient has nausea or abdominal distress. 9. Patient has trembling or shaking of hands or limbs. 10. Patient has sweating, e.g., palms. 11. Patient feels very cold. 12. Patient has hot flushes. 13. Patient has fear of dying. 14. Patient has fear of going crazy or fear of losing emotional control. 15. Patient feels that things are not real. 16. Patient feels that people are not real.	
Panic scale score	

(continued)

SCIP Phobia Scale

PHOB1. Social phobia	*Score*
Have you been afraid and anxious when you do things in front of people, such as eating or speaking in public? ***Do you avoid social situations or endure with intense fear?*** 0 Patient had no social phobia. 1 Patient had social phobia. . Not sure *or* not applicable *or* missing.	
PHIB2. Panic attacks with social phobia 0 Patient had no panic attacks with social phobia. 1 Patient had panic attacks only with social phobia. 2 Patient had panic attacks with social phobia and other phobias. . Not sure or not applicable or missing.	
PHOB3. Autonomic symptoms with panic attacks **(Enter the number of positive symptoms)** 1. Patient cannot catch breath and has feeling of being smothered. 2. Patient has chest pain or discomfort. 3. Patient has feeling of choking. 4. Patient feels heart is pounding, missing beats, or beating faster. 5. Patient feels dizzy, unsteady, light-headed, or faint. 6. Patient has numbness or tingling sensations in face or fingers. 7. Patient has dry mouth or difficulty swallowing. 8. Patient has nausea or abdominal distress. 9. Patient has trembling or shaking of hands or limbs. 10. Patient has sweating, e.g., palms. 11. Patient feels very cold. 12. Patient has hot flushes. 13. Patient has fear of dying. 14. Patient has fear of going crazy or fear of losing emotional control. 15. Patient feels that things are not real. 16. Patient feels that people are not real.	

Social phobia score

PHOB4. Agoraphobias	*Score*
Have you been afraid of being alone (at home or outside of the home), traveling in a car, train, or plane, being in an open space (e.g., park) or being in a closed space (e.g., store), or being in crowds? ***Do you avoid these situations, or require a companion, or endure with intense fear?*** 0 Patient had no agoraphobia. 1 Patient had agoraphobia. . Not sure or not applicable or missing	
PHOB5. Panic attacks with agoraphobia 0 Patient had no panic attacks with agoraphobia. 1 Patient had panic attacks only with agoraphobia. 2 Patient had panic attacks with agoraphobia and other phobias. . Not sure or not applicable or missing.	

(continued)

Appendix II (continued)

PHOB6. <u>Autonomic symptoms with panic attacks</u> **(Enter the number of positive symptoms)** 1. Patient cannot catch breath and has feeling of being smothered. 2. Patient has chest pain or discomfort. 3. Patient has feeling of choking. 4. Patient feels heart is pounding, missing beats, or beating faster. 5. Patient feels dizzy, unsteady, light-headed, or faint. 6. Patient has numbness or tingling sensations in face or fingers. 7. Patient has dry mouth or difficulty swallowing. 8. Patient has nausea or abdominal distress. 9. Patient has trembling or shaking of hands or limbs. 10. Patient has sweating, e.g., palms. 11. Patient feels very cold. 12. Patient has hot flushes. 13. Patient has fear of dying. 14. Patient has fear of going crazy or fear of losing emotional control. 15. Patient feels that things are not real. 16. Patient feels that people are not real.	

Agoraphobias score

PHOB7. Specific phobias	***Score***
Have you had strong fears of certain objects or situations (e.g., heights, animals, spiders, snakes, seeing blood, receiving injections)? ***Do you avoid objects or situations or endure with intense fear?*** 0 Patient had no specific phobias. 1 Patient had a specific phobia. . Not sure or not applicable or missing.	
PHOB8. <u>Panic attacks with specific phobias</u> 0 Patient had no panic attacks with specific phobias. 1 Patient had panic attacks only with specific phobias. 2 Patient had panic attacks with specific phobias and other phobias. . Not sure or not applicable or missing.	
PHOB9. <u>Autonomic symptoms with panic attacks</u> **(Enter the number of positive symptoms)** 1. Patient cannot catch breath and has feeling of being smothered. 2. Patient has chest pain or discomfort. 3. Patient has feeling of choking. 4. Patient feels heart is pounding, missing beats, or beating faster. 5. Patient feels dizzy, unsteady, light-headed, or faint. 6. Patient has numbness or tingling sensations in face or fingers. 7. Patient has dry mouth or difficulty swallowing. 8. Patient has nausea or abdominal distress. 9. Patient has trembling or shaking of hands or limbs. 10. Patient has sweating, e.g., palms. 11. Patient feels very cold. 12. Patient has hot flushes. 13. Patient has fear of dying. 14. Patient has fear of going crazy or fear of losing emotional control. 15. Patient feels that things are not real. 16. Patient feels that people are not real.	

Specific phobias score

(continued)

Appendix II (continued)

SCIP Obsessive-Compulsive Scale

<u>Codes for OCD</u>	
0 Absent or nonsignificant.	
1 Symptom present.	
. Not sure *or* not applicable *or* missing.	
Questions apply to <u>the past week,</u> unless otherwise specified by the interviewer.	
<u>Obsessions</u> ***OCD1. Do you ever have an intrusive thought or image that does not make sense and keeps coming back to your mind even when you try to avoid the thought or the image?***	**Score**
0 No. 1 Yes, less than 1 hour/day. 2 Yes, 1–4 hours/day. 3 Yes, more than 4 hours/day. . Not sure *or* not applicable *or* missing.	
OCD2. During a one-week period, on how many days do you have obsessive thoughts on average (please write down the number of days from 0 to 7 in the space provided)?	
OCD3. Aggressive obsessions ***<u>Potential examples:</u> fears of harming oneself, fears of unintentionally hurting someone, urges to stab someone, thoughts of "losing control" and hurting a partner or significant other***	
0 No. 1 Yes. . Not sure *or* not applicable *or* missing.	
OCD4. Contamination obsessions ***<u>Potential examples:</u> fear of contamination in public bathrooms, outdoors, or public places, fear of what might happen after touching one's own bodily secretions, fear of getting germs or viruses from others***	
0 No. 1 Yes. . Not sure *or* not applicable *or* missing.	
OCD5. Sexual obsessions ***<u>Potential examples:</u> disturbing thoughts about sex, unwanted images of sexual acts toward strangers, family members or children, fear of being found with pornography***	
0 No. 1 Yes. . Not sure *or* not applicable *or* missing.	
OCD6. Religious obsessions ***<u>Potential examples</u>: fear of having blasphemous or "sinful" thoughts, concerns for engaging in sinful or forbidden behavior, feeling the need to complete a certain number of prayers or "good deeds"***	
0 No. 1 Yes. . Not sure *or* not applicable *or* missing.	

(continued)

Appendix II (continued)

OCD7. Somatic obsessions ***<u>Potential examples:</u> worries about having an undiagnosed illness like cancer or heart disease, fear of contracting a deadly disease, images of your own death***	
0 No. 1 Yes. . Not sure *or* not applicable *or* missing.	
OCD8. Appearance obsessions ***<u>Potential examples:</u> worries about the size of certain body parts (ears, nose, mouth), fears of certain body parts being disgusting to others***	
0 No. 1 Yes. . Not sure *or* not applicable *or* missing.	
OCD9. Other obsessions	
0 No. 1 Yes. . Not sure *or* not applicable *or* missing.	

Obsession score			
Severity of obsession	**1**	**Mild**	**1–3**
	2	**Moderate**	**4–8**
	3	**Severe**	**9 or more**

	Score
<u>Compulsions</u> ***OCD10. Do you find that you have to do things over and over, that is, a compulsive behavior like checking things you have already done (such as washing your hands even if they are clean, checking doors, or repeating mental acts such as counting or praying)?*** ***Do you get very anxious or tense if you do not repeat the act over and over?***	
0 No. 1 Yes, less than 1 hour/day. 2 Yes, 1–4 hours/day. 3 Yes, more than 4 hours/day. . Not sure *or* not applicable *or* missing.	
OCD11. During a one-week period, on how many days do you have a compulsive behavior on average (please write down the number of days from 0 to 7 in the space provided)?	
OCD12. Checking compulsions ***<u>Potential examples:</u> checking door locks, switches, or appliances many times before leaving the house, checking one's appearance for an excessive amount of time before leaving the house***	
0 No. 1 Yes. . Not sure *or* not applicable *or* missing.	
OCD13. Cleaning/washing compulsions ***<u>Potential examples:</u> excessively changing your clothes, excessive handwashing, tooth brushing, showering, scrubbing surfaces***	
0 No. 1 Yes. . Not sure *or* not applicable *or* missing.	

(continued)

Appendix II (continued)

OCD14. Repeating compulsions ***<u>Potential examples</u>: rereading text out of concerns that one "missed something," rewriting or retracing words, reentering buildings or living spaces, retying one's shoes***	
0 No. 1 Yes. . Not sure *or* not applicable *or* missing.	
OCD15. Ordering/arranging compulsions ***<u>Potential examples:</u> rearranging one's pantry or refrigerator, spending excessive amounts of time organizing one's desk or workspace***	
0 No. 1 Yes. . Not sure *or* not applicable *or* missing.	
OCD16. Hoarding/collecting compulsions ***<u>Potential examples:</u> picking up, collecting or buying useless things, owning an excessive amount of items, and being unable to donate or get rid of them***	
0 No. 1 Yes. . Not sure *or* not applicable *or* missing.	
OCD17. Mental compulsions ***<u>Potential examples:</u> repetitively counting certain numbers or avoiding certain "bad" numbers,*** ***repeating certain words, counting senseless things (e.g., ceiling tiles), reciting prayers or statements***	
0 No. 1 Yes. . Not sure *or* not applicable *or* missing.	
OCD18. Other compulsions	
0 No. 1 Yes. . Not sure *or* not applicable *or* missing.	

Compulsion score/severity of compulsion		
1	**Mild**	**1–3**
2	**Moderate**	**4–8**
3	**Severe**	**9 or more**

Appendix II (continued)

SCIP Posttraumatic Stress Scale

Codes for PTSD
0 Absent or nonsignificant.
1 Symptom present.
. Not sure *or* not applicable *or* missing.

PTSD1. Witness or experience traumatic events	***Score***
Have you ever witnessed or experienced a traumatic event that involved actual or threatened death or serious injury to you or someone else (e.g., physical or sexual abuse, rape, terrorist attack, natural disaster, war)? ***Did you feel intense fear and helplessness?*** 0 Patient had no traumatic events. 1 Patient has experienced one traumatic event. 2 Patient has experienced several traumatic events. . Not sure *or* not applicable *or* missing.	
During the past month (or during a specified period)	
PTSD2. Distressing recollection of events	
Did you have recurrent upsetting memories (distressing recollection) of the event? 0 Patient had no significant symptom. 1 Patient has recurrent upsetting memories (distressing recollection) of the event. . Not sure *or* not applicable *or* missing.	
PTSD3. Bad dreams or nightmares	
Did you have recurrent upsetting dreams or nightmares of the event? 0 Patient had no significant symptom. 1 Patient has recurrent upsetting dreams and nightmares of the event. . Not sure *or* not applicable *or* missing.	
PTSD4. Flashbacks	
Did you have a sense or feeling that the event was happening again: the sense of reliving the event (flashbacks), auditory/visual hallucinations related to the event, or body/somatosensory experiences of the event? 0 Patient had no significant symptom. 1 Patient has a sense or feeling that the event is happening again, the sense of reliving the event (flashbacks). . Not sure *or* not applicable *or* missing.	
PTSD5. Avoidance of thoughts or feelings	
Did you try to avoid thoughts and feelings associated with the event? 0 Patient had no significant symptom. 1 Patient tries not to think about the event. . Not sure *or* not applicable *or* missing.	
PTSD6. Avoidance of people, places, activities	
Did you try to avoid things that reminded you of the event (such as certain people, certain places, or some activities)? 0 Patient had no significant symptom. 1 Patient avoids things that are reminders of the event (such as certain people, certain places or some activities). . Not sure *or* not applicable *or* missing.	

(continued)

Appendix II (continued)

PTSD7. Amnesia	
Did you have difficulty remembering some or all important aspects of the event? 0 Patient had no significant symptom. 1 Patient has difficulty remembering some or all important aspects of the event. . Not sure *or* not applicable *or* missing.	
PTSD8. Diminished social interest (asociality)	
Did you spend less time or show less interest in activities with friends/family or hobbies that you used to enjoy due to the event? 0 Patient had no significant symptom. 1 Patient spends less time or shows less interest in activities with friends/family or hobbies due to the event. . Not sure *or* not applicable *or* missing.	
PTSD9. Detachment and isolation	
Did you feel distant, cut off, or isolated from other people due to the event? 0 Patient had no significant symptom. 1 Patient feels distant, cut off, or isolated from other people due to the event. . Not sure *or* not applicable *or* missing.	
PTSD10. Diminished emotional feelings (diminished experience of emotions)	
Did you feel emotionally numb? ***Did you have trouble experiencing feelings (happiness, love feelings) due to the event?*** 0 Patient had no significant symptom. 1 Patient feels emotionally numb. Patient has trouble experiencing feelings (such as happiness or love feelings) due to the event. . Not sure *or* not applicable *or* missing.	
PTSD11. Insomnia	
Did you have difficulty falling or staying asleep due to the event? 0 Patient had no significant symptom. 1 Patient has difficulty falling or staying asleep due to the event. . Not sure *or* not applicable *or* missing.	
PTSD12. Anger	
Did you have periods of irritability or sudden outbursts of anger due to the event? 0 Patient had no significant symptom. 1 Patient has periods of irritability or sudden outbursts of anger due to the event. . Not sure *or* not applicable *or* missing.	
PTSD13. Attention impairment/poor concentration	
Did you have difficulty concentrating due to the event? 0 Patient had no significant symptom. 1 Patient has difficulty concentrating due to the event. . Not sure *or* not applicable *or* missing.	
PTSD14. Hypervigilance	
Did you feel very alert or watchful of things going on around you even when there was no need to be? 0 Patient had no significant symptom. 1 Patient feels very alert or watchful of things going on around even when there is no need to be. . Not sure *or* not applicable *or* missing.	

(continued)

Appendix II (continued)

PTSD15. Startle response	
Did you feel jumpy and easily startled? ***Were you easily scared or did you make a sudden movement or jump when you heard noises or if you were caught by surprise?*** 0 Patient had no significant symptom. 1 Patient feels jumpy and has a startle response. . Not sure *or* not applicable *or* missing.	
PTSD16. Other PTSD symptoms	
0 No. 1 Yes (specify). . Not sure *or* not applicable *or* missing.	

PTSD score			
Severity of PTSD	**1**	**Mild**	**1–3**
	2	**Moderate**	**4–8**
	3	**Severe**	**9 or more**

SCIP Depression Scale

Codes for depression
Unless otherwise specified in the question, the rating of a symptom is as follows:
0 Absent or nonsignificant.
1 Symptom present < 50% of the time or <50% of times.
2 Symptom present > 50% of the time or >50% of times.
. Not sure *or* not applicable *or* missing.

Questions apply to the present episode, typically the past month, unless otherwise specified by the interviewer.

D1. Depressed mood	*Score*
Have you been feeling sad, depressed, or in low spirits? 0 Patient has no depressed mood. 1 Patient has depressed mood less than half the time. 2 Patient has depressed mood more than half the time. . Not sure *or* not applicable *or* missing.	
Duration of depressed mood in days	
D2. Anhedonia (loss of pleasure and interest)	
Have you been unable to experience pleasure and enjoy things that you used to enjoy like exercising, enjoying your hobbies, or socializing with friends? 0 Patient has no anhedonia. 1 Patient has anhedonia less than half the time. 2 Patient has anhedonia more than half the time. . Not sure *or* not applicable *or* missing.	
Duration of anhedonia in days	

D3. Hopelessness	
Have you felt hopeless about your future? 0 Patient is not hopeless. 1 Patient feels hopeless less than half the time. 2 Patient feels hopeless more than half the time. . Not sure *or* not applicable *or* missing.	
D4. Attention impairment/poor concentration	
Have you found that your concentration has decreased and you are unable to complete a task (e.g., at work, reading an article, reading a book, or watching a movie), even though you were able to do that before? 0 Patient has no concentration problems. 1 Patient has difficulty concentrating less than half the time. 2 Patient has difficulty concentrating more than half the time. . Not sure *or* not applicable *or* missing.	
D5. Psychomotor slowing/retardation	
Have you felt as though you were talking or moving more slowly than normal for you when depressed? 0 Patient has normal activity. 1 Patient has psychomotor retardation less than half the time. 2 Patient has psychomotor retardation more than half the time. . Not sure *or* not applicable *or* missing.	

(continued)

Appendix II (continued)

D6. Worthlessness (low self-esteem)	
Have you felt that you are a worthless person in the society or a failure? 0 Patient has no feeling of worthlessness. 1 Patient feels worthless less than half the time. 2 Patient feels worthless more than half the time. . Not sure *or* not applicable *or* missing.	
D7. Excessive guilt	
Have you felt guilty or ashamed of yourself for something you have done or thought? 0 Patient has no feeling of guilt. 1 Patient feels guilty less than half the time. 2 Patient feels guilty more than half the time. . Not sure *or* not applicable *or* missing.	
D8. Other depressive symptoms	
0 Absent. 1 Present (specify). . Not sure *or* not applicable *or* missing.	
D9. Suicidal ideation during the past month	
Have you had thoughts about harming or killing yourself? ***Have you had thoughts you would not care if you didn't wake in the morning?*** ***Have you had thoughts you would be better off dead?*** 0 Patient had no suicidal ideation. 1 Patient had suicidal ideation. . Not sure *or* not applicable *or* missing.	
D10. Suicidal intention during the past month	
Have you had the intention to carry out the suicidal thoughts? 0 Patient had no suicidal intention. 1 Patient had suicidal intention. . Not sure *or* not applicable *or* missing.	
D11. Suicidal plans during the past month	
Have you had specific suicidal plans during the past month? 0 Patient had no suicidal plans. 1 Patient had suicidal plans. . Not sure *or* not applicable *or* missing.	
D12. Suicidal attempt during the past month	
Have you made a suicide attempt during the past month? 0 Patient made no suicide attempt during the past month. 1 Patient made one recent suicide attempt during the past month. 2 Patient made two or more recent suicide attempts during the past month. . Not sure *or* not applicable *or* missing.	
D13. Delusions associated mainly with depressed mood	
0 Absent. 1 Present. . Not sure *or* not applicable *or* missing.	
D14. Hallucinations associated mainly with depressed mood	
0 Absent. 1 Present. . Not sure *or* not applicable *or* missing.	

Depression score			
Severity of depression	**1**	**Mild**	**1–4**
	2	**Moderate**	**5–8**
	3	**Severe**	**9 or more**

SCIP Mania Scale

Codes for Mania
Unless otherwise specified in the question, the rating of a symptom is as follows:
0 Absent or nonsignificant.
1 Symptom present < 50% of the time or <50% of times.
2 Symptom present > 50% of the time or >50% of times.
. Not sure *or* not applicable *or* missing.

M1. Expansive (elated) mood	***Score***
Have you sometimes felt very happy, elated, or on top of the world without much reason? 0 Patient has no elated mood. 1 Patient has elated mood less than half the time. 2 Patient has elated mood more than half the time. . Not sure *or* not applicable *or* missing.	
Duration of elated mood in days	
M2. Irritable mood	
Have you sometimes felt that you were easily irritated without reason? ***Have you found yourself so irritable that you shout at people or start arguments or actually become aggressive?*** 0 Patient has no irritable mood. 1 Patient has irritable mood less than half the time. 2 Patient has irritable mood more than half the time. . Not sure *or* not applicable *or* missing.	
Duration of irritable mood in days	
M3. Mixed mood (mood lability)	
Have you had mixed mood swings: periods of depression and elation or irritability on the same day? 0 Patient has no mixed mood swings. 1 Patient has mixed mood less than half the time. 2 Patient has mixed mood more than half the time. . Not sure *or* not applicable *or* missing.	
Duration of mixed mood in days	
M4. Racing thoughts (observed as flight of ideas)	
Have you felt that you had too many different thoughts racing through your mind compared with normal? 0 Patient has no racing thoughts. 1 Patient has racing thoughts less than half the time. 2 Patient has racing thoughts more than half the time. . Not sure *or* not applicable *or* missing.	
M5. Pressured speech	
Have you been talking faster than usual during this time (for example, people said that they were unable to understand you because you were speaking too fast or you felt a pressure to continue talking)? 0 Patient has normal speech. 1 Patient has pressured speech less than half the time. 2 Patient has pressured speech more than half the time. . Not sure *or* not applicable *or* missing.	

(continued)

Appendix II (continued)

M6. Distraction (attention is distracted by environmental noises)	
Do you find yourself easily distracted by unimportant activities or things happening around you? 0 Patient has no distraction. 1 Patient has been easily distracted by external stimuli less than half the time. 2 Patient has been easily distracted by external stimuli more than half the time. . Not sure *or* not applicable *or* missing.	
M7. Increase in activities	
Have you been more active and had more energy than usual? ***Did you do more things than usual at work, school, or socially?*** 0 Patient has no increased energy. 1 Patient has too much energy less than half the time. 2 Patient has too much energy more than half the time. . Not sure *or* not applicable *or* missing.	
M8. Grandiosity	
Have you felt more self-confident than usual? ***Have you felt that you have special powers or special abilities?*** 0 Patient has no grandiosity. 1 Patient has grandiose thoughts, but not of a delusional quality. . Not sure *or* not applicable *or* missing.	
M9. Overspending (poor judgment in new activities)	
Have you done something that you regretted later (e.g., spending a lot of money that you could not afford, writing bad checks, investing money foolishly, or sexual indiscretions)? 0 Patient did not go on a spending spree. 1 Patient went on a spending spree during manic phase. . Not sure *or* not applicable *or* missing.	
M10. Decreased sleep	
Have you needed less sleep than usual and without getting tired? 0 Patient has normal sleep. 1 Patient sleeps four hours or less (in a 24-hour period including naps) and feels rested. . Not sure *or* not applicable *or* missing.	
M11. Other symptoms (e.g., hypersexuality, aggressive driving, illegal drug use, or gambling)	
0 Absent. 1 Present (specify). . Not sure *or* not applicable *or* missing.	
M12. Delusions associated mainly with manic episode	
0 Absent. 1 Present. . Not sure *or* not applicable *or* missing.	
M13. Hallucinations associated mainly with manic episode	
0 Absent. 1 Present. . Not sure *or* not applicable *or* missing.	

Mania score			
Severity of mania	**1**	**Mild**	**1–3**
	2	**Moderate**	**4–8**
	3	**Severe**	**9 or more**

(continued)

SCIP Hallucinations Scale

Questions apply to the present episode, typically the past month, unless otherwise specified by the interviewer.

Hallucinations

HAL1. Auditory hallucinations	***Score***
Do you hear noises (like music, whispering sounds) or voices talking to you when there is no one around? ***Are the voices like a real voice or just thoughts in your mind?*** 0 Patient has no auditory hallucinations. 1 Patient has auditory hallucinations. 2 Patient has auditory hallucinations with command. . Not sure *or* not applicable *or* missing.	
HAL2. Frequency of auditory hallucinations	
How often do you hear noises (like music, whispering sounds) or voices talking to you when there is no one around? 0 Patient has no auditory hallucinations. 1 Patient has auditory hallucinations (1–4 days/month). 2 Patient has auditory hallucinations (5–15 days/month). 3 Patient has auditory hallucinations (>15 days/month). . Not sure *or* not applicable *or* missing.	
HAL3. Hallucination duration	
On days when you hear noises or voices, how often do you hear them? 0 Patient has no auditory hallucinations. 1 Patient has auditory hallucinations (less than 1 hour/day). 2 Patient has auditory hallucinations (1–4 hours/day). 3 Patient has auditory hallucinations (more than 4 hours/day). . Not sure *or* not applicable *or* missing.	
HAL4. Audible thoughts	
Do you think that your thoughts are so loud that someone close to you can hear what you are thinking? 0 Patient has no audible thoughts. 1 Patient has audible thoughts. . Not sure *or* not applicable *or* missing.	
HAL5. Voices arguing	
Do you hear two or more voices that argue about what you are doing or thinking? 0 Voices do not argue with the patient. 1 Voices argue about what the patient is doing or thinking. . Not sure *or* not applicable *or* missing.	
HAL6. Voices commenting	
Do you hear a voice or voices commenting on what you are doing or thinking? 0 Voices do not comment about the patient. 1 Voices comment on what the patient is doing or thinking. . Not sure *or* not applicable *or* missing.	
HAL7. Visual hallucinations	
Do you see things other people cannot see (e.g., shadows, objects, or people)? 0 Patient has no visual hallucinations. 1 Patient has visual hallucinations. . Not sure *or* not applicable *or* missing.	

(continued)

Appendix II (continued)

HAL8. Observed hallucinations	
0 Patient has not been observed talking to self. 1 Patient has been observed talking to self, talking to a mirror, or running a conversation with unseen person. . Not sure *or* not applicable *or* missing.	
HAL9. Other hallucinations (olfactory, gustatory, tactile)	
Do you sometimes notice unusual smells that other people do not notice, experience strange tastes in your mouth, or feel strange sensations on your body? 0 Patient has no other hallucinations. 1 Patient has other hallucinations (olfactory, gustatory, or tactile hallucinations). . Not sure *or* not applicable *or* missing.	

Hallucination score			
Severity of hallucinations	**1**	**Mild**	**1–3**
	2	**Moderate**	**4–8**
	3	**Severe**	**9 or more**

SCIP Delusions Scale

DEL1. Somatic passivity (bizarre delusions associated with somatic sensations)	*Score*
Do you feel or have a bodily sensation (e.g., something is crawling under your skin) and think it is caused by an outside person or force? 0 Patient has no somatic passivity. 1 Patient has somatic passivity. . Not sure *or* not applicable *or* missing.	
DEL2. Delusions of thought insertion	
Do you think that thoughts in your mind are not your own thoughts and that they were inserted into your mind by an outside person or force? 0 Patient has no delusions of thought insertion. 1 Patient has delusions of thought insertion. . Not sure *or* not applicable *or* missing.	
DEL3. Delusions of thought withdrawal	
Do you think that your thoughts were taken out of your mind by an outside person or force? 0 Patient has no delusions of thought withdrawal. 1 Patient has delusions of thought withdrawal. . Not sure *or* not applicable *or* missing.	
DEL4. Delusions of thought broadcasting	
Do you think that your thoughts are broadcast so that people are able to know what you are thinking, even if they are in different places? 0 Patient has no delusions of thought broadcast. 1 Patient has delusions of thought broadcast. . Not sure *or* not applicable *or* missing.	
DEL5. Paranoid/persecutory delusions	
Have you felt that people are against you, talking about you, or laughing at you? Do you think someone is trying to harm you (e.g., trying to poison your food or trying to kill you)? 0 Patient has no paranoid/persecutory delusions. 1 Patient has paranoid/persecutory delusions some of the time. 2 Patient has paranoid/persecutory delusions most of the time. . Not sure *or* not applicable *or* missing.	
DEL6. Delusions of conspiracy	
Do you think there is a plot or a conspiracy against you by anyone (e.g., a person, FBI, CIA)? 0 Patient has no delusions of conspiracy. 1 Patient has delusions of conspiracy some of the time. 2 Patient has delusions of conspiracy most of the time. . Not sure *or* not applicable *or* missing.	
DEL7. Delusions of reference	
When you are watching TV, listening to the radio, or reading the newspaper, do you think that special messages are intended specifically for you? 0 Patient has no delusions of reference. 1 Patient has delusions of reference some of the time. 2 Patient has delusions of reference most of the time. . Not sure *or* not applicable *or* missing.	

(continued)

Appendix II (continued)

DEL8. Other delusions	
Do you have any other strange thoughts or beliefs that other people do not have? 0 Patient has no other delusions. 1 Patient has other delusions. . Not sure *or* not applicable *or* missing.	
DEL9. Bizarreness of delusions (delusions are bizarre if they are completely impossible (e.g., patient believes he/she was born on Mars and brought to earth on a spaceship))	
0 Patient has no bizarre delusions. 1 Patient has bizarre delusions. . Not sure *or* not applicable *or* missing.	

Delusion score			
Severity of delusions	**1**	**Mild**	**1–3**
	2	**Moderate**	**4–5**
	3	**Severe**	**6 or more**

SCIP Disorganization Scale

DIS1. Derailment (looseness of association)	*Score*
0 Normal speech. 1 Patient has derailment (looseness of association): speech shifts to different topics, related or unrelated, but eventually comes back to the main topic. 2 Patient has severe derailment (looseness of association): speech shifts to different topics, mostly unrelated and never comes back to main topic. . Not sure *or* not applicable *or* missing.	
DIS2. Tangentiality	
0 Normal speech. 1 Patient has some tangentiality: replying to a question is related in some distant way. 2 Patient has severe tangentiality: replying to a question is totally unrelated. . Not sure *or* not applicable *or* missing.	
DIS3. Incoherent speech	
0 Normal speech. 1 Patient has incoherent speech: each sentence by itself makes sense, however, the first sentence is unrelated to the next sentence. . Not sure *or* not applicable *or* missing.	
DIS4. Other disorganized thoughts (e.g., illogical speech, word salad)	
0 Thoughts are organized. 1 Patient has other disorganized thoughts. . Not sure *or* not applicable *or* missing.	

Disorganization score			
Severity of disorganization	**1**	**Mild**	**1–2**
	2	**Moderate**	**3–4**
	3	**Severe**	**5–6**

SCIP Aggression Scale

AG1. Verbal agitation	***Score***
0 Patient has no verbal agitation. 1 Patient is verbally agitated causing people to **feel annoyed** (e.g., makes loud noises, shouts angrily, constant whining or constant attention seeking). . Not sure *or* not applicable *or* missing.	
AG2. Verbal aggression	
0 Patient has no verbal aggression. 1 Patient is verbally aggressive causing people to **feel insulted or scared** (e.g., cursing or using foul language, makes threats to others or self). . Not sure *or* not applicable *or* missing.	
AG3. Physical agitation	
0 Patient has no physical agitation. 1 Patient is **physically agitated towards self** (e.g., pacing up and down or disrobing). . Not sure *or* not applicable *or* missing.	
AG4. Destructiveness to objects	
0 Patient is not destructive to objects. 1 Patient is destructive to objects (e.g., slams doors, throws clothes or objects, kicks wall or furniture, breaks objects, smashes windows). . Not sure *or* not applicable *or* missing.	
AG5. Violence towards people	
0 Patient is not violent towards people. 1 Patient is physically violent and threatening **towards people without touching** (e.g., makes threatening gesture, swings at people). 2 **Patient is physically violent and touches victims with or without resulting injury** (e.g., grabs at clothes, strikes, kicks, pulls hair, attacks). . Not sure *or* not applicable *or* missing.	
AG6. Frequency of destructive or violent episodes	
0 Patient has no destructive or violent episodes. 1 Patient had one destructive episode to objects. 2 Patient had one violent episode towards people. 3 Patient had two destructive or violent episodes. 4 Patient had three or more destructive or violent episodes. . Not sure *or* not applicable *or* missing.	

Severity of aggression	**1**	**Mild**	**1–3**
	2	**Moderate**	**4–8**
	3	**Severe**	**9 or more**

SCIP Negative Symptoms Scale

Note to interviewer rate only if negative symptoms are not caused by medications, mood disorders, catatonia or any other known causes.

NEG1. Anhedonia (loss of pleasure and interest)	Score
Have you been unable to experience pleasure and enjoy things that you used to enjoy like exercising, enjoying hobbies, or socializing with friends? 0 Patient has no anhedonia. 1 Patient has anhedonia less than half the time. 2 Patient has anhedonia more than half the time. . Not sure *or* not applicable *or* missing.	
NEG2. Blunted/flat affect (decrease in affective expression) ***Decreased facial expression, e.g., not smiling or laughing at a joke, poor eye contact, indifference to things around, loss of emotional reaction and indifference***	
0 Patient has broad affect. 1 Patient has blunted affect. 2 Patient has flat affect. . Not sure *or* not applicable *or* missing.	
NEG3. Avolition (decrease in goal-directed activities) ***Decrease in the three main goal-directed activities in life: school or work, or social activities with other people***	
0 Patient has normal activities. 1 Patient has avolition less than half time. 2 Patient has avolition more than half time. . Not sure *or* not applicable *or* missing.	
NEG4. Alogia ***Poverty of speech, poverty of content of speech***	
0 Patient has normal speech. 1 Patient has alogia less than half time. 2 Patient has alogia more than half time. . Not sure *or* not applicable *or* missing.	
NEG5. Psychomotor slowing (psychomotor retardation) ***Patient is moving slow, patient is talking slow, or patient is usually sitting or lying down***	
0 Patient has normal activities. 1 Patient has psychomotor slowing less than half time. 2 Patient has psychomotor slowing more than half time. . Not sure *or* not applicable *or* missing.	
NEG6. Poor self-care ***Patient does not wear proper clothes for the weather, does not shower regularly, does not eat properly, very dirty, and disheveled***	
0 Patient has proper self-care. 1 Patient has poor self-care less than half time. 2 Patient has poor self-care more than half time. . Not sure *or* not applicable *or* missing.	

Negative symptoms score			
Severity of negative symptoms	**1**	**Mild**	**1–3**
	2	**Moderate**	**4–8**
	3	**Severe**	**9 or more**

SCIP Core Schizophrenia Scale (CSS-22)

Codes: Unless otherwise specified in the question, the rating of a symptom is as follows:	
0	**Absent or nonsignificant**
1	**Symptom present < 50% of the time or <50% of times**
2	**Symptom present > 50% of the time or >50% of times**
(A positive rating of 1or 2 implies that the patient has the symptom more than most people, or has at least some distress, or seeks professional help).	
.	**Not sure *or* not applicable *or* missing.**

Questions apply to the present episode, typically the past month, unless otherwise specified by the interviewer.

Hallucinations

1_HAL1. Auditory hallucinations	*Score*
Do you hear noises (like music, whispering sounds) or voices talking to you when there is no one around? ***Are the voices like a real voice or just thoughts in your mind?*** 0 Patient has no auditory hallucinations. 1 Patient has auditory hallucinations. 2 Patient has auditory hallucinations with command. . Not sure *or* not applicable *or* missing.	
2_HAL2. Frequency of auditory hallucinations	
How often do you hear noises (like music, whispering sounds) or voices talking to you when there is no one around? 0 Patient has no auditory hallucinations. 1 Patient has auditory hallucinations (1–4 days/month). 2 Patient has auditory hallucinations (5–15 days/month). 3 Patient has auditory hallucinations (>15 days/month). . Not sure *or* not applicable *or* missing.	
3_HAL3. Hallucination duration	
On days when you hear noises or voices, how often do you hear them? 0 Patient has no auditory hallucinations. 1 Patient has auditory hallucinations (less than 1 hour/day). 2 Patient has auditory hallucinations (1–4 hours/day). 3 Patient has auditory hallucinations (more than 4 hours/day). . Not sure *or* not applicable *or* missing.	
4_HAL4. Audible thoughts	
Do you think that your thoughts are so loud that someone close to you can hear what you are thinking? 0 Patient has no audible thoughts. 1 Patient has audible thoughts. . Not sure *or* not applicable *or* missing.	
5_HAL5. Voices arguing	
Do you hear two or more voices that argue about what you are doing or thinking? 0 Voices do not argue with the patient. 1 Voices argue about what the patient is doing or thinking. . Not sure *or* not applicable *or* missing.	
6_HAL6. Voices commenting	
Do you hear a voice or voices commenting on what you are doing or thinking? 0 Voices do not comment about the patient. 1 Voices comment on what the patient is doing or thinking. . Not sure *or* not applicable *or* missing.	

(continued)

Appendix II (continued)

7_HAL7. Visual hallucinations	
Do you see things other people cannot see (e.g., shadows, objects, or people)? 0 Patient has no visual hallucinations. 1 Patient has visual hallucinations. . Not sure *or* not applicable *or* missing.	
8_HAL8. Observed hallucinations	
0 Patient has not been observed talking to self. 1 Patient has been observed talking to self, talking to a mirror, or running a conversation with unseen person. . Not sure *or* not applicable *or* missing.	
9_HAL9. Other hallucinations (olfactory, gustatory, tactile)	
Do you sometimes notice unusual smells that other people do not notice, experience strange tastes in your mouth, or feel strange sensations on your body? 0 Patient has no other hallucinations. 1 Patient has other hallucinations (olfactory, gustatory, or tactile hallucinations). . Not sure *or* not applicable *or* missing.	
Delusions	
10_DEL1. Somatic passivity (bizarre delusions associated with somatic sensations)	***Score***
Do you feel or have a bodily sensation (e.g., something is crawling under your skin) and think it is caused by an outside person or force? 0 Patient has no somatic passivity. 1 Patient has somatic passivity. . Not sure *or* not applicable *or* missing.	
11_DEL2. Delusions of thought insertion	
Do you think that thoughts in your mind are not your own thoughts and that they were inserted into your mind by an outside person or force? 0 Patient has no delusions of thought insertion. 1 Patient has delusions of thought insertion. . Not sure *or* not applicable *or* missing.	
12_DEL3. Delusions of thought withdrawal	
Do you think that your thoughts were taken out of your mind by an outside person or force? 0 Patient has no delusions of thought withdrawal. 1 Patient has delusions of thought withdrawal. . Not sure *or* not applicable *or* missing.	
13_DEL4. Delusions of thought broadcasting	
Do you think that your thoughts are broadcast so that people are able to know what you are thinking, even if they are in different places? 0 Patient has no delusions of thought broadcast. 1 Patient has delusions of thought broadcast. . Not sure *or* not applicable *or* missing.	
14_DEL5. Paranoid/persecutory delusions	
Have you felt that people are against you, talking about you, or laughing at you? Do you think someone is trying to harm you (e.g., trying to poison your food or trying to kill you)? 0 Patient has no paranoid/persecutory delusions. 1 Patient has paranoid/persecutory delusions some of the time. 2 Patient has paranoid/persecutory delusions most of the time. . Not sure *or* not applicable *or* missing.	

(continued)

Appendix II (continued)

15_DEL6. Delusions of conspiracy	
Do you think there is a plot or a conspiracy against you by anyone (e.g., a person, FBI, CIA)? 0 Patient has no delusions of conspiracy. 1 Patient has delusions of conspiracy some of the time. 2 Patient has delusions of conspiracy most of the time. . Not sure *or* not applicable *or* missing.	
16_DEL7. Delusions of reference	
When you are watching TV, listening to the radio, or reading the newspaper, do you think that special messages are intended specifically for you? 0 Patient has no delusions of reference. 1 Patient has delusions of reference some of the time. 2 Patient has delusions of reference most of the time. . Not sure *or* not applicable *or* missing.	
17_DEL8. Other delusions	
Do you have any other strange thoughts or beliefs that other people do not have? 0 Patient has no other delusions. 1 Patient has other delusions. . Not sure *or* not applicable *or* missing.	
18_DEL9. Bizarreness of delusions (delusions are bizarre if they are completely impossible (e.g., patient believes he/she was born on Mars and brought to earth on a spaceship))	
0 Patient has no bizarre delusions. 1 Patient has bizarre delusions. . Not sure *or* not applicable *or* missing.	

Disorganization

19_DIS1. Derailment (looseness of association)	***Score***
0 Normal speech. 1 Patient has derailment (looseness of association): speech shifts to different topics, related or unrelated, but eventually comes back to the main topic. 2 Patient has severe derailment (looseness of association): speech shifts to different topics, mostly unrelated and never comes back to main topic. . Not sure *or* not applicable *or* missing.	
20_DIS2. Tangentiality	
0 Normal speech. 1 Patient has some tangentiality: replying to a question is related in some distant way. 2 Patient has severe tangentiality: replying to a question is totally unrelated. . Not sure *or* not applicable *or* missing.	3
21_DIS3. Incoherent speech	
0 Normal speech. 1 Patient has incoherent speech: each sentence by itself makes sense, however, the first sentence is unrelated to the next sentence. . Not sure *or* not applicable *or* missing.	
22_DIS4. Other disorganized thoughts (e.g., illogical speech, word salad)	
0 Thoughts are organized. 1 Patient has other disorganized thoughts. . Not sure *or* not applicable *or* missing.	

SCIP Alcohol Scale

Codes for alcohol use disorder
0 Absent or nonsignificant.
1 Symptom present.
. Not sure *or* not applicable *or* missing.
Questions apply to the past year, unless otherwise specified.

Questions apply to the past year, unless otherwise specified by the interviewer. "Over the past year…."

How often do you drink alcohol?

0	Never or monthly or less.
1	2–4 times a month.
2	2–4 times a week.
3	5 or more times a week.

On a typical day when you drink alcohol, how many drinks do you usually have?

0	1–2 drinks a day.
1	3–5 drinks a day.
2	6 or more drinks a day.

When was the last time you had a drink containing alcohol?

ALC1. Tolerance	*Score*
Did you use a lot more alcohol than you previously used to get the same effect (compared when you first started to drink)? ***Did you notice that the same amount of alcohol you take now has less effect than before (compared when you first started to drink)?*** 0 Patient had no tolerance to alcohol. 1 Patient had tolerance to alcohol. . Not sure *or* not applicable *or* missing.	
ALC2. Withdrawal	
When you stopped or cut down on alcohol use, did you have withdrawal symptoms? (Interviewer gives examples of alcohol withdrawal symptoms) 0 Patient had no withdrawal symptoms from alcohol. 1 Patient had withdrawal symptoms from alcohol. . Not sure *or* not applicable *or* missing.	
ALC3. Failure to fulfill major obligations	
Did alcohol use result in failure to fulfill major role obligations (work, school, or home)? 0 Alcohol had no effect on work, school or social obligations. 1 Alcohol had negative effect on work, school or social obligations. . Not sure *or* not applicable *or* missing.	
ALC4. Social, interpersonal problems due to alcohol	
Did alcohol cause any social or interpersonal problems (e.g., work problems, school problems, relationship problems, family problems, legal problems, physical fights)? 0 Alcohol caused no social or interpersonal problems. 1 Alcohol caused social or interpersonal problems. . Not sure *or* not applicable *or* missing.	

(continued)

Appendix II (continued)

ALC5. Alcohol use in spite of problems	
Did you continue to use alcohol even though you had problems? 0 Patient had no alcohol problems. 1 Patient continued to use alcohol even though alcohol caused problems. . Not sure *or* not applicable *or* missing.	
ALC6. Alcohol use in hazardous situations	
Did you use alcohol in a situation, in which it was physically hazardous (e.g., driving a car or operating machinery)? 0 Patient did not use alcohol in hazardous situations. 1 Patient used alcohol in hazardous situations. . Not sure *or* not applicable *or* missing.	
ALC7. Alcohol blackout	
Did you have a blackout after drinking so much alcohol that the next day you could not remember what you said or did? 0 Patient had no blackout. 1 Patient had blackout. . Not sure *or* not applicable *or* missing.	
ALC8. Other alcohol problems	
Did you have any other problems due to alcohol use? 0 No. 1 Yes (specify). . Not sure *or* not applicable *or* missing.	

Alcoholism score = Severity of alcoholism		
1	**Mild**	**1–3**
2	**Moderate**	**4–5**
3	**Severe**	**6 or more**

SCIP Drug Scale

Codes for drug use disorder
0 Absent or nonsignificant.
1 Symptom present.
. Not sure *or* not applicable *or* missing.
Questions apply to the past year, unless otherwise specified.

Name of the drug

Questions apply to the past year, unless otherwise specified by the interviewer.
"Over the past year…."

How often do you use the drug?

0	Never or monthly or less.
1	2–4 times a month.
2	2–4 times a week.
3	5 or more times a week.

When was the last time you used the drug?

DRUG1. Tolerance	***Score***
Did you use a lot more of the drug than you previously used to get the same effect (compared when you first started to use the drug)? ***Did you notice that the same amount of the drug you take now has less effect than before (compared when you first started to use the drug)?*** 0 Patient had no tolerance to the drug. 1 Patient had tolerance to the drug. . Not sure *or* not applicable *or* missing.	
DRUG2. Withdrawal	
When you stopped or cut down on the drug use, did you have withdrawal symptoms? (Interviewer gives examples of the drug withdrawal symptoms) 0 Patient had no withdrawal symptoms from the drug. 1 Patient had withdrawal symptoms from the drug. . Not sure *or* not applicable *or* missing.	
DRUG3. Failure to fulfill major obligations	
Did the drug use result in failure to fulfill major role obligations at work, school, or home? 0 Drug use had no effect on work, school or social obligations. 1 Drug use had a negative effect on work, school or social obligations. . Not sure *or* not applicable *or* missing.	
DRUG4. Social, interpersonal problems due to drug	
Did the drug cause any social or interpersonal problems (e.g., work problems, school problems, relationship problems, family problems, legal problems, physical fights)? 0 Drug caused no social or interpersonal problems. 1 Drug caused social or interpersonal problems. . Not sure *or* not applicable *or* missing.	
DRUG5. Drug use in spite of problems	
Did you continue to use the drug even though you had problems? 0 Patient had no problems from the drug use. 1 Patient continued to use the drug even though the drug caused problems. . Not sure *or* not applicable *or* missing.	

(continued)

Appendix II (continued)

DRUG6. Drug use in hazardous situations	
Did you use the drug in a situation, in which it was physically hazardous (e.g., driving a car or operating machinery)? 0 Patient did not use the drug in hazardous situations. 1 Patient used the drug in hazardous situations. . Not sure *or* not applicable *or* missing.	
DRUG7. Other drug problems	
Did you have any other problems due to drug use? 0 No. 1 Yes (specify). . Not sure *or* not applicable *or* missing.	

Drug abuse score			
Severity of drug abuse	**1**	**Mild**	**1–3**
	2	**Moderate**	**4–5**
	3	**Severe**	**6 or more**

SCIP ADHD Scale (Long) (Past month)

Codes for ADHD	
0 Absent or nonsignificant.	
1 Symptom present.	
. Not sure *or* not applicable *or* missing.	
Questions apply to the past month, unless otherwise specified.	
Attention deficit	
ATT1. Attention impairment/poor concentration	***Score***
Do you have difficulty paying attention and concentrating when reading an article, watching a TV show or a movie, or doing your work or school assignments? 0 Absent or nonsignificant. 1 Patient has poor attention and concentration. . Not sure *or* not applicable *or* missing.	
ATT2. Sustained attention impairment	
Do you have difficulty concentrating on one thing for a long time (e.g., reading a book, writing a letter)? 0 Absent or nonsignificant. 1 Patient has difficulty concentrating for a long period of time. . Not sure *or* not applicable *or* missing.	
ATT3. Avoiding sustained attention tasks	
Do you avoid tasks that require a lot of concentration at work, school, or home (e.g., reading a book, writing a letter)? 0 Absent or nonsignificant. 1 Patient avoids tasks that require sustained mental effort. . Not sure *or* not applicable *or* missing.	
ATT4. Attention when spoken to	
Do you have difficulty concentrating on what people say to you, even when they are speaking to you directly? 0 Absent or nonsignificant. 1 Patient has difficulty concentrating on what people say. . Not sure *or* not applicable *or* missing.	
ATT5. Organization and meeting deadlines	
Do you have difficulty with tasks that require organization and keeping track of many things all at once (e.g., planning and organizing your work or household chores)? Do you have difficulty managing your time (e.g., usually fail to meet deadlines)? 0 Absent or nonsignificant. 1 Patient has difficulty with tasks that require organization or meeting deadlines. . Not sure *or* not applicable *or* missing.	
ATT6. Changing activities	
Do you change from one activity to another without finishing the first? 0 Absent or nonsignificant. 1 Patient changes from one activity to another without finishing the first. . Not sure *or* not applicable *or* missing.	
ATT7. Distraction (attention is distracted by environmental noises)	
Are you easily distracted from tasks by activity or noise around you? 0 Absent or nonsignificant. 1 Patient is easily distracted from tasks by activity or noise. . Not sure *or* not applicable *or* missing.	

(continued)

Appendix II (continued)

ATT8. Misplacing things	
Do you lose or misplace things more often than others do (e.g., wallets, keys, cell phones)? 0 Absent or nonsignificant. 1 Patient loses or misplaces things more often than others do. . Not sure *or* not applicable *or* missing.	
ATT9. Forgetting daily activities	
Do you forget daily activities more often than others do (e.g., appointments, paying bills, returning phone calls)? 0 Absent or nonsignificant. 1 Patient forgets daily activities more often than others do. . Not sure *or* not applicable *or* missing.	
ATT10. Losing track	
Do you lose track of what you are doing (e.g., forget why you went to get something)? 0 Absent or nonsignificant. 1= Patient loses track of what he or she is doing. . Not sure *or* not applicable *or* missing.	

Attention problem score			
Severity of attention problems	**1**	**Mild**	**1–3**
	2	**Moderate**	**4–8**
	3	**Severe**	**9 or more**

Hyperactivity

HYP1. Fidgety	***Score***
Do you have difficulty remaining seated (fidget with hands and feet, squirm, or wiggle in seat) when expected to remain seated (e.g., in a meeting or a church service)? 0 Absent or nonsignificant. 1 Patient has difficulty remaining seated when expected to. . Not sure *or* not applicable *or* missing.	
HYP2. Leaving seats	
Do you leave your seat in meetings or other situations (e.g., during an appointment or a church service) where you are expected to remain seated? 0 Absent or nonsignificant. 1 Patient leaves seat in meetings or other situations when expected to remain seated. . Not sure *or* not applicable *or* missing.	
HYP3. Restlessness/moving	
Do you feel restless, fidgety, and that you must get up and move around? 0 Absent or nonsignificant. 1 Patient feels restless, fidgety and must move around. . Not sure *or* not applicable *or* missing.	
HYP4. Hyperactivity	
Do you feel overly active and compelled to do things, like you are driven by a motor? 0 Absent or nonsignificant. 1 Patient feels overly active and compelled to do things. . Not sure *or* not applicable *or* missing.	
HYP5. Waiting in line	
Is it difficult for you to wait in line for your turn when the situation calls for it? 0 Absent or nonsignificant. 1 Patient has difficulty waiting in line. . Not sure *or* not applicable *or* missing.	
HYP6. Talking too much	
Do you think you talk too much? ***Do others say that you talk too much?*** 0 Absent or nonsignificant. 1 Patient talks too much. . Not sure *or* not applicable *or* missing.	
HYP7. Loud and noisy	
Do you think that you are a loud and noisy person? ***Do other people sometimes ask you to quiet down or lower your voice?*** 0 Absent or nonsignificant. 1 Patient or others feel the patient is loud and noisy. . Not sure *or* not applicable *or* missing.	
HYP8. Impulsivity	
Are you impulsive (e.g., act before you think adequately about consequences of actions)? 0 Absent or nonsignificant. 1 Patient is impulsive. . Not sure *or* not applicable *or* missing.	

(continued)

Appendix II (continued)

HYP9. Disturbing others
Do you disturb others or intrude on others (e.g., when people are talking or when people are involved in activities?) 0 Absent or nonsignificant. 1 Patient disturbs others or intrudes on others. . Not sure *or* not applicable *or* missing.
HYP10. Blurt out answers
Do you have tendency to blurt out the answer before another person has finished asking the question? 0 Absent or nonsignificant. 1 Patient blurts out the answers. . Not sure *or* not applicable *or* missing.

Hyperactivity score			
Severity of hyperactivity	**1**	**Mild**	**1–3**
	2	**Moderate**	**4–8**
	3	**Severe**	**9 or more**

SCIP ADHD Scale (Short) (Past month)

Attention deficit

ATT1. Attention impairment/poor concentration	***Score***
Do you have difficulty paying attention and concentrating when reading an article, watching a TV show or a movie, or doing your work or school assignments? 0 Absent or nonsignificant. 1 Patient has poor attention and concentration. . Not sure *or* not applicable *or* missing.	
ATT2. Sustained attention impairment	
Do you have difficulty concentrating on one thing for a long time (e.g., reading a book, writing a letter)? 0 Absent or nonsignificant. 1 Patient has difficulty concentrating for a long period of time. . Not sure *or* not applicable *or* missing.	
ATT3. Attention when spoken to	
Do you have difficulty concentrating on what people say to you, even when they are speaking to you directly? 0 Absent or nonsignificant. 1 Patient has difficulty concentrating on what people say. . Not sure *or* not applicable *or* missing.	
ATT4. Changing activities	
Do you change from one activity to another without finishing the first? 0 Absent or nonsignificant. 1 Patient changes from one activity to another without finishing the first. . Not sure *or* not applicable *or* missing.	
ATT5. Distraction (attention is distracted by environmental noises)	
Are you easily distracted from tasks by activity or noise around you? 0 Absent or nonsignificant. 1 Patient is easily distracted from tasks by activity or noise. . Not sure *or* not applicable *or* missing.	

Hyperactivity

HYP1. Fidgety	***Score***
Do you have difficulty remaining seated (fidget with hands and feet, squirm, or wiggle in seat) when expected to remain seated (e.g., in a meeting or a church service)? 0 Absent or nonsignificant. 1 Patient has difficulty remaining seated when expected to. . Not sure *or* not applicable *or* missing.	
HYP2. Leaving seats	
Do you leave your seat in meetings or other situations (e.g., during an appointment or a church service) where you are expected to remain seated? 0 Absent or nonsignificant. 1 Patient leaves seat in meetings or other situations when expected to remain seated. . Not sure *or* not applicable *or* missing.	
HYP3. Restlessness/moving	
Do you feel restless, fidgety, and that you must get up and move around? 0 Absent or nonsignificant. 1 Patient feels restless, fidgety and must move around. . Not sure *or* not applicable *or* missing.	

(continued)

HYP4. Hyperactivity	
Do you feel overly active and compelled to do things, like you are driven by a motor? 0 Absent or nonsignificant. 1 Patient feels overly active and compelled to do things. . Not sure *or* not applicable *or* missing.	
HYP5. Impulsivity	
Are you impulsive (e.g., act before you think adequately about consequences of actions)? 0 Absent or nonsignificant. 1 Patient is impulsive. . Not sure *or* not applicable *or* missing.	

SCIP Anorexia Nervosa Scale

Codes for eating disorders
0 Absent or nonsignificant.
1 Symptom present.
. Not sure *or* not applicable *or* missing.
Questions apply to the past THREE months, unless otherwise specified.

A. How tall are you? ____feet _____ inches
B. How much do you weigh now? ____lbs.
C. What has been your highest weight ever (when not pregnant)? ____lbs.
When was that? ____________________________
D. What has been your lowest weight ever (when not physically ill)? ____lbs.
When was that? ____________________________

Anorexia nervosa

EATING1. Being underweight	*Score*
***Have you ever** been very thin and could not maintain a minimal normal weight? **Have people ever** said you weighed much less than normal?* 0 Absent or nonsignificant. 1 Symptoms present. . Not sure *or* not applicable *or* missing.	
EATING2. Weight affects feeling	
Do you feel that your weight and shape are very important and affect how you feel about yourself to the point that you do not worry about the health risks of being so little? 0 Absent or nonsignificant. 1 Symptoms present. . Not sure *or* not applicable *or* missing.	
EATING3. Fear of weight gain	
Do you have an intense fear of gaining weight or becoming fat, even though you are underweight? 0 Absent or nonsignificant. 1 Symptoms present. . Not sure *or* not applicable *or* missing.	
EATING4. Losing weight by fasting	
Do you try to lose weight by fasting (not eating anything at all for at least 24 hours)? 0 Absent or nonsignificant. 1 Symptoms present. . Not sure *or* not applicable *or* missing.	
EATING5. Losing weight by exercise	
Do you try to lose weight by exercising too much (more than one hour a day for at least one week)? 0 Absent or nonsignificant. 1 Symptoms present. . Not sure *or* not applicable *or* missing.	

(continued)

Appendix II (continued)

EATING6. Losing weight by using diet pills	
Do you try to lose weight by using diet pills? 0 Absent or nonsignificant. 1 Symptoms present. . Not sure *or* not applicable *or* missing.	
EATING7. Losing weight by vomiting	
Do you try to lose weight by inducing vomiting? 0 Absent or nonsignificant. 1 Symptoms present. . Not sure *or* not applicable *or* missing.	
EATING8. Losing weight by laxatives	
Do you try to lose weight by taking laxatives or using enemas? 0 Absent or nonsignificant. 1 Symptoms present. . Not sure *or* not applicable *or* missing.	
EATING9. Losing weight by other methods	
Do you try to lose weight by taking diuretics? ***Do you try to lose weight by other methods?*** 0 Absent or nonsignificant. 1 Symptoms present. . Not sure *or* not applicable *or* missing.	
Anorexia nervosa score ***(Add EATING1 to EATING 9)***	

SCIP Binge and Bulimia Scale

Codes for eating disorders
0 Absent or nonsignificant.
1 Symptom present.
. Not sure *or* not applicable *or* missing.
Questions apply to the past TH

REE months, unless otherwise specified.

E. How tall are you? ____feet _____ inches
F. How much do you weigh now? ____lbs.
G. What has been your highest weight ever (when not pregnant)? ____lbs.
When was that? ______________________________
H. What has been your lowest weight ever (when not physically ill)? ____lbs.
When was that? ______________________________

Binge eating

EATING1. Binge eating	*Score*
Do you have episodes of binge eating (eating within one or two-hour period what most people would consider an unusually large amount of food)? 0 Absent or nonsignificant. 1 Symptoms present. . Not sure *or* not applicable *or* missing.	
EATING2. Binge eating frequency	
0 None. 1 1–3 times per month. 2 At least once a week for 3 months. . Not sure *or* not applicable *or* missing.	
EATING3. Losing control with binge eating	
During the episodes of binge eating, did you feel that you had lost control and could not stop eating? 0 Absent or nonsignificant. 1 Symptoms present. . Not sure *or* not applicable *or* missing.	
EATING4. Eating fast during binge eating	
During the episodes of binge eating, did you eat much more rapidly than usual? 0 Absent or nonsignificant. 1 Symptoms present. . Not sure *or* not applicable *or* missing.	
EATIG5. Eating until uncomfortably full during binge eating	
During the episodes of binge eating, did you eat until you felt uncomfortably full? 0 Absent or nonsignificant. 1 Symptoms present. . Not sure *or* not applicable *or* missing.	
EATING6. Eating when not hungry during binge eating	
During the episodes of binge eating, did you eat a large amount of food when you did not feel physically hungry? 0 Absent or nonsignificant. 1 Symptoms present. . Not sure *or* not applicable *or* missing.	

(continued)

Appendix II (continued)

EATING7. Eating alone during binge eating	
During the episodes of binge eating, did you eat alone because you were embarrassed by how much you were eating? 0 Absent or nonsignificant. 1 Symptoms present. . Not sure *or* not applicable *or* missing.	
EATING8. Feeling disgusted and guilty during binge eating	
***During the episodes of binge eating, did you feel disgusted with yourself, depressed or guilty by your overeating*?** 0 Absent or nonsignificant. 1 Symptoms present. . Not sure *or* not applicable *or* missing.	
EATING9. Distressed by overeating during binge eating	
During the episodes of binge eating, did you feel quite upset or very distressed by your overeating? 0 Absent or nonsignificant. 1 Symptoms present. . Not sure *or* not applicable *or* missing.	
Binge eating score ***(Add EATING1 to EATING9)***	
Bulimia nervosa	
EATING10. Fasting after binge eating	
After binge eating episodes, did you try to lose weight by fasting (not eating anything at all for at least 24 hours)? 0 = Absent or nonsignificant. 1 = Symptoms present. . Not sure *or* not applicable *or* missing.	
EATING11. Exercise after binge eating	
After binge eating episodes, did you try to lose weight by exercising too much (more than one hour a day for at least one week)? 0 = Absent or nonsignificant. 1 = Symptoms present. . Not sure *or* not applicable *or* missing.	
ATING12. Using diet pills after binge eating	
After binge eating episodes, did you try to lose weight by using diet pills? 0 Absent or nonsignificant. 1 Symptoms present. . Not sure *or* not applicable *or* missing.	
EATING13. Vomiting after binge eating	
After binge eating episodes, did you try to lose weight by inducing vomiting? 0 Absent or nonsignificant. 1 Symptoms present. . Not sure *or* not applicable *or* missing.	
EATING14. Taking laxatives after binge eating	
After binge eating episodes, did you try to lose weight by taking laxatives or enemas? 0 = Absent or nonsignificant. 1 = Symptoms present. . Not sure *or* not applicable *or* missing.	

(continued)

Appendix II (continued)

EATING15. Other losing weight methods after binge eating	
After binge eating episodes, did you try to lose weight by taking diuretics? ***Do you try to lose weight by other methods?*** 0 = Absent or nonsignificant. 1 = Symptoms present. . Not sure *or* not applicable *or* missing.	
Bulimia nervosa score ***(Add EATING1 to EATING 15)***	

Appendix III

The SCIP Self-Administered (SA) Scales

	Self-administered (SA) scales	Number of items	Reliability	Validity
1	**Anxiety**	**7**	**Yes**	**Yes**
2	**Panic**	**5**	**Yes**	**Yes**
3	**Phobia**	**9**	**Not studied**	**Not studied**
4	**OCD**	**18**	**Not studied**	**Not studied**
5	**PTSD**	**16**	**Yes**	**Yes**
6	**Depression**	**12**	**Yes**	**Yes**
7	**Mania**	**11**	**Yes**	**Yes**
8	**Hallucinations**	**9**	**Yes**	**Poor validity**
9	**Delusions**	**9**	**Yes**	**Poor validity**
10	**Alcohol**	**8**	**Yes**	**Yes**
11	**Drug**	**7**	**Yes**	**Yes**
12	**ADHD**	**20**	**Yes**	**Yes**
13	**Anorexia Nervosa**	**9**	**Not studied**	**Not studied**
14	**Binge and Bulimia**	**15**	**Not studied**	**Not studied**
15	**Intake self-administered**	**18**	**Yes**	**Yes**

(continued)

SCIP Generalized Anxiety Scale (Self-Administered)

Instructions Circle the number that best describes how you have felt either during the past month OR since your last visit.

<u>During the past month OR since your last visit…</u>

1. Have you had excessive worry and anxiety for long periods of time (e.g., for hours each day, lasting several months), <u>not</u> just during panic attacks?

0 No, *or* Some anxiety, but it does not bother me.
1 Yes.
. Not sure *or* not applicable *or* missing.

2. Have you felt restless, keyed up, or on edge when anxious?

0 No.
1 Yes.
. Not sure *or* not applicable *or* missing.

3. Have you felt tense in your muscles when anxious?

0 No.
1 Yes.
. Not sure *or* not applicable *or* missing.

4. Have you felt tired or easily exhausted even without work when anxious?

0 No.
1 Yes.
. Not sure *or* not applicable *or* missing.

5. Have you had difficulty concentrating when anxious?

2 No.
3 Yes.
. Not sure *or* not applicable *or* missing.

6. Have you felt irritable when anxious?

2 No.
3 Yes.
. Not sure *or* not applicable *or* missing.

7. Have you had difficulty falling asleep or staying asleep when anxious?

2 No.
3 Yes.
. Not sure *or* not applicable *or* missing.

Generalized anxiety score

Severity of anxiety	**1**	**Mild**	**1–3**
	2	**Moderate**	**4–5**
	3	**Severe**	**6 or more**

SCIP Panic Scale (Self-Administered)

Instructions Please circle the number that best describes how you felt **during the past month.**

1a. Did you have a panic attack, when you suddenly become anxious and frightened for a short period of time (up to 60 minutes)?

3 *No.*
4 *Yes.*
. *Not sure or not applicable or missing.*

1b. During that time, did you feel that your heart was racing or pounding, or did you start shaking or sweating, or did you feel you were choking?

0 *No.*
1 *Yes.*
. *Not sure or not applicable or missing.*

2. Please write down the frequency of panic attacks you have per week in the space provided below.

3a. After a panic attack, do you worry about having another attack?

0 No.
1 Yes.
. Not sure *or* not applicable *or* missing.

3***b. Do you worry about the effects of panic attacks (e.g., losing control, having a heart attack or going crazy)?***

0 No.
1 Yes.
. Not sure *or* not applicable *or* missing.

4a. Did you have to do something to end the panic attack, like leaving a store, calling someone, taking deep breaths?

0 No.
1 Yes.
. Not sure *or* not applicable *or* missing.

4b. Do you do anything to prevent panic attacks (like avoiding places that trigger the panic attacks)?

0 No.
1 Yes.
. Not sure *or* not applicable *or* missing.

5. Please circle all of the symptoms (listed in the space below) that you experience while having a panic attack.

1. Patient cannot catch breath and has feeling of being smothered.
2. Patient has chest pain or discomfort.
3. Patient has feeling of choking.
4. Patient feels heart is pounding, missing beats, or beating faster.
5. Patient feels dizzy, unsteady, light-headed, or faint.
6. Patient has numbness or tingling sensations in face or fingers.
7. Patient has dry mouth or difficulty swallowing.
8. Patient has nausea or abdominal distress.
9. Patient has trembling or shaking of hands or limbs.
10. Patient has sweating, e.g., palms.
11. Patient feels very cold.
12. Patient has hot flushes.
13. Patient has fear of dying.
14. Patient has fear of going crazy or fear of losing emotional control.
15. Patient feels that things are not real.
16. Patient feels that people are not real.

Panic scale score =

SCIP Phobia Scale (Self-Administered)

Instructions Please circle the number that best describes how you felt **during the past month.**

Social phobia

1a. Have you been afraid and anxious when you do things in front of people, such as eating or speaking in public?

0 No.
1 Yes.
. Not sure or not applicable or missing.

1b. Do you avoid social situations that involves other people or endure them with intense fear?

0 No.
1 Yes.
. Not sure *or* not applicable *or* missing.

2. Have you ever experienced panic attacks because of your fear/anxiety of doing things in front of people?

0 No.
1 Yes.
. Not sure or not applicable or missing.

3. If you answered YES to question 2, please circle all of the symptoms (listed in the space below) that you experience while having a panic attack.

1. Patient cannot catch breath and has feeling of being smothered.
2. Patient has chest pain or discomfort.
3. Patient has feeling of choking.
4. Patient feels heart is pounding, missing beats, or beating faster.
5. Patient feels dizzy, unsteady, light-headed, or faint.
6. Patient has numbness or tingling sensations in face or fingers.
7. Patient has dry mouth or difficulty swallowing.
8. Patient has nausea or abdominal distress.
9. Patient has trembling or shaking of hands or limbs.
10. Patient has sweating, e.g., palms.
11. Patient feels very cold.
12. Patient has hot flushes.
13. Patient has fear of dying.
14. Patient has fear of going crazy or fear of losing emotional control.
15. Patient feels that things are not real.
16. Patient feels that people are not real.

Social phobia score

Agoraphobia

4a. Have you been afraid of being alone (at home or outside of the home), traveling in a car/ train/plane, being in an open space (e.g., park) or being in a closed space (e.g., store), or being in crowds?

0 No.
1 Yes.
. Not sure or not applicable or missing.

4b. Do you avoid these situations, or require a companion, or endure with intense fear?

0 No.
1 Yes.
. Not sure or not applicable or missing.

(continued)

Appendix III (continued)

5. Do you experience panic attacks because of your fear of being alone, traveling in a car/train/ plan, being in an open space (e.g., park), being in a closed space (e.g., store), or being in crowds?

0 No.
1 Yes.
. Not sure or not applicable or missing.

6. If you answered YES to question 5, please circle all of the symptoms (listed in the space below) that you experience while having a panic attack.

1. Patient cannot catch breath and has feeling of being smothered.
2. Patient has chest pain or discomfort.
3. Patient has feeling of choking.
4. Patient feels heart is pounding, missing beats, or beating faster.
5. Patient feels dizzy, unsteady, light-headed, or faint.
6. Patient has numbness or tingling sensations in face or fingers.
7. Patient has dry mouth or difficulty swallowing.
8. Patient has nausea or abdominal distress.
9. Patient has trembling or shaking of hands or limbs.
10. Patient has sweating, e.g., palms.
11. Patient feels very cold.
12. Patient has hot flushes.
13. Patient has fear of dying.
14. Patient has fear of going crazy or fear of losing emotional control.
15. Patient feels that things are not real.
16. Patient feels that people are not real.

Agoraphobia score

Specific phobia

7a. Have you had strong fears of certain objects or situations (e.g., heights, animals, spiders, snakes, seeing blood, receiving injections)?

0 No.
1 Yes.
. Not sure or not applicable or missing.

7b. Do you avoid objects or situations or endure with intense fear?

0 No.
1 Yes.
. Not sure or not applicable or missing.

8. Have you ever experienced a panic attack because of the object/situation you have a strong fear of?

0 No.
1 Yes.
. Not sure or not applicable or missing.

(continued)

Appendix III (continued)

9. <u>If you answered YES to question 8,</u> please circle all of the symptoms (listed in the space below) that you experience while having a panic attack.
1. Patient cannot catch breath and has feeling of being smothered. 2. Patient has chest pain or discomfort. 3. Patient has feeling of choking. 4. Patient feels heart is pounding, missing beats, or beating faster. 5. Patient feels dizzy, unsteady, light-headed, or faint. 6. Patient has numbness or tingling sensations in face or fingers. 7. Patient has dry mouth or difficulty swallowing. 8. Patient has nausea or abdominal distress. 9. Patient has trembling or shaking of hands or limbs. 10. Patient has sweating, e.g., palms. 11. Patient feels very cold. 12. Patient has hot flushes. 13. Patient has fear of dying. 14. Patient has fear of going crazy or fear of losing emotional control. 15. Patient feels that things are not real. 16. Patient feels that people are not real.
Specific phobia score

SCIP Obsessive-Compulsive Scale (Self-Administered)

Instructions Please circle the number that best describes how you felt **<u>during the past week.</u>**

Obsessions

1. "Obsessive thoughts" are thoughts or images in your mind that do not make sense and keep coming back to your mind even when you try to avoid them.
In the past week, did you have obsessive thoughts?

2 No.
3 Yes, for less than 1 hour/day.
4 Yes, for 1–4 hours/day.
5 Yes, for more than 4 hours/day.
. Not sure *or* not applicable *or* missing.

2. In the past week, on approximately how many days did you have obsessive thoughts?

0 1 2 3 4 5 6 7

3. In the past week, did you have obsessive thoughts related to aggression?
<u>Potential examples:</u> fears of harming oneself, fears of unintentionally hurting someone, urges to stab someone, thoughts of "losing control" and hurting a partner or significant other.

0 No.
1 Yes.
. Not sure *or* not applicable *or* missing.

4. In the past week, did you have obsessive thoughts related to contamination, germs, or sickness?
<u>Potential examples:</u> fear of contamination in public bathrooms, outdoors, or public places, fear of what might happen after touching one's own bodily secretions, fear of getting germs or viruses from others.

0 No.
1 Yes.
. Not sure *or* not applicable *or* missing.

5. In the past week, did you have obsessive thoughts related to sex or sexuality?
<u>Potential examples:</u> disturbing thoughts about sex, unwanted images of sexual acts toward strangers, family members or children, fear of being found with pornography.

0 No.
1 Yes.
. Not sure *or* not applicable *or* missing.

6. In the past week, did you have obsessive thoughts related to religion?
<u>Potential examples:</u> fear of having blasphemous or "sinful" thoughts, concerns for engaging in sinful or forbidden behavior, feeling the need to complete a certain number of prayers or "good deeds"

0 No.
1 Yes.
. Not sure *or* not applicable *or* missing.

7. In the past week, did you have obsessive thoughts related to your health?
<u>Potential examples:</u> worries about having an undiagnosed illness like cancer or heart disease, fear of contracting a deadly disease, images of your own death

(continued)

Appendix III (continued)

0 No.
1 Yes.
. Not sure *or* not applicable *or* missing.

8. In the past week, did you have obsessive thoughts about your physical appearance?
***Potential examples:** worries about the size of certain body parts (ears, nose, mouth), fears of certain body parts being disgusting to others*

0 No.
1 Yes.
. Not sure *or* not applicable *or* missing.

9. In the past week, did you have obsessive thoughts about anything else that was not mentioned yet?

0 No.
1 Yes.
. Not sure *or* not applicable *or* missing.

Obsession score

Severity of obsession	**1**	**Mild**	**1–3**
	2	**Moderate**	**4–8**
	3	**Severe**	**9 or more**

Compulsions

10a. ***"Compulsive behaviors" are things you feel you must do over and over, such as washing your hands even if they are clean, checking doors and windows more than once, or repeating mental acts such as counting or praying.***
In the past week, did you have compulsive behaviors?

0 No.
1 Yes, for less than 1 hour/day.
2 Yes, for 1–4 hours/day.
3 Yes, for more than 4 hours/day.
. Not sure *or* not applicable *or* missing.

10b. Do you get very anxious or tense if you did not repeat the behaviors?

0 No.
1 Yes.
. Not sure *or* not applicable *or* missing.

11. In the past week, on approximately how many days did you engage in a compulsive behavior?

0 1 2 3 4 5 6 7

12. In the past week, did you check things over and over again?
***Potential examples:** checking door locks, switches, or appliances many times before leaving the house, checking one's appearance for an excessive amount of time before leaving the house*

0 No.
1 Yes.
. Not sure *or* not applicable *or* missing.

13. In the past week, did you clean or wash things over and over again?
***Potential examples:** excessively changing your clothes, excessive handwashing, tooth brushing, showering, scrubbing surfaces*

3 No.
4 Yes.
. Not sure *or* not applicable *or* missing.

(continued)

Appendix III (continued)

14. In the past week, did you repeat things many times?
<u>Potential examples</u>: rereading text out of concerns that one "missed something," rewriting or retracing words, reentering buildings or living spaces, retying one's shoes

0 No.
1 Yes.
. Not sure *or* not applicable *or* missing.

15. In the past week, did you arrange and rearrange things, order and reorder items over and over again?
<u>Potential examples:</u> rearranging one's pantry or refrigerator, spending excessive amounts of time organizing one's desk or workspace

0 No.
1 Yes.
. Not sure *or* not applicable *or* missing.

16. In the past week, did you feel the need to collect and/or hoard things?
<u>Potential examples:</u> picking up, collecting or buying useless things, owning an excessive amount of items and being unable to donate or get rid of them

0 No.
1 Yes.
. Not sure *or* not applicable *or* missing.

17. In the past week, did you engage in any repetitive counting or rituals in your mind?
<u>Potential examples:</u> repetitively counting certain numbers or avoiding certain "bad" numbers, repeating certain
words, counting senseless things (e.g., ceiling tiles), reciting prayers or statements

0 No.
1 Yes.
. Not sure *or* not applicable *or* missing.

18. In the past week, did you engage in any other repetitive behaviors that were not yet mentioned in order to manage or avoid distress?

0 No.
1 Yes.
. Not sure *or* not applicable *or* missing.

Compulsions score/severity of compulsion		
1	**Mild**	**1–3**
2	**Moderate**	**4–8**
3	**Severe**	**9 or more**

SCIP Posttraumatic Scale (Self-Administered)

Instructions Please circle the number that best describes how you felt **during the past month.**

***1a. Have you ever witnessed or experienced** a traumatic event that involved actual or threatened death or serious injury to you or someone else (e.g., physical or sexual abuse, rape, terrorist attack, natural disaster, war)?*
0 I have not experienced any traumatic events. 1 I have experienced **one traumatic event.** 2 I have experienced **several traumatic events.** . Not sure or not applicable or missing.
1b. Did you feel intense fear and helplessness?
0 No. 1 Yes. . Not sure or not applicable or missing.
2. Did you have recurrent upsetting memories (distressing recollection) of the event?
0 No. 1 Yes. . Not sure or not applicable or missing.
3. Did you have recurrent upsetting dreams or nightmares of the event?
0 No. 1 Yes. . Not sure or not applicable or missing.
4. Did you have a sense or feeling that the event was happening again, the sense of reliving the event (flashbacks)?
0 No. 1 Yes. . Not sure or not applicable or missing.
5. Did you try to avoid thoughts and feelings associated with the event?
0 No. 1 Yes. . Not sure or not applicable or missing.
6. Did you try to avoid things that reminded you of the event (such as certain people, certain places, or some activities)?
0 No. 1 Yes. . Not sure or not applicable or missing.
7. Did you have difficulty remembering some or all important aspects of the event?
0 No. 1 Yes. . Not sure or not applicable or missing.
8. Did you spend less time or show less interest in activities with friends/family or hobbies that you used to enjoy due to the event?
0 No. 1 Yes. . Not sure or not applicable or missing.

(continued)

Appendix III (continued)

9. Did you feel distant, cut off, or isolated from other people due to the event?

0 No.
1 Yes.
. Not sure or not applicable or missing.

10a. Did you feel emotionally numb?

0 No.
1 Yes.
. Not sure or not applicable or missing.

10b. Did you have trouble experiencing feelings (happiness, love feelings) due to the event?

0 No.
1 Yes.
. Not sure or not applicable or missing.

11. Did you have difficulty falling or staying asleep due to the event?

0 No.
1 Yes.
. Not sure or not applicable or missing.

12. Did you have periods of irritability or sudden outbursts of anger due to the event?

0 No.
1 Yes.
. Not sure or not applicable or missing.

13. Did you have difficulty concentrating due to the event?

0 No.
1 Yes.
. Not sure *or* not applicable *or* missing.

14. Did you feel very alert or watchful of things going on around you even when there was no need to be?

0 No.
1 Yes.
. Not sure or not applicable or missing.

15a. Did you feel easily startled?

0 No.
1 Yes.
. Not sure *or* not applicable *or* missing.

15b. Were you easily scared or did you make a sudden movement or jump when you heard noises or if you were caught by surprise?

0 No.
1 Yes.
. Not sure *or* not applicable *or* missing.

16. Did you have any other symptoms due to the event that are troubling you?

0 No.
1 Yes (please specify in the space provided below):

PTSD score

Severity of PTSD	**1**	**Mild**	**1–3**
	2	**Moderate**	**4–8**
	3	**Severe**	**9 or more**

(continued)

SCIP Depression Scale (Self-Administered)

Instructions Circle the number that best describes how you have felt either during the past month OR since your last visit.

During the past month OR since your last visit…

1. Have you felt sad, depressed, or in low spirits?

0 No.
1 Yes, some of the time.
2 Yes, most of the time.
. Not sure *or* not applicable *or* missing.

2. Did you lose interest in things, or not enjoy things you normally would?

0 No.
1 Yes, some of the time.
2 Yes, most of the time.
. Not sure *or* not applicable *or* missing.

3. Did you feel hopeless about the future?

0 No.
1 Yes, some of the time.
2 Yes, most of the time.
. Not sure *or* not applicable *or* missing.

4. Did you have trouble concentrating to complete a task, read an article, or watch a show?

0 No.
1 Yes, some of the time.
2 Yes, most of the time.
. Not sure *or* not applicable *or* missing.

5. Did you talk or move very slowly?

0 No.
1 Yes, some of the time.
2 Yes, most of the time.
. Not sure *or* not applicable *or* missing.

6. Did you feel worthless or like a failure?

0 No.
1 Yes, some of the time.
2 Yes, most of the time.
. Not sure *or* not applicable *or* missing.

7. Did you feel very guilty or ashamed for something you have done or thought?

0 No.
1 Yes, some of the time.
2 Yes, most of the time.
. Not sure *or* not applicable *or* missing.

8. Any other depressive symptoms (for example, appetite changes, sleep changes, or losing interest in sex)?

0 No.
1 Yes.
. Not sure *or* not applicable *or* missing.

9. Did you have thoughts of killing yourself?

0 No.
1 Yes.
. Not sure *or* not applicable *or* missing.

(continued)

Appendix III (continued)

10. Did you intend to carry out the suicidal thoughts in the past month?

0 No.
1 Yes.
. Not sure *or* not applicable *or* missing.

11. Did you make a specific plan to kill yourself in the past month?

0 No.
1 Yes.
. Not sure *or* not applicable *or* missing.

12. Did you make a suicide attempt in the past month?

0 No, I did not make a suicide attempt in the past month.
1 Yes, one suicide attempt in the past month.
2 Yes, two or more suicide attempts in the past month.
. Not sure *or* not applicable *or* missing.

Depression score

Severity of depression	**1**	**Mild**	**1–4**
	2	**Moderate**	**5–8**
	3	**Severe**	**9 or more**

SCIP Mania Scale (Self-Administered)

Instructions Circle the number that best describes how you have felt either during the past month OR since your last visit.

<u>During the past month OR since your last visit…</u>

1. Did you feel extremely happy, elated, or on top of the world?

0 No.
1 Yes, some of the time.
2 Yes, most of the time.
. Not sure *or* not applicable *or* missing.

2. Did you feel irritable without a reason (for example, shouting at people, starting an argument, or becoming aggressive)?

0 No.
1 Yes, some of the time.
2 Yes, most of the time.
. Not sure *or* not applicable *or* missing.

3. Did you experience quick changes in mood or mood swings (depressed and happy or depressed and irritable) <u>on the same day?</u>

0 No.
1 Yes, some of the time.
2 Yes, most of the time.
. Not sure *or* not applicable *or* missing.

4. Did you have racing thoughts going through your mind?

0 No.
1 Yes, some of the time.
2 Yes, most of the time.
. Not sure *or* not applicable *or* missing.

5. Did you notice that you were speaking very quickly or that other people told you that you were speaking very fast?

0 No.
1 Yes, some of the time.
2 Yes, most of the time.
. Not sure *or* not applicable *or* missing.

6. Were you easily distracted by noises?

0 No.
1 Yes, some of the time.
2 Yes, most of the time.
. Not sure *or* not applicable *or* missing.

7. Did you have too much energy and start more projects than usual at work, school, or socially?

0 No.
1 Yes, some of the time.
2 Yes, most of the time.
. Not sure *or* not applicable *or* missing.

8. Did you feel very self-confident or that you have special abilities others do not have?

0 No.
1 Yes.
. Not sure *or* not applicable *or* missing.

(continued)

Appendix III (continued)

9. Did you spend a lot of money, even if you couldn't afford it?			
0 No.			
1 Yes.			
. Not sure *or* not applicable *or* missing.			
10. Did you feel rested after sleeping 4 hours or less (in a 24-hour period including naps)?			
0 No.			
1 Yes, some days.			
. Not sure *or* not applicable *or* missing.			
11. Did you engage in a risky behavior that is out of character for you (for example, being hypersexual, aggressive driving, illegal drug use, or gambling)?			
0 No.			
1 Yes.			
. Not sure *or* not applicable *or* missing.			
Mania score			
Severity of mania	**1**	**Mild**	**1–3**
	2	**Moderate**	**4–8**
	3	**Severe**	**9 or more**

SCIP Hallucinations Scale (Self-Administered)

Instructions Circle the number that best describes how you have felt either during the past month OR since your last visit.

During the past month OR since your last visit…

1. Do you hear noises (for example, music or whispering sounds) or voices talking to you when there is no one around? Do voices sometimes give you commands to do things?	
0	No.
1	Yes, but without voices telling me to do things.
2	Yes, with voices telling me do things.
.	Not sure *or* not applicable *or* missing.
2. How often did you hear these sounds or voices (hallucinations)?	
0	Never.
1	1–4 days out of the last month.
2	5–15 days out of the last month.
3	More than 15 days out of the last month.
.	Not sure *or* not applicable *or* missing.
3. How long do these sounds or voices (hallucinations) last on days when you hear them (on average)?	
0	I don't hear these sounds or voices.
1	Less than 1 hour per day.
2	1–4 hours per day.
3	More than 4 hours per day.
.	Not sure *or* not applicable *or* missing.
4. Do you think that your thoughts are so loud that someone close to you can hear what you are thinking?	
0	No.
1	Yes.
.	Not sure *or* not applicable *or* missing.
5. Do you hear two or more voices that argue about what you are doing or thinking?	
0	No.
1	Yes.
.	Not sure *or* not applicable *or* missing.
6. Do you hear a voice or voices commenting on what you are doing or thinking?	
0	No.
1	Yes.
.	Not sure *or* not applicable *or* missing.
7. Do you see things other people cannot see (for example, shadows, objects, or people)?	
0	No.
1	Yes.
.	Not sure *or* not applicable *or* missing.
8. Do people sometimes say that they observe you talking to yourself or talking to unseen?	
0	No.
1	Yes.
.	Not sure *or* not applicable *or* missing.

(continued)

Appendix III (continued)

9. Do you notice unusual smells you cannot explain?
Do experience strange tastes in your mouth?
Do you feel strange sensations on your body?

0 No.
1 Yes.
. Not sure *or* not applicable *or* missing.

Hallucination score

Severity of hallucinations	**1**	**Mild**	**1–3**
	2	**Moderate**	**4–8**
	3	**Severe**	**9 or more**

SCIP Delusions Scale (Self-Administered)

Instructions Circle the number that best describes how you have felt either **during the past month OR since your last visit.**

During the past month OR since your last visit.

1. Do you feel or have a bodily sensation (e.g., something is crawling under your skin) and think it is caused by an outside person or force?

0 No.
1 Yes.
. Not sure *or* not applicable *or* missing.

2. Do you think that thoughts in your mind are not your own thoughts and that they were inserted into your mind by an outside person or force?

0 No.
1 Yes.
. Not sure *or* not applicable *or* missing.

3. Do you think that your thoughts have been taken out of your mind by an outside person or force?

0 No.
1 Yes.
. Not sure *or* not applicable *or* missing.

4. Do you think that your thoughts are broadcast so that people are able to know what you are thinking, even if they are in different places?

0 No.
1 Yes.
. Not sure *or* not applicable *or* missing.

5. Do you think that someone or some group of people are after you, spying on you, or even trying to harm you?

0 No.
1 Yes, some of the time.
2 Yes, most of the time.
. Not sure *or* not applicable *or* missing.

6. Do you think there is a plot or a conspiracy against you by an outside person or force or agency (e.g., a person, FBI, CIA)?

0 No.
1 Yes, some of the time.
2 Yes, most of the time.
. Not sure *or* not applicable *or* missing.

7. Do you think the TV, the radio, or the newspaper are sending special messages that are intended specifically for you?

0 No.
1 Yes, some of the time.
2 Yes, most of the time.
. Not sure *or* not applicable *or* missing.

(continued)

Appendix III (continued)

8. Do you have other thoughts or beliefs that other people say they are not real?

2 No.
3 Yes.
. Not sure *or* not applicable *or* missing.

9. Do you have other thoughts or beliefs that other people say they are very strange or bizarre?

0 No.
1 Yes.
. Not sure *or* not applicable *or* missing.

Delusion score			
Severity of delusions	**1**	**Mild**	**1–3**
	2	**Moderate**	**4–5**
	3	**Severe**	**6 or more**

SCIP Alcohol Scale (Self-Administered)

Over the past year, how often do you drink alcohol (please circle one)?

0	Never or monthly or less.
1	2–4 times a month.
2	2–4 times a week.
3	5 or more times a week.

On a typical day when you drink alcohol, how many drinks do you usually have (please circle one)?

0	1–2 drinks a day.
1	3–5 drinks a day.
2	6 or more drinks a day.

When was the last time you had a drink containing alcohol (please write your answer in the space provided below)?

Instructions For the remaining questions, please circle the number that best describes how you felt **during the past year.**

1a. Did you use a lot more alcohol than you previously used to get the same effect (compared when you first started to drink)?

0 No.
1 Yes.
. Not sure *or* not applicable *or* missing.

1b. Did you notice that the same amount of alcohol you take now has less effect than before (compared when you first started to drink)?

0 No.
1 Yes.
. Not sure *or* not applicable *or* missing.

2. When you stopped or cut down on alcohol use, did you have withdrawal symptoms (e.g., shakes, hand tremors, sweating, seizure)?

0 No.
1 Yes.
. Not sure *or* not applicable *or* missing.

3. Did alcohol use result in failure to fulfill major role obligations (work, school, or home)?

0 No.
1 Yes.
. Not sure *or* not applicable *or* missing.

4. Did alcohol cause any social or interpersonal problems (e.g., work problems, school problems, relationship problems, family problems, legal problems, physical fights)?

0 No.
1 Yes.
. Not sure *or* not applicable *or* missing.

5. Did you continue to use alcohol even though you had problems?

0 No, *or* I did not have any problems.
1 Yes, I continued to use alcohol even though alcohol caused problems.
. Not sure *or* not applicable *or* missing.

(continued)

6. Did you use alcohol in a situation, in which it was physically hazardous (e.g., driving a car or operating machinery)?

0 No.
1 Yes.
. Not sure *or* not applicable *or* missing.

7. Did you have a blackout after drinking so much alcohol that the next day you could not remember what you said or did?

0 No.
1 Yes.
. Not sure *or* not applicable *or* missing.

8. Did you have any other problems due to alcohol use?

0 No.
1 Yes (please specify in the space provided below):

Alcohol use score

Severity of alcohol use score	**1**	**Mild**	**1–3**
	2	**Moderate**	**4–5**
	3	**Severe**	**6 or more**

SCIP Drug Scale (Self-Administered)

Please write in the provided space below the name of the drug causing you the most problems or that is the focus of the visit today:

Over the past year, how often did you use the drug (please circle one)?

0 Never or monthly or less.
1 2–4 times a month.
2 2–4 times a week.
3 5 or more times a week.

When was the last time you used the drug (please write your answer in the space below)?

Instructions For the remaining questions, please circle the number that best describes how you felt **during the past year.**

1a. Did you use a lot more of the drug than you previously used to get the same effect (compared when you first started to use the drug)?

0 No.
1 Yes.
. Not sure *or* not applicable *or* missing.

1b. Did you notice that the same amount of the drug you take now has less effect than before (compared when you first started to use the drug)?

0 No.
1 Yes.
. Not sure *or* not applicable *or* missing.

2. When you stopped or cut down on the drug use, did you have withdrawal symptoms?

0 No.
1 Yes.
. Not sure *or* not applicable *or* missing.

3. Did the drug use result in failure to fulfill major role obligations at work, school, or home?

0 No.
1 Yes.
. Not sure *or* not applicable *or* missing.

4. Did the drug cause any social or interpersonal problems (e.g., work problems, school problems, relationship problems, family problems, legal problems, physical fights)?

0 No.
1 Yes.
. Not sure *or* not applicable *or* missing.

5. Did you continue to use the drug even though you had problems?

0 No, *or* the drug use did not cause me any problems.
1 Yes.
. Not sure *or* not applicable *or* missing.

6. Did you use the drug in a situation, in which it was physically hazardous (e.g., driving a car or operating machinery)?

0 No.
1 Yes.
. Not sure *or* not applicable *or* missing.

7. Did you have any other problems due to drug use?

0 No.
1 Yes (please specify in the space provided below):

Severity of drug abuse	**1**	**Mild**	**1–3**
	2	**Moderate**	**4–5**
	3	**Severe**	**6 or more**

SCIP Attention Deficit Scale (Self-Administered)

Instructions *Circle the number that best describes how you have felt either* ***during the past month OR since your last visit.***

1. Do you have difficulty paying attention and concentrating when reading an article, watching a TV show or a movie, or doing your work or school assignments?

0 No, *or* sometimes, but it does not bother me.
1 Yes.
. Not sure *or* not applicable *or* missing.

2. Do you have difficulty concentrating on one thing for a long time (for example, reading a book, writing a letter)?

0 No, *or* sometimes, but it does not bother me.
1 Yes.
. Not sure *or* not applicable *or* missing.

3. Do you avoid tasks that require a lot of concentration at work, school, or home (for example, reading a book or writing a letter)?

0 No, *or* sometimes, but it does not bother me.
1 Yes.
. Not sure *or* not applicable *or* missing.

4. Do you have difficulty concentrating on what people say to you, even when they are speaking to you directly?

0 No, *or* sometimes, but it does not bother me.
1 Yes, even when they are speaking to me directly.
. Not sure *or* not applicable *or* missing.

5a. Do you have difficulty with tasks that require organization and keeping track of many things all at once (for example, planning and organizing your work or household chores)?

0 No, *or* sometimes, but it does not bother me.
1 Yes.
. Not sure *or* not applicable *or* missing.

5b. Do you have difficulty managing your time (for example, usually fail to meet deadlines)?

0 No, *or* sometimes, but it does not bother me.
1 Yes.
. Not sure *or* not applicable *or* missing.

6. Do you change from one activity to another without finishing anything?

0 No, *or* sometimes, but it does not bother me.
1 Yes.
. Not sure *or* not applicable *or* missing.

7. Are you easily distracted by activity or noise around you?

0 No, *or* sometimes, but it does not bother me.
1 Yes.
. Not sure *or* not applicable *or* missing.

8. Do you lose or misplace things more often than others do (for example, wallets, keys, cell phones)?

0 No, *or* sometimes, but it does not bother me.
1 Yes.
. Not sure *or* not applicable *or* missing.

9. Do you forget daily activities more often than others do (for example, appointments, paying bills, returning phone calls)?	
0	No, *or* sometimes, but it does not bother me.
1	Yes.
.	Not sure *or* not applicable *or* missing.
10. Do you lose track of what you are doing (for example, forget why you went to get something)?	
0	No, *or* sometimes, but it does not bother me.
1	Yes, I lose track of what I am doing.
.	Not sure *or* not applicable *or* missing.

Attention problems score			
Severity of attention problems	**1**	**Mild**	**1–3**
	2	**Moderate**	**4–8**
	3	**Severe**	**9 or more**

SCIP Hyperactivity Scale (Self-Administered)

Instructions Circle the number that best describes how you have felt either **during the past month OR since your last visit.**

1. Do you have difficulty remaining seated (fidget with hands and feet, squirm, or wiggle in seat) when expected to remain seated (for example, in a meeting or a church service)?

0 No, *or* sometimes, but it does not bother me.
1 Yes.
. Not sure *or* not applicable *or* missing.

2. Do you leave your seat in meetings or other situations (for example, during an appointment or a church service) where you are expected to remain seated?

0 No, *or* sometimes, but it does not bother me.
1 Yes.
. Not sure *or* not applicable *or* missing.

3. Do you feel restless, fidgety, and you must get up and move around?

0 No, *or* sometimes, but it does not bother me.
1 Yes.
. Not sure *or* not applicable *or* missing.

4. Do you feel overly active and you must do things, like you are driven by a motor?

0 No, *or* sometimes, but it does not bother me.
1 Yes.
. Not sure *or* not applicable *or* missing.

5. Is it difficult for you to wait in line for your turn when the situation calls for it?

0 No, *or* sometimes, but it does not bother me.
1 Yes.
. Not sure *or* not applicable *or* missing.

6. Do you think you talk too much? Do others say that you talk too much?

0 No, *or* sometimes, but it does not bother me.
1 Yes.
. Not sure *or* not applicable *or* missing.

7a. Do you think that you are a loud and noisy person?

0 No, *or* sometimes, but it does not bother me or others.
1 Yes.
. Not sure *or* not applicable *or* missing.

7b. Do other people sometimes ask you to quiet down or lower your voice?

0 No, *or* sometimes, but it does not bother me or others.
1 Yes.
. Not sure *or* not applicable *or* missing.

8. Are you impulsive (in other words, act before you think)?

0 No, *or* sometimes, but it does not bother me.
1 Yes.
. Not sure *or* not applicable *or* missing.

9. Do you disturb others or intrude on others (for example, when people are talking or when people are involved in activities?)

0 No, *or* sometimes, but it does not bother me or others.
1 Yes.
. Not sure *or* not applicable *or* missing.

10. Do you have tendency to blurt out the answer before another person has finished asking the question?

0 No, *or* sometimes, but it does not bother me.
1 Yes.
. Not sure *or* not applicable *or* missing.

Hyperactivity score

Severity of hyperactivity	**1**	**Mild**	**1–3**
	2	**Moderate**	**4–8**
	3	**Severe**	**9 or more**

SCIP Anorexia Nervosa Scale (Self-Administered)

Instructions Please fill in the information requested for the following questions.

A. How tall are you? ____feet _____ inches
B. How much do you weigh now? ____lbs.
C. What has been your highest weight ever (when not pregnant)? ____lbs.
When was that? ______________________________
D. What has been your lowest weight ever (when not physically ill)? ____lbs.
When was that? ______________________________

1a. Have you ever been very thin and could not maintain a minimal normal weight?

0 No.
1 Yes.
. Not sure *or* not applicable *or* missing.

1b. Have people ever said you weighed much less than normal?

0 No.
1 Yes.
. Not sure *or* not applicable *or* missing.

Instructions For the remaining questions, please circle the number that best describes how you felt **during the past three months.**

2. Do you feel that your weight and shape are very important and affect how you feel about yourself to the point that you do not worry about the health risks of being so little?

0 No.
1 Yes.
. Not sure *or* not applicable *or* missing.

3. Do you have an intense fear of gaining weight or becoming fat, even though you are underweight?

0 No.
1 Yes.
. Not sure *or* not applicable *or* missing.

4. Do you try to lose weight by fasting (not eating anything at all for at least 24 hours)?

0 No.
1 Yes.
. Not sure *or* not applicable *or* missing.

5. Do you try to lose weight by exercising too much (more than one hour a day for at least one week)?

0 No.
1 Yes.
. Not sure *or* not applicable *or* missing.

6. Do you try to lose weight by using diet pills?

0 No.
1 Yes.
. Not sure *or* not applicable *or* missing.

7. Do you try to lose weight by inducing vomiting?

0 No.
1 Yes.
. Not sure *or* not applicable *or* missing.

8. Do you try to lose weight by taking laxatives or using enemas?

0 No.
1 Yes.
. Not sure *or* not applicable *or* missing.

9. Do you try to lose weight by taking diuretics or by other methods?

0 No.
1 Yes.
. Not sure *or* not applicable *or* missing.

Anorexia nervosa score = sum of items 1 through 9

SCIP Binge and Bulimia Scale (Self-Administered)

Instructions Please fill in the information requested for the following questions.

E. How tall are you? ____feet _____ inches
F. How much do you weigh now? ____lbs.
G. What has been your highest weight ever (when not pregnant)? ____lbs.
When was that? ______________________________
H. What has been your lowest weight ever (when not physically ill)? ____lbs.
When was that? ______________________________

Binge eating

1. Do you have episodes of binge eating (eating within one or two-hour period what most people would consider an unusually large amount of food)?

0 No.
1 Yes.
. Not sure *or* not applicable *or* missing.

2. Please circle the number that best represents the frequency in which you binge eat (on average):

0 None.
1 **1–3** times per month.
2 at least once per week for the past 3 months.
. Not sure *or* not applicable *or* missing.

3. During the episodes of binge eating, did you feel that you had lost control and could not stop eating?

0 No.
1 Yes.
. Not sure *or* not applicable *or* missing.

4. During the episodes of binge eating, did you eat much more rapidly than usual?

0 No.
1 Yes.
. Not sure *or* not applicable *or* missing.

5. During the episodes of binge eating, did you eat until you felt uncomfortably full?

0 No.
1 Yes.
. Not sure *or* not applicable *or* missing.

6. During the episodes of binge eating, did you eat a large amount of food when you did not feel physically hungry?

0 No.
1 Yes.
. Not sure *or* not applicable *or* missing.

7. During the episodes of binge eating, did you eat alone because you were embarrassed by how much you were eating?

0 No.
1 Yes.
. Not sure *or* not applicable *or* missing.

8. During the episodes of binge eating, did you feel disgusted with yourself, depressed or guilty by your overeating?	
0	No.
1	Yes.
.	Not sure *or* not applicable *or* missing.
9. During the episodes of binge eating, did you feel quite upset or very distressed by your overeating?	
0	No.
1	Yes.
.	Not sure *or* not applicable *or* missing.

Binge eating score = Sum of items 1 through 9

Bulimia nervosa

10. After binge eating episodes, did you try to lose weight by fasting (not eating anything at all for at least 24 hours)?	
0	No.
1	Yes.
.	Not sure *or* not applicable *or* missing.
11. After binge eating episodes, did you try to lose weight by exercising too much (more than one hour a day for at least one week)?	
0	No.
1	Yes.
.	Not sure *or* not applicable *or* missing.
12. After binge eating episodes, did you try to lose weight by using diet pills?	
0	No.
1	Yes.
.	Not sure *or* not applicable *or* missing.
13. After binge eating episodes, did you try to lose weight by inducing vomiting?	
0	No.
1	Yes.
.	Not sure *or* not applicable *or* missing.
14. After binge eating episodes, did you try to lose weight by taking laxatives or enemas?	
0	No.
1	Yes.
.	Not sure *or* not applicable *or* missing.
15. After binge eating episodes, did you try to lose weight by taking diuretics or other methods?	
0	No.
1	Yes.
.	Not sure *or* not applicable *or* missing.

Bulimia nervosa score = sum of items 1 through 15

SCIP Intake Scale (Self-Administered)

Instructions Circle the number that best describes how you have felt either during the past month OR since your last visit.

During the past month OR since your last visit…

1. Did you have excessive worry and anxiety for long periods of time (e.g., for hours each day, lasting several months), not just during panic attacks?

0 No, *or* Some anxiety, but it does not bother me.
1 Yes.
. Not sure *or* not applicable *or* missing.

2. Did you have a panic attack, when you suddenly become anxious and frightened for a short period of time (up to 60 minutes)?
During that time, did you feel that your heart was racing or pounding, did you start shaking or sweating, or did you feel you were choking?

0 No.
1 Yes.
. *Not sure or not applicable or missing.*

3. "Obsessive thoughts" are thoughts or images in your mind that do not make sense and keep coming back to your mind even when you try to avoid them.
In the past month, did you have obsessive thoughts?

0 No.
1 Yes.
. Not sure *or* not applicable *or* missing.

4. "Compulsive behaviors" are things you feel you must do over and over, such as washing your hands even if they are clean, checking doors and windows more than once, or repeating mental acts such as counting or praying.
In the past month, did you have compulsive behaviors?

0 No.
1 Yes.
. Not sure *or* not applicable *or* missing.

5. Have you ever witnessed or experienced a traumatic event that involved actual or threatened death or serious injury to you or someone else (e.g., physical or sexual abuse, rape, terrorist attack, natural disaster, war)?

0 I have not experienced any traumatic events.
1 I have experienced **one traumatic event.**
2 I have experienced **several traumatic events.**
. Not sure *or* not applicable *or* missing.

6. Over the past month, have you re-experienced the event in a distressing way (e.g., flashbacks, nightmares, bad dreams)?
0 Absent or nonsignificant.
1 Symptom present.
. Not sure *or* not applicable *or* missing.

7. Did you feel sad, depressed, or in low spirits?

0 No.
1 Yes, some of the time.
2 Yes, most of the time.
. Not sure *or* not applicable *or* missing.

8. Did you have thoughts of killing yourself?

0 No.
1 Yes.
. Not sure *or* not applicable *or* missing.

9. Did you feel extremely happy, elated, or on top of the world without much reason?

0 No.
1 Yes, some of the time.
2 Yes, most of the time.
. Not sure *or* not applicable *or* missing.

10. Did you experience quick changes in mood or mood swings (depressed and happy or depressed and irritable) <u>on the same day?</u>

0 No.
1 Yes, some of the time.
2 Yes, most of the time.
. Not sure *or* not applicable *or* missing.

11. Did you experience hearing voices or noises that other people cannot hear?
0 Absent.
1 Symptom present.
. Not sure *or* not applicable *or* missing.

12. Did you feel that someone is spying on you or trying to harm you or has a plot or conspiracy against you?
0 Absent or nonsignificant.
1 Symptom present.
. Not sure *or* not applicable *or* missing.

<u>13. During the past year,</u> did alcohol cause problems for you at work or school, problems with family or friends, legal problems, or other problems such as getting in physical fights?
0 Absent or nonsignificant.
1 Symptom present.
. Not sure *or* not applicable *or* missing.

<u>14. During the past year,</u> did drug use (___________) cause problems for you at work or school, problems with family or friends, legal problems, or other problems such as getting in physical fights?
0 Absent or nonsignificant.
1 Symptom present.
. Not sure *or* not applicable *or* missing.

15. Have you worried about gaining weight to the point that you did things such as self-induced vomiting, using diet pills, laxatives, or heavy exercise?
0 Absent or nonsignificant.
1 Symptom present.
. Not sure *or* not applicable *or* missing.

16. Do you have episodes of binge eating (eating within one or two-hour period what most people would consider an unusually large amount of food)?
0 Absent or nonsignificant.
1 Symptom present.
. Not sure *or* not applicable *or* missing.

17. Did you have difficulty concentrating on one task for a sustained period of time (e.g., reading a book, writing a letter)?
0 Absent or nonsignificant.
1 Patient has difficulty concentrating for a long period of time.
. Not sure *or* not applicable *or* missing.

18. Did you have difficulty remaining seated (e.g., did you find yourself fidgeting with hands and feet, squirming or wiggling in seat, etc.) during a time when you were expected to remain seated (e.g., during a meeting or a church service)?
0 Absent or nonsignificant.
1 Patient fidgets with hands and feet, or wiggles in seat.
. Not sure *or* not applicable *or* missing.

Appendix IV

Measurement-Based Care (MBC)

Competency Test

Read the questions and circle the correct answers. ***<u>Some questions may have more than one correct answer.</u>***

1. Psychiatric assessment includes the following:

   A. Interviewing the patient
   B. Determining etiology
   C. Diagnosis
   D. All of the above

2. Approaches to psychiatric diagnosis include the following:

   A. "Top-down" approach
   B. "Bottom-up" approach
   C. "Bottom first then top (BFTT)" approach
   D. All of the above

3. A classic example of the top-down approach is:

   A. The Structured Clinical Interview for DSM-IV Axis I Disorders (SCID-I)
   B. The Schedules for Clinical Assessment in Neuropsychiatry (SCAN)
   C. The Mini-International Neuropsychiatric Interview (M.I.N.I.)
   D. The Standard for Clinicians' Interview in Psychiatry (SCIP)
   E. None of the above

4. A classic example of the bottom-up approach is:

   A. The Structured Clinical Interview for DSM-IV Axis I Disorders (SCID-I)
   B. The Schedules for Clinical Assessment in Neuropsychiatry (SCAN)
   C. The Mini-International Neuropsychiatric Interview (M.I.N.I.)
   D. The Standard for Clinicians' Interview in Psychiatry (SCIP)
   E. None of the above

5. True or False: The Standard for Clinicians' Interview in Psychiatry (SCIP) follows the "bottom first then top (BFTT)" approach.

   A. True
   B. False

6. Clinical assessment of symptoms includes evaluation of:

   A. Symptom severity (mild, moderate, severe)
   B. Symptom duration
   C. Symptom effect on functioning
   D. Symptom frequency
   E. All of the above

7. True or False: Psychological signs can affect psychiatric diagnosis.

   A. True
   B. False

8. True or False: MBC involves the systematic administration of measures and the use of measures to drive clinical decision making at the level of the individual patient.

   A. True
   B. False

9. The SCIP principles for creating reliable dimensions recommend considering the following **except:**

   A. Reliability of symptoms and signs
   B. Significance of symptoms and signs
   C. Maximizing the number of symptom subcategories
   D. Frequency of symptoms and signs

10. Symptom evaluation includes the following:

    A. Presence of the symptom
    B. Frequency of the symptom
    C. Duration of the symptom
    D. Distress to the patient
    E. Function of the patient
    F. All of the above
    G. Only A: the presence of the symptom

11. Types of descriptive psychopathology include:

    A. Qualitative
    B. Quantitative
    C. Etiologic
    D. Experimental
    E. All of the above

12. True or False: Tools of MBC need to be useful for the clinician to make decisions at the individual level.

    A. True
    B. False

13. True or False: Rating scales, when designed properly for measurement-based care (MBC), can be very useful tools for the clinicians.

    A. True
    B. False

14. The SCIP principles for creating reliable dimensions recommend considering the following:

    A. Duration of symptoms
    B. Recency of symptoms
    C. Quality of symptoms
    D. The summation principle

15. Psychological dimensions are formulated based upon:

    A. Existing classification systems (DSM, ICD)
    B. Experts' opinions
    C. Statistical analyses
    D. All of the above

16. Advantages of measurement-based care (MBC) include:

    A. Improving accuracy of diagnoses
    B. Improving outcomes in psychotherapy
    C. Improving function, quality of care, and quality of life
    D. Enhance communications between providers and patients
    E. All of the above

17. The widespread use of DSM-III after its publication in 1980 resulted in the following, **except:**

    A. Improvement in the reliability of psychiatric diagnosis
    B. Improvement in the validity of psychiatric diagnosis
    C. Promotion of the top-down approach
    D. Promotion of clinical research such as clinical trials

18. Psychiatrists do not use rating scales in clinical settings because:

    A. Psychiatrists do not have adequate training in using scales
    B. Scales are time-consuming
    C. Scales are designed for research and not designed for clinical use by psychiatrists
    D. Scales interfere with establishing rapport with patients
    E. All of the above
    F. None of the above

19. Barriers to measurement-based care (MBC) include:

    A. Measures are time-consuming
    B. Measures are designed for research
    C. Measures interfere with establishing rapport with patients
    D. Lack of formal training in using measures
    E. All of the above

20. True or False: The principle of the least subcategories of symptom severity (LSSS) leads to an efficient interview.

    A. True
    B. False

21. Which of the following is a **fully structured diagnostic interview:**

    A. WHO Composite International Diagnostic Interview (CIDI)
    B. Diagnostic Interview Schedule (DIS)
    C. Mini International Neuropsychiatric Interview (MINI)
    D. Schedules for Clinical Assessment in Neuropsychiatry (SCAN)
    E. Structured Clinical Interview for DSM-IV Axis I Disorders (SCID-I)
    F. The Standard for Clinicians' Interview in Psychiatry (SCIP)

22. Which of the following is a **semi-structured diagnostic interview:**

    A. WHO Composite International Diagnostic Interview (CIDI)
    B. Diagnostic Interview Schedule (DIS)
    C. Mini International Neuropsychiatric Interview (MINI)
    D. Schedules for Clinical Assessment in Neuropsychiatry (SCAN)
    E. Structured Clinical Interview for DSM-IV Axis I Disorders (SCID-I)
    F. The Standard for Clinicians' Interview in Psychiatry (SCIP)

23. True or False: The WHO Composite International Diagnostic Interview (CIDI) and the Diagnostic Interview Schedule (DIS) are designed to be used by lay interviewers.

    A. True
    B. False

24. The depression dimension of the SCIP includes the following **EXCEPT:**

    A. Depressed mood
    B. Anhedonia
    C. Self-injurious behavior
    D. Suicidal ideation and plan
    E. Hopelessness

25. True or False: Reliability is the consistency and stability of a measure:

    A. True
    B. False

26. True or False: Validity is the approximate truth or falsity of a scientific proposition:

    A. True
    B. False

27. True or False: Criterion validity is the degree of correlation between a new measure and an established gold standard measure:

    A. True
    B. False

28. True or False: Sensitivity is the ability of a test to correctly identify those who have a disease:

    A. True
    B. False

29. True or False: Specificity is the ability of a test to correctly identify those who do not have the disease:

    A. True
    B. False

30. Types of reliability include:

    A. Cronbach's alpha
    B. Inter-rater
    C. Test-retest
    D. All of the above
    E. All of the above except A

Important Note to the Readers

If you are interested in having a formal MBC trainer certificate and 12 Continuing Medical Education (CME) credits, please contact the American Academy of Clinical Psychiatrists (AACP): 7 Century Drive, Suite 301, Parsippany, NJ 07054.

Email: clinicalpsychiatrists@gmail.com

Measurement-Based Care (MBC)
Competency Test Answers

Question Number	Answer
1	D
2	D
3	A,C
4	B
5	A
6	E
7	A
8	A
9	C
10	F

Question Number	Answer
11	E
12	A
13	A
14	A,B,C,D
15	D
16	E
17	B
18	E
19	E
20	A
21	A,B,C
22	D,E,F
23	A
24	C
25	A
26	A
27	A
28	A
29	A
30	D

Index

A. S. Aboraya, *Manual for the Standard for Clinicians' Interview in Psychiatry (SCIP)*, Advances in Mental Health and Addiction,
https://doi.org/10.1007/978-3-030-94930-3